Master the UCAT

By the Top 1%

Edited by:

Aayesha Malik
Syed Aqib Bukhari

Publisher: Independent Publishing Network
Publication date: 2nd March 2021
ISBN: 978-1-80049-511-1
Author: MedicHut.
Email: team@medichut.com
Website: https://www.medichut.com
Cover design and illustration: Zarwa Malik
First Paperback Edition

Dedicated to our parents who have always supported us.

About the Authors

Editors

Aayesha Malik is a fifth-year medical student at The University of Leeds. She has a keen interest in medical teaching, writing, leadership, and project management.

Syed Bukhari is a fifth-year medical student at The University of Leeds. He has been teaching his juniors and peers for over ten years, including medicine-related content since 2016.

Contributors

Taylor Burdett is a first-year medical student at University College London. His contributions helped shape the Verbal Reasoning section of this book, as well as numerous test questions.

Emery Shen is a first-year medical student at The University of Sheffield. Her contributions helped shape the Quantitative Reasoning section of this book.

Rishab Bharadwaj is a first-year medical student at The University of Manchester. His contributions helped shape the Abstract Reasoning and Decision Making sections of this book.

Thank you to Maxim Iwanskyj and Stefan Palade who also contributed questions to this book. Thank you to Zarwa Malik who designed the book cover. Other contributors wished to remain anonymous, though their contributions will remain forever valued in the creation of this book.

Table of Contents

Introduction

The University Clinical Aptitude Test (UCAT) is an admissions test used by the majority of medical schools in the UK and has recently been taken up by medical schools in Australia and New Zealand. It is conducted on a computer, usually in a test centre, but the option to sit the UCAT at home was presented in 2020 due to COVID-19. There are many test centres around the world, although some international applicants may need to travel to nearby places to access a test centre.

The UCAT is defined as an aptitude test, but it has long since been proven that preparation and hard work can significantly improve an individual's score. There is no prior knowledge that is required, but a range of key strategies will allow you to answer the questions with ease and efficiency. The main difficulty of the UCAT is the time pressure – there are a number of seconds given for each question, and you must learn to adapt to answering questions in the given time.

Sections of the UCAT

Verbal Reasoning

This is the first section of the UCAT. There are 44 questions that must be answered in 21 minutes, providing an average of 28 seconds per question. This section tests your speed-reading, critical-thinking, and evaluation skills when presented with a lengthy block of text. Verbal reasoning is a crucial skill to have, both while studying at university and while working as a doctor. At university, the ability to read large sections of text quickly, while digesting the general meaning of the text and recognising the relevant sections, will help you to cover the content of the course to the best of your ability. This is particularly relevant to those studying Medicine or Dentistry, as these courses are very content-heavy. Thus, the ability to read and understand information quickly and accurately will be essential in preparation for exams and working life. It is also important as a doctor to be able to recognise unqualified assumptions and illogical conclusions, both in the context of patient treatment and scientific writing.

Decision Making

This is the second section of the UCAT. There are 29 questions that must be answered in 31 minutes, providing an average of 64 seconds per question. Some questions will take less time, while others will take more. This section assesses your ability to make sound decisions and judgements using complex information. The variety in question types is greater than any other section, and topics from Verbal Reasoning and Quantitative Reasoning present in slightly altered formats. As a clinician, you will often be required to interpret information and analyse data to make quick, thoughtful decisions within a short time span. Your ability to make decisions can directly impact a patient's wellbeing, so this is an important skill to have.

Quantitative Reasoning

This is the third section of the UCAT. There are 36 questions that must be answered in 24 minutes, providing an average of roughly 40 seconds per question. This section assesses your ability to critically evaluate information presented in numerical form. You do not need to be excellent at mathematics to score well in this section, as the main aim is to test your problem-solving and analysis skills using simple maths. This is important for doctors as medicine is a discipline that involves statistics and graphical analysis. A qualified doctor should excel in these skills in order to interpret data given regarding patients in their care, as well as data found in research papers.

Abstract Reasoning

This is the fourth section of the UCAT. There are 55 questions that must be answered in 13 minutes, providing an average of 16 seconds per question. This section assesses your ability to find various types of patterns within sets of shapes. This demonstrates your ability to develop ideas and hypotheses and utilise them to predict outcomes within a short period of time. It is often the most difficult section for students to understand at first, as pattern recognition is not as readily taught in schools as other subjects like reading comprehension and mathematics. However, with practice, Abstract Reasoning can become second nature. Doctors are required to recognise patterns in symptom presentation in order to make diagnoses. As such, it is not possible for someone to diagnose a disease based on a list of symptoms, but someone who is highly qualified and has the experience of recognising patterns with symptom presentation is able to more accurately make this decision. Thus, pattern recognition is a key skill that is required of clinicians.

Situational Judgement Test

The final section of the UCAT is a separate test of its own, so its scoring system is not included in the average of all of the other sections. There are 69 questions that must be answered in 26 minutes, providing an average of 23 seconds per question. It assesses your ability to make decisions in clinical and non-clinical environments, considering the General Medical Council's (GMC) standards for doctors. Scoring is given as Band 1, 2, 3 or 4, where Band 1 is the best and Band 4 is the worse. When assessing applications, universities use the Situation Judgement Test in various ways, such as:

- Some universities will assign a specific number of points to each applicant depending on which band they achieve.
- Some universities have a cut-off band. For example, anyone with less than Band 2 may automatically be rejected.
- Some universities may use this only to differentiate between two equally remarkable candidates.
- Some do not give any importance to the band achieved by their applicants.

Timing

As the UCAT is highly time-pressured, you need to ensure that you are finishing the correct number of questions within the given timeframe. It can be very time-consuming to constantly check the timer and work out how much time you have left. A more sufficient way to keep track of your time is to learn the "halfway point" for each section. Once you know each halfway point, you should use these while doing practice questions to get accustomed to this method. For example: The halfway point for Verbal Reasoning is around 11 minutes. When you check the time around 11 minutes into the section, you should have completed 5 sets of questions and be on or around question 21. This means that for the first half of the section, your speed was perfect, and you need to continue working at the same speed. If you have flagged a lot of questions that you need to come back to, you should ensure that you are ahead of the halfway marker listed for the section.

	Time	Number of Questions	Average Time Per Question	Halfway Point
Verbal Reasoning	21 minutes	44 (11 sets)	29 seconds	11 minutes; question 21
Decision Making	31 minutes	29	64 seconds	15 minutes; question 15
Quantitative Reasoning	24 minutes	36 (9 sets)	40 seconds	12 minutes; question 17
Abstract Reasoning	13 minutes	55	14 seconds	7 minutes; question 26
Situational Judgement Test	26 minutes	69	23 seconds	13 minutes; question 35

Scoring

Each of the first four sections, Verbal Reasoning, Decision Making, Quantitative Reasoning, and Abstract Reasoning, are scored together. The lowest score you can achieve in each section is 300, and the maximum is 900. The scores are added up to give a total score out of 3600. You do not necessarily need to answer each question correctly to gain full marks in a section, as the scores are skewed slightly each year. This is similar to the way that grade boundaries work in GCSEs and A-levels. It is a useful method to ensure that the scoring is fair for all students, especially in case of particularly difficult papers. The Situational Judgement Test is scored in bands, as explained previously. After you complete your exam, you can compare it to the scores of others on the UCAT website here:
https://www.ucat.ac.uk/ucat/results/test-statistics/

A competitive score is normally ≥2800, or an average of ≥700 in each section. This score will ensure that you exceed the UCAT requirements for the majority of UK universities, thus drastically increasing your chances of being accepted for an interview. It is important to remember that universities will use your overall average when assessing you. Therefore, if you happen to perform poorly in one section, you should stay calm, regain focus, and know that you can make up for it in the next section.

The average scores in each of the first four sections from 2016-2020 can be found in the table below.

	2020	**2019**	**2018**	**2017**	**2016**
Verbal Reasoning	570	565	567	570	573
Decision Making	625	618	624	647	N/A
Quantitative Reasoning	664	662	658	695	690
Abstract Reasoning	653	638	637	629	630

Source: https://www.ucat.ac.uk/results/test-statistics/

The average score in the Situational Judgement Test is Band 2. A competitive application may have a score of Band 1, although many universities will not consider it as such. Below is a table showing the percentage of students scoring within each band of the Situational Judgement Test from 2016-2020.

	2020	2019	2018	2017	2016
Band 1	30%	17%	21%	28%	26%
Band 2	36%	40%	34%	42%	44%
Band 3	24%	33%	32%	21%	22%
Band 4	9%	10%	13%	9%	9%

Source: https://www.ucat.ac.uk/results/test-statistics/

Universities

The majority of medical schools in the UK require applicants to undertake the UCAT prior to applying. An application missing a UCAT score, for a university that requires the UCAT, will automatically be rejected. Each university has its own unique admissions process, and therefore, each university will use the UCAT in a distinct way. Some universities may have a cut-off score, meaning only applicants above a certain score will be considered, but scores higher than the cut-off will not have additional benefit. Others may include a candidate's UCAT score within an overall average of their other admissions criteria, such as GCSE grades, A-level predictions, and personal statement. This is often done by giving a set number of points for each of the criteria, then ranking candidates based on their points. This would mean that a higher UCAT score would provide an applicant with a greater number of points, thus putting them in a better position than others with a lower score. In other universities, perhaps UCAT score does not play a large role in admissions, but may be used to select one out of two similar candidates.

Tactical Applications

Universities usually describe on their website how they use the UCAT to score candidates, but if you are unsure, you should contact your desired university to ask their admissions staff directly. Knowing how your desired universities use the UCAT in their admissions criteria will help you to apply tactically.

- If you achieve a very high UCAT score, you will be able to maximise your chances by applying to a university with a very high cut-off score. Many students will not be able to meet a high cut-off, so this can be used to your advantage. It would be unwise to apply to a university that places little emphasis on UCAT if you have a very high UCAT score, as you would not be using the highlights of your application to your advantage.
- If your UCAT score is very low, you should stay away from universities that highly value the UCAT.
- If you do not meet the cut-off score for a particular university, it is clear that you should not apply to that university.
- Some universities may not consider the Situational Judgement Test, so if you scored poorly on it, look for these universities. Alternatively, if you did incredible on it, you can use your score to your advantage elsewhere.

Registration

You can register for the UCAT on their website as follows:
https://www.ucat.ac.uk/ucat/registration-booking/

The fee is £75 for tests taken within the UK and European Union, and £120 for tests taken outside the UK and the European Union.

Bursaries

Bursaries are available for students who may not be able to afford the cost, such as those receiving free school meals, or who have a parent receiving Universal Credit. For the full list of criteria, please see https://www.ucat.ac.uk/ucat/bursary-scheme/. You must be able to provide evidence of the criteria that you fulfil.

After applying, a decision is usually made within 5 working days and you will receive a decision via email. If your bursary application is accepted and you have already paid for the UCAT, you will be eligible for a refund.

It is important to note that if you book a test using a bursary, and you do not intend to sit the test, you must arrange for it to be cancelled. Otherwise, UCAT reserves the right to charge you for the missed test.

UCATSEN and Access Arrangements

The alternative UCAT tests are known as: UCATSEN, UCATSA, UCATSENSA and UCATSEN50. These are reserved for students who require extended time due to dyslexia, autism, ADHD, ADD, or a variety of other social, psychological, and physical disabilities. The test content will remain the same, but students will either be allocated more time to complete each section, 5-minute breaks before each section, or both. Besides these alternative tests, students are able to apply for other access arrangements such as:

1. An individual room in a test centre
2. Food or drink at the workstation that is necessary due to a medical condition

For more details on access arrangements, view the UCAT website here: https://www.ucat.ac.uk/ucat/access-arrangements/.

To apply for access arrangements, fill in the form here: https://www.ucat.ac.uk/access-arrangements

The approval process can take up to 5 working days, but it is recommended that you apply well in advance if you feel that you may need any additional support.

Preparing for the UCAT

Firstly, you must book your UCAT test date. You need to know how much time you have in order to plan your revision effectively. Secondly, download our free UCAT planner from our website at https://www.medichut.com/product-page/2020-ucat-planner. This will help you to formulate a revision timetable, focussing on every stage of your learning and preparation.

As a summary of our planner, we recommend that you spend around 6 weeks preparing. These 6 weeks are divided into stages as follows:

1. Planning your timetable
2. Learning strategies to tackle each type of question
3. Practicing questions
4. Intense practice and official mocks prior to exam date

You should aim to spend around 2 hours a day on revision, and increase the amount of time you spend closer to the exam date. In the last week before your exam, you should attempt the official UCAT mock exams, as found on the UCAT website at: https://www.practice.ucat.ac.uk

Aside from completing this book and working through the practice questions, we highly recommend booking in with an expert UCAT tutor who can help transform your UCAT score. Our team will gauge your exact requirements to find you the most suitable tutor to help you every step of the way. All of our tutors have scored in the top decile in their own UCAT exams, are DBS-cleared, and will go above and beyond to help *you* improve your score. Booking a tutor can make the biggest difference between an average or good score and an *excellent* score that guarantees you interviews. You can find more information on https://www.medichut.com/ucat.

We also highly recommend our 5-star rated Live UCAT Masterclass for students looking to cover all of the important UCAT strategies in a single intensive day, while having expert instructors on hand to answer any questions. You can find more information and registration dates on https://www.medichut.com/ucat.

Analysing Mistakes

While practicing, it is important to keep a reflective journal in a format that suits you. For every question you answer incorrectly, you need to evaluate what you did wrong. *Why* did you answer it incorrectly? What error did you make in your judgement? Was it simply a lack of time, and so you need to work on improving your speed? Or are there equations that you have forgotten, and so you need to remind yourself? Is it a lack of understanding of certain concepts and strategies? Whatever it is, you need to recognise it and work on fixing it. If you continue to do practice questions and mock exams without reflecting on the mistakes you make, you will be strengthening the bad habits that you have created and will struggle to improve your score.

It may be helpful to use labels for your mistakes, such as:

1. Careless: You can use this label for questions where you made careless errors. This should push you to increase your focus when answering questions.
2. Understanding: You can use this label when you did not understand a question properly. Questions are not always worded in a simple format, so it is important to read thoroughly and ensure that you understand what the question is asking for.
3. Skill: You can use this label if you did not know how to solve the question. For example, in Quantitative Reasoning, you may have been unaware of the necessary formula. You would then be prompted to review the formula that was required to answer the question in order to avoid making the same mistake in future questions.

Flagging Questions

Each question is worth the same number of marks, so spending minutes on a single difficult question at the expense of perhaps five easy questions will be detrimental to your UCAT score. You need to be aware of how much time you have and how well you are on track for the given amount of time – refer to halfway markers (page 3). It is highly recommended that you become comfortable with the idea of not answering each question in the exam. You must learn to skip questions that are too difficult or are taking too much time. Some questions are purposely placed in the UCAT to waste your time, and the majority of students will fall in this trap. Through practice, you will recognise which types of questions take too long and therefore should be flagged rather than attempted. If you are presented with a very long and complicated question, you may be able to quickly discard some of the options and make a more educated guess before moving on. Sometimes, you will not spend any time on it at all, as you simply do not have the time. Either way, you can guess one of the answers, flag the question, and move on. If you do not guess before you move on, you may run out of time at the end. By guessing, you provide yourself with a 25% chance of getting a mark for that question.

Psychological Readiness

With a large number of questions and a limited amount of time, the UCAT is a test that requires a lot of mental stamina and strength – skills that are developed through practice. You will be tested on your ability to display mental endurance from section to section, with only a short break in between each. In a section like Abstract Reasoning, where you have on average 14 seconds per question, you endurance must function at its peak capacity. As such, it is paramount to maintain your nerves and keep a positive spirit. It is difficult to function well under pressure, especially when clouded with any form of negativity. If you are unable to answer a question, make sure that you are comfortable with moving on to the next question. If you underperform in a whole section, or are unable to complete all of the questions, ensure that you are comfortable with this. Know that you must stay calm and stay positive, as your ability to perform well in the next section can significantly improve your overall score. If you begin to panic, or allow one section to impact you negatively, your overall score may suffer. As such, you must practice questions under time pressure, and practice controlling your nerves.

Remember, the UCAT is not the be-all or end-all. Having a good UCAT score will help you to get a place in medical or dental school, but it is not the only thing that admissions tutors look at. There are thousands of places in medical schools across the UK each year, so thousands of students must get accepted each year. It is possible to get into medical school with an average or even a low score. Ensure that you tactically apply (page 5). Further, students with incredible UCAT scores are not guaranteed to get a place in medical school. It is possible to obtain four interviews based on an amazing UCAT scores, but not get accepted due to underperforming in A-levels or interviews. Likewise, it is possible to underperform in the UCAT, manage to obtain at least one interview due to a good personal statement and tactical application, and achieve an offer after performing well in the interview. You should recognise that the medical school application process consists of many steps. As such, you should not let the UCAT take all of your energy. Stay positive, work hard, and do your best each step of the way!

We hope that this book will provide you great insight into the UCAT and allow you to maximise your score through the various strategies taught. If you have any questions about any of the content, please do not hesitate to contact us at team@medichut.com.

SECTION 1

Verbal Reasoning

INTRODUCTION

Verbal Reasoning is the first section that you will be tested on in the UCAT. It is usually considered the most difficult section to score highly in. The average score for the 2020 testing cycle was 570, compared to the other three sections which averaged between 625 and 653. This section consists of 11 passages of text that are 200-400 words in length, each with 4 associated questions, giving a total of 44 questions. You will have 21 minutes to complete this entire section, giving you an average of 29 seconds per question. This section is designed to test your logical thinking skills when asked to read and understand a block of text, so none of the questions require any prior knowledge. Often, using your own prior knowledge on a topic covered in the exam can lead you to the wrong answer as it can distract you from the focus of the question.

In this section, we will teach you how to unlearn some bad habits that slow down your reading speed, as well as learn new habits that can increase your reading speed. You'll also be taught how to scan for keywords, make inferences from passages, avoid faulty logic, and a tonne of other useful techniques! There are various examples throughout that will help you understand the techniques taught, followed by a mock test of 44 Verbal Reasoning questions at the end of the section.

Types of Questions

In this section of the UCAT, you will come across two main types of questions:

1) True, False, Can't Tell questions
2) Statement-based questions

True, False, Can't Tell

You will be given a statement and asked to determine which category it belongs to. The categories can be defined as follows:

True: Based on the information given in the passage, this statement is true.
False: Based on the information given in the passage, this statement is false.
Can't Tell: The information given in the passage is not enough to tell whether this statement is true or false.

When it comes to "Can't Tell", you always need to think – If you were given more information, would that change the answer? Is it possible that it could be true or false, but there is not enough evidence to suggest either?

Statement-Based Questions

You will be given a question, such as "Which of the following can be deduced from the passage?" followed by four statements. Most of these questions are inference (see page 39) questions, meaning that you are required to "read between the lines", so it is vital to have a general understanding of the full passage. This type of question is more difficult and so requires excellent reading speed and comprehension. There is only **one** right answer for these questions.

The majority of passages in Verbal Reasoning will involve statement-based questions. No passage will have a mixture of question types – they will either be True, False, Can't Tell or statement-based.

Basic Strategy

True, False, Can't Tell

The best way to answer this type of question is by "selective reading". The strategy for this is as follows:

1. Skip the passage and go straight to question 1.
2. Read the question and identify keywords (see page 20)
3. Scan the text for the relevant keywords.
4. When a keyword is found, read the sentence containing the keyword as well as the sentence **before** and **after**.
5. Continue to scan the passage for further mentions of the keyword and repeat step 4 if any are found.
6. Answer the question based on this selective reading.
7. Follow steps 2-6 for the rest of the questions in the passage.
8. Aim to complete all 4 questions in a passage within 1 minute to allow more time for the more challenging questions.

Statement-Based Questions

For each passage with statement-based questions, you will have 16 statements divided between 4 questions. The general strategy is as follows:

1. Read the first question to identify that this is a statement-based question.
2. Read the entire passage once, ensuring that you focus on everything you are reading.
    - You may not understand and remember the whole passage at this stage, but by reading it once, you will have a general understanding of where topics are located within the passage.
3. Go to the first question. Read statement A. Based on your knowledge of the text you have just read, decide whether this is the correct answer.
    - If you are unsure, quickly locate and read the relevant information in the passage.
4. If it is not the correct answer, try statement B. If B is correct, **do not** move on to statement C or D. Stop there and move on to the next question.
5. If statement B is incorrect, try the next statement, and repeat until you find the correct answer.
6. Follow steps 3-5 for the rest of the questions in the passage.

Exceptions to the Strategies

These rules are not set in stone. You should only read the entire passage if:

1. You have time to do so, or
2. There are inference-based questions, and so you require a general understanding of the passage, or

3. The passage seems very complex, and so you require a general understanding of the passage.

Some statement-based questions can be answered by simply following the same scanning and selective reading strategy used in True, False, Can't Tell questions. The scenarios for this are as follows:

1. A very *short and straight-forward* passage that does not require thorough reading and general understanding, or
2. Search-and-retrieve type questions (i.e. the statements are present in the passage almost word-for-word and do not require you to make any inferences).

The UCAT has some difficult questions and some easy questions. If you have an extremely long and complex passage with statement-based questions that all require you to make difficult inferences, you may spend a lot of time trying to read, understand and answer all of the questions. These types of passages are inserted purposefully, as the question-writers would like for you to waste time on them. Here, we would advise that you flag and move on to easier questions, coming back at the end to attempt the more difficult ones.

With enough practice under timed conditions, you will be able to identify such time-consuming questions. Make sure you train yourself to make an educated guess, flag the question and move on – this will give you at least a 25% chance of getting the answer right.

Here are two separate passages that you might find in the UCAT. Determine which passage you should scan and read selectively, and which one you should read thoroughly. You can attempt to answer the questions if you wish.

Example 1

China has warned students to reconsider travelling to Australia to study because of a string of "incidents of discrimination" targeting people of Asian descent. China's ministry of education said in a statement on Tuesday that students preparing to study abroad should do a "good risk assessment" and "exercise caution" in choosing to go to or return to Australia for study. "During the pandemic, Australia has seen multiple incidents of discrimination targeting those of Asian descent."

The warning comes as ties between China and Australia have reached their lowest point in years. Australia led calls for an independent inquiry into the origins of the coronavirus outbreak, which was first detected in China in December before spreading to the rest of the world.

In response to Australia's push for an investigation, China had warned its citizens could boycott of Australian goods and services. China's culture and tourism ministry issued a travel alert on Friday, warning Chinese travellers from going to Australia where they might be the target of racially motivated attacks, caused by anger over the pandemic.

Chinese experts have accused Australia of "smearing China" over the pandemic and thus encouraging discriminatory attitudes. "The Australian side should recognise the real problem rather than hiding its head in the sand," Chen Hong, director of the Australian Studies Centre at East China Normal University in Shanghai told the state-run Global Times.

Australia has also criticised Beijing's decision to force controversial national security laws on Hong Kong. China has placed tariffs on Australian barley as well as blocked imports of Australian beef, moves that Beijing has said are not related to Australia's push for an inquiry.

Source: https://www.newsbreak.com/news/0PHhbwSX/china-warns-students-toreconsider-travel-to-australia-for-study

According to the text, which statement can be correctly inferred?

A. Relations between Australia and China are friendly
B. China does not want its students travelling to Australia to study
C. China's new security laws being put in place in Hong Kong were met with global support
D. Australia's call for an independent inquiry into the origins of the coronavirus outbreak were supported by China

Example 2

Some people are more sensitive than others – and around half of these differences can be attributed to our genes, new research has found.

The study, led by Queen Mary University of London, compared pairs of identical and non-identical 17-year-old twins to see how strongly they were affected by positive or negative experiences -- their 'sensitivity' level. The aim was to tease out how much of the differences in sensitivity could be explained by either genetic or environmental factors during development: nature or nurture.

Twins who are brought up together will mostly experience the same environment. But only identical twins share the same genes: non-identical twins are like any other sibling. If identical twins show no more similarity in their levels of sensitivity than non-identical twins, then genes are unlikely to play a role.

Using this type of analysis, the team found that 47 percent of the differences in sensitivity between individuals were down to genetics, leaving 53 percent accounted for by environmental factors. The research, from Queen Mary University of London and Kings College London, is the first to show this link conclusively in such a large study. The findings are published in *Molecular Psychiatry*.

Michael Pluess, Professor of Developmental Psychology at Queen Mary University of London and study lead, said: "We are all affected by what we experience -- sensitivity is something we all share as a basic human trait. But we also differ in how much of an impact our experiences have on us. Scientists have always thought there was a genetic basis for sensitivity, but this is the first time we've been able to actually quantify how much of these differences in sensitivity are explained by genetic factors."

Source: https://www.qmul.ac.uk/media/news/2020/se/study-in-twins-finds-oursensitivity-is-partly-in-our-genes.html

The study showed that 53% of differences in sensitivity are due to genetic factors.

A. True
B. False
C. Can't Tell

Answer 1

Based on the first question, we can tell that all of the questions from this passage will be statement-based. Further, the question is asking you to make an inference, so other questions will likely be of a similar standard. This will require a general understanding of the passage, so the general strategy for statement-based questions, i.e. reading the entire passage, should be utilised.

The answer for the question was B, as demonstrated by the first sentence.

Answer 2

The first question is a True, False, Can't Tell question, meaning that the other three questions on this passage will be the same. As we do not need to read between the lines in these types of questions, it is not necessary to have a deep understanding of the text. Therefore, the strategy to utilise here is scanning and selective reading.

The correct answer is "False". This is backed up by the sentence "Using this type of analysis, the team found that 47 percent of the differences in sensitivity between individuals were down to genetics, leaving 53 percent accounted for by environmental factors."

Reading: Speed and Comprehension

Now that you've seen the basic strategies, we'll go in-depth on how to execute these strategies. Excellent reading speed and comprehension are vital for statement-based questions, as you are required to speed read. This is different to skimming, which is the best strategy for True, False, Can't Tell questions.

The following techniques will help you to break bad habits and learn how to read quickly while still digesting all of the crucial information in a passage.

1. Eliminating subvocalisation
2. Reducing fixations
3. Eliminating backtracking

Let's take a look at these sections in more detail.

Subvocalisation

Subvocalisation, also known as silent speech, is the habit of reading a chunk of text word-by-word, in your head, or subtly with your mouth. Your larynx, which is the organ used for speech, is also stimulated during this process. Most readers have this habit – it is the way we are taught to understand full sentences when we first learn to read. However, this limits our reading speed to our speaking speed, which is roughly 150-200 words per minute. Ideally, in a highly time-pressured exam, you should be reading at minimum of 400-500 words per minute to understand the passage as quickly as possible and start answering the questions. This can be achieved by **seeing** and **understanding** the text without physically saying each word in your head.

The first step to overcoming subvocalisation is to recognise that you do it! Practice reading longer sections of text, such as newspaper articles or books, and look out for any subvocalisation.

If subvocalisation does affect you, the following methods may help to break the habit:

1) **Follow the text with your finger as you read.** This stops your brain from reading it back to you to "keep your place" as your finger is doing the same job. Doing this for a while can help to break the habit, and once you are accustomed to reading without subvocalising, you will no longer need your finger.

2) **Distract yourself while you read.** Listening to something in the background or chewing gum can be very effective. Of course, you will not be able to do this in the actual exam, but beating the habit of subvocalisation in the first place is the primary goal.
3) **Put a pencil between your lips** if you move your lips while reading. It may sound odd, but it helps prevent you from mouthing or saying the words, which is the first step to shutting off the voice in your head.

Fixations

The next topic is a natural progression from stopping subvocalisation: reducing the number of "fixations" you have per sentence.

A fixation is a point where your eyes rest on the page while reading a sentence.

When you subvocalise, you fixate on various words as you read a sentence. By reducing subvocalisation, you will naturally reduce the number of fixations per line, allowing your eyes to read the text at a faster speed. However, it is still essential to ensure that your eyes rest on the page long enough to take in all of the information.

Once again, the first part of breaking this habit is to become aware of it. How many times are you resting your eyes on each line? Ideally, you should have 2-3 fixations per line to get the best speed while still understanding the text. This is where **chunking** text together comes into play. Instead of focusing on every word, break the sentence up into naturally forming chunks of 3-4 words. Your brain will naturally group words that go together, such as an adverb or adjective with the target verb or noun. Here is an example:

- "Technology is advancing at a rate faster than we have ever seen before."

If we were to break this into chunks, we'd read it as follows:

- "Technology is advancing / at a rate faster than / we have ever seen before"

By grouping the sentence like this instead of taking every word individually, your eyes only have to flick between "targets" three times, increasing your reading speed while maintaining a solid understanding of the sentence. Practicing reading like this will help you reform your reading habits, leading to faster reading times.

The next method for reducing the number of fixations is similar, but instead of chunking words together, you only read every second or third word. Your brain is able to see things that you are not focussing on and fill in any gaps. To better understand this concept, think about where you're looking right now – perhaps at your computer screen while reading this book. Your peripheral vision might be seeing the cup of tea next to you, or your notebook on the other side of your desk. Although you are not focussing on these items, your eyes are able to see them, and your brain is able to process that they are there. It is a similar concept with reading – if you read every few words in a sentence, your eyes and your brain will process the words you skip and still understand the sentence. Use the following example:

- "The man went to his kitchen in the morning and had a cup of tea, then he made himself some buttered toast for breakfast."

This can, instead, be read as such:

- "Man kitchen morning cup tea himself buttered toast breakfast."

If, instead of saying each word in your head, you say the words listed above, your eyes will have skimmed over the rest of the words in between and allow your brain to understand the rest of the sentence.

Whichever method you prefer for reducing fixations will require practice. Whenever you are reading, try to implement these techniques to improve your reading speed.

Backtracking

Backtracking, or regression, means to go backwards in text to re-read a sentence. This is usually a learned habit – people re-read sections of text to ensure full understanding. However, this habit can be detrimental. By backtracking, your reading time will be longer and the flow of text may be lost, often resulting in some level of confusion.

You can fight backtracking the same way you would fight subvocalisation: increasing concentration and using your finger to trace the text. By increasing your concentration, you are more likely to be certain of what you have read and have confidence in your reading abilities. This will reduce the likelihood of backtracking. Likewise, by tracing the text with your fingers, you keep your place in the text and maintain greater focus on what you are reading.

By practicing these techniques from the *beginning* of your UCAT preparation, you will have formed excellent reading habits by the time you sit the exam.

Scanning: Keywords

Types of keywords

When deciding what to selectively read, there are two main categories of words to look for:

1. Numbers (e.g. dates, measurements, percentages, years, etc.)
2. Nouns

If there is a number or date in the question, it is likely that the number will also be present in the text. Numbers stand out in a block of text and are easy to find, so looking for these straight away can quickly help locate the section of the passage you need to read. Dates and years should be your first port of call when looking for numbers, as these usually do not change between the question and the passage. When a question contains a measurement, such as "160 kilometres", you can either search for the number "160" or the unit "kilometres" – both are equally effective. Sometimes, the number can change between the question and the passage, so if you are unable to find the number in the passage, you can move on to scanning for nouns.

Proper nouns, such as names and places, will also stand out in a block of text due to capitalisation of the first letter. However, if a city or country's name is mentioned in the question, it may be featured in the passage multiple times. If this is the case, you would want to isolate a more specific keyword that will only appear in the section of the passage relevant to the question.

If there are no capitalised nouns, looking for **unique** nouns will be helpful. A unique noun is a world that you would not see in the average sentence and is not present multiple times throughout the passage.

Take a look at the following passage:

"The amount of time teenagers spend on social networking sites has risen 62.5 percent since 2012 and continues to grow. Just last year, the average time teenagers spent on social media was estimated as 2.6 hours per day. Critics have claimed that more screen time is increasing depression and anxiety in teenagers.
However, new research led by Sarah Coyne, a professor of family life at Brigham Young University, found that the amount of time spent on social media is not directly increasing anxiety or depression in teenagers."

Source: https://www.sciencedaily.com/releases/2019/10/191022174406.htm

If you were given the statement, “A professor found that social media is not linked to the high levels of depression and anxiety in teenagers,” you would not want to scan the passage for any of the commonly mentioned words, such as: teenage, social media/network, depression, or anxiety. You may not be able to immediately identify common words, however, a quick glance at the passage will show you that the main purpose of the passage is to discuss social media in relation to depression and anxiety in teenagers – therefore, any of these words will not be useful in helping you identify the relevant part of the passage for selective reading. Instead, a unique word that you could scan for is “professor”.

Dispersed key words

When scanning for keywords, do not stop at the first occurrence of a keyword. Ensure that you continue to scan the rest of the passage, as examiners will often try to disperse keywords throughout the passage to increase difficulty. For example, you may find one relevant part of the answer in the first paragraph, but the missing information does not appear until the last paragraph. Even if the first set of selective reading seems to answer your question, you may find a contradiction or extra relevant information later in the text. For these reasons, you always need to scan the entire passage to look for any more occurrences of your keywords.

Synonyms

Sometimes, rather than using the same word in the passage and in the question, you may find that there are similar words or synonyms used. There is no clear strategy to tackle this, as it is not possible to learn every synonym of every word that may appear, but it is vital to know that synonyms may be used. Thus, you need to be very observant when skimming the text and keep an eye out for different words with the same meaning.

Superlatives and Comparative Adjectives

A superlative is an adjective that describes the highest degree of a quality, e.g. greatest, furthest, highest, lowest, nearest.

A comparative adjective directly compares two nouns, although not to the highest degree, e.g. greater, further, higher, lower, nearer.

When a superlative is present in a statement, this becomes the focus of the statement.

- E.g. “Ahmed has the highest salary in the team.”

Yes, we could look for “Ahmed”, “salary”, or “team”, but you will not find the answer to the question until you can identify whether or not Ahmed’s salary is the high<u>est</u>. The passage may use another synonym such as most or greatest. If you find a comparative word, or a different adjective to describe Ahmed's salary, such as "similar", "higher", "greater", the answer would usually "Can't Tell." For example, if the passage states that he has a "higher" salary than someone else, it is *possible* that his salary is the highest, however, there is no clear evidence to back this up, nor is there something to refute it. Therefore, if your question contains a superlative but you are unable to find one in the passage, you will not usually be able to determine whether the statement is "True" or "False".

If you are unable to identify any numbers, nouns, or superlatives to use as keywords, comparative adjectives can be used as a final option.

To bring all this together, let us take a look at two statements:

1. **Globalisation is having a greater impact on our environment than ever before.**
2. **The Soviet Union sought to use the reunification of Germany in 1990 to push Germany out of NATO.**

In statement 1, there are no proper nouns (i.e. nouns with capitals), so we should turn our attention to the other available nouns: globalisation and environment. Although we have not been given a passage here, it is likely that the theme of the passage is to do with globalisation and the environment. So, if these words are part of a common theme, they would not be classified as unique nouns, and so, it would not be useful to scan the text for them. We can use the backup strategy of comparative adjectives. One noun (globalisation) is having a "greater" impact on another noun (environment). If you scan the text for comparative words, you should be able to isolate the relevant section and conduct your selective reading.

In statement 2, there are three proper nouns (Germany, Soviet Union and NATO) and one date (1990). As we mentioned earlier, numbers are usually better keywords than nouns, as it is likely that proper nouns will come up more than once. Therefore, the first keyword to scan for would be "1990".

Try the following questions. One of them will be a passage which you should read, and the other will be a passage you should scan. Ensure that you use the correct techniques for each question.

Example 3

For the first time in history, NASA astronauts have launched from American soil in a commercially built and operated American crew spacecraft on its way to the International Space Station. The SpaceX Crew Dragon spacecraft carrying NASA astronauts Robert Behnken and Douglas Hurley lifted off at 3:22 p.m. EDT Saturday on the company's Falcon 9 rocket from Launch Complex 39A at NASA's Kennedy Space Center in Florida.

Known as NASA's SpaceX Demo-2, the mission is an end-to-end test flight to validate the SpaceX Crew Transportation System, including launch, in-orbit, docking and landing operations. This is SpaceX's second spaceflight test of its Crew Dragon and its first test with astronauts aboard, which will pave the way for its certification for regular crew flights to the station as part of NASA's Commercial Crew Program.

"Today a new era in human spaceflight begins as we once again launched American astronauts on American rockets from American soil on their way to the International Space Station, our national lab orbiting Earth," said NASA Administrator Jim Bridenstine.

For operational missions, Crew Dragon will be able to launch as many as four crew members at a time and carry more than 220 pounds of cargo, allowing for an increased number crew members aboard the space station and increasing the time dedicated to research in the unique microgravity environment, as well as returning more science back to Earth.

Source: https://www.sciencedaily.com/releases/2020/05/200530172612.htm

1. According to the passage, which of the following statements is true?
    A. The launch of the Crew Dragon spacecraft on Saturday was the first test of this spacecraft
    B. Robert Behnken was the lead engineer for this project
    C. This is the first time that NASA astronauts have launched from American soil
    D. The International Space Station orbits the Earth
2. What statement can be inferred from the passage?
    A. Using the Crew Dragon will increase the amount of new scientific discoveries made in space
    B. SpaceX have never sent a spacecraft into space before
    C. The SpaceX Demo-2 is certified for regular crew flights to the ISS
    D. SpaceX are part-owned by NASA
3. Which of the following is not listed as an advantage of using Crew Dragon?
    A. The ability to launch four crew members at a time
    B. The ability to carry over 220 pounds of cargo
    C. Lower launch costs
    D. Increased research time on the ISS
4. What is the purpose of the SpaceX Demo-2 launch?
    A. To conduct research in microgravity
    B. To test NASA's Kennedy Space Center
    C. To validate the Crew Transportation System

D. To commercialize space travel

Answer 3

Strategy: Read the text, then answer the questions. This is a standard example of a statement-based question. The text is slightly complex, and the questions ask for inferences, so it is important to have a general understanding of the passage.

1. The correct answer is D. This is evidenced by the statement "...on their way to the International Space Station, our national lab orbiting Earth".
2. The correct answer is A. From the content in paragraph 4, we can infer that an increased amount of research taking place in space would increase the amount of scientific discoveries being made in space.
3. The correct answer is C. After reading the whole text, it should be easier to remember that A, B and D were all mentioned but C was not.
4. The correct answer is C. This is evidenced by the statement "Known as NASA's SpaceX Demo-2, the mission is an end-to-end test flight to validate the SpaceX Crew Transportation System, including launch, in-orbit, docking and landing operations."

Example 4

It happened more than two centuries ago, but its impact remains enormous. Historians have credited the infamous "year without a summer" of 1816, at least indirectly, with the invention of the bicycle and the writing of the classic novel "Frankenstein."

In April of 1815, Mount Tambora exploded in a powerful eruption that killed tens of thousands of people on the Indonesian island of Sumbawa. The following year became known as the "year without a summer" when unusually cold, wet conditions swept across Europe and North America.

Since 1913, researchers have suggested that the two events were linked. Now a new study shows that the cold summer temperatures of 1816 wouldn't have been possible without the volcanic eruption. The research was published Tuesday in the journal Environmental Research Letters.

The immediate effects of the volcano resulted in mass destruction. The eruption, the flows that came from it and the related tsunamis destroyed homes and claimed 10,000 lives. Another 80,000 would die from disease that spread in the aftermath.

"The eruption of Mount Tambora in April 1815 was among the most explosive of the last millennium," said Andrew Schurer, lead study author and research associate at the University of Edinburgh's School of Geosciences. "It had an enormous impact locally, devastating the island of Sumbawa."

Source: https://edition.cnn.com/2019/09/17/world/tambora-eruption-year-without-summer-scn/index.html

1. The Mount Tambora eruption occurred in the year 1816.
   A. True
   B. False
   C. Can't Tell
2. The cold temperatures in the summer were caused by the volcanic eruption.
   A. True
   B. False
   C. Can't Tell
3. 90,000 lives were lost as a consequence of the volcanic eruption.
   A. True
   B. False
   C. Can't Tell
4. The Mount Tambora eruption was the strongest volcanic eruption ever.
   A. True
   B. False
   C. Can't Tell

Answer 4

Strategy: Scan and read selectively. Because it is a True, False, Can't Tell passage, your overall understanding of the text does not need to be as high as it would in a statement-based passage, as you are not required to make inferences to answer these questions.

1. The correct answer is B. If you scanned for the number 1816, you would have found information about the "year without summer" which is irrelevant to the question. This scanning did not work, so you should then scan for the proper noun "Mount Tambora", leading you to the sentence "In April of 1815, Mount Tambora exploded in a powerful eruption that killed tens of thousands of people on the Indonesian island of Sumbawa."
2. The correct answer is A. You have already seen the mention of "volcanic eruption" from the question, scanning, and selective reading prior to this. Therefore, we would not use "volcanic eruptions" again, and would instead use "cold temperatures" as the keyword/phrase. You should find this sentence: "Now a new study shows that the cold summer temperatures of 1816 wouldn't have been possible without the volcanic eruption."
3. The correct answer is A. As discussed previously, if you cannot see the number in the passage, you look for the unit of measurement. Here, the unit is "lives lost" so

synonyms like "deaths", "lives" or "fatalities" would work. This would lead you to the fourth paragraph, where the importance of reading around the key words is highlighted. It would be very easy to just take the "10,000 lives lost" by itself. However, when you read on, it becomes clear that the 80,000 lives mentioned in the next sentence is relevant too, making our total 90,000.

4. The correct answer is C. As we cannot find a superlative along the lines of "strongest" in the passage, we should assume that it is either B or C. However, scanning for other superlatives would help us find the line "The eruption of Mount Tambora in April 1815 was among the **most** explosive of the last millennium." Because of the word "among" it is possible that it *is* the strongest, and it is also possible that it is not the strongest. We need more information, so the answer is "Can't Tell."

Use of Language

In reading comprehension, understanding the use of language is vital to achieving a high score. This topic will help you understand how question writers may attempt to trick the reader with the use of language.

Subjective vs Objective Statements

It is common for a student to be caught out by the use of subjective and objective statements.

A subjective statement is a statement made by the writer which cannot be verified by factual or scientific sources.

Essentially, it is the expression of the writer's opinion. However, these statements will not always appear to be just an opinion. Sometimes it may be stated as a fact, but it is evident from the context that it is influenced by the speaker's bias.

A subjective statement will sometimes include words such as:

- according
- believed
- said
- thought

An objective statement is one which is completely unbiased and based purely on factual evidence.

An objective statement can usually be discernible by the use of definitive words such as:

- know

- proved
- calculated

This is because the objective words all have basis in fact, whereas the subjective words infer a bias or a belief, rather than fact.

Why is this relevant? Certain questions in the UCAT will ask you to determine which statement out of four is "best supported" or "true". In these cases, the answer will always be an objective statement. They can also ask questions such as "Which of the following four statements does the author agree with?" whereby you should seek a subjective statement.

Try the examples below to see this in practice.

Example 5

New research was published this week highlighting the associations between teenage cannabis use and a range of mental health problems. The results suggested that use of the drug was associated with an increased risk of depression and a significantly higher risk of suicide attempts.

As usual in a study based on survey data, the authors noted that a clear line of causation from cannabis use to the reported effects cannot be drawn. There are always other potential mechanisms in action. Young people who use cannabis regularly may already be experiencing mental health issues that make drug use more likely; or be facing adverse life experiences that influence both their mental health and drug consumption.

Nevertheless, we cannot ignore evidence of a relationship between cannabis use among young people and mental health harms, especially as the strains of cannabis on the market become more potent. The question is how we can best address this challenge in ways that reduce harm.

The temptation is to call for more stringent enforcement of the law. The idea that we can deter use and restrict supply with tough policing has instinctive appeal. However, in reality, this approach has exacerbated and added to the harms we see. Prohibition has instead contributed to the market dominance of riskier high-THC, low-CBD products, and the continued linking of cannabis use to a wider illegal drug market that draws young people into criminalised environments. These both increase the risk of arrest, and of exposure to other drugs, as well as exploitation, including the more violent world of "county lines".

Source: https://www.theguardian.com/commentisfree/2019/feb/15/legalisation-cannabis-protect-users-mental-health

1. Which of the following statements is best supported by the text?
    A. The use of cannabis in teenage years causes depression and higher risk of suicide attempts.
    B. Stricter law enforcement would drive down risks associated with cannabis use.
    C. In the past, stricter law enforcement has harmed young people.
    D. The main threat of cannabis use is that the more people use it, the stronger strains on the market become.

2. According to the article, policing cannabis use will most likely lead to:
    A. A reduction in the use of cannabis in teenagers.
    B. More strain being put on the police force's budget.
    C. A reduction in mental health issues in teenagers.
    D. An increase in the risk of exploitation of young people.

3. Which statement can be correctly inferred from the passage?
    A. The speaker doesn't believe that cannabis use will lead to mental health conditions.
    B. The speaker doesn't believe that stricter law enforcement would be the right way to reduce harm in youth.
    C. The speaker believes that low-THC products are more dangerous than high-THC products.
    D. THC is a safer compound than CBD.

4. Which of the following is not listed as a potential reason for risks of depression associated with cannabis use?
    A. Cannabis interfering with brain pathways.
    B. Young people who use cannabis may already be experiencing mental health issues.
    C. Young people who use cannabis may be more likely to be exploited through county lines and other criminal environments.
    D. Young people who use cannabis may have external factors, leading to both mental health conditions and heavier cannabis use.

Answer 5

1. The correct answer is C. All of the other statements are either untrue or subjective. Statement A would be considered untrue as the word "cause" is used, and correlation does not equal causation. B is subjective – at the start of the fourth paragraph, the speaker briefly mentions this idea but provides no evidence to back it up, and instead,

shows evidence to the contrary. C has clear evidence – the speaker lists visible effects of increased policing surrounding cannabis, backing up the idea that it has caused increased harm to young people.

2. The correct answer is D. This is mentioned in the fourth paragraph: "These both increase the risk of arrest, and of exposure to other drugs, as well as exploitation, including the more violent world of 'county lines'."
3. The correct answer is B. This is a similar question to the previous two, and so having read the text it should be clear that this is what the reader believes. Note how three out of the four statements use the word 'believe', and so in order for any of those statements to be correct the relevant section of text does not need to have a factual basis, as the purpose is to demonstrate the author's views.
4. The correct answer is A. This is a simple "search and retrieve" question. All of the other reasons can be found in the second and fourth paragraphs.

Qualifiers of Necessity and Possibility

Another language device to be cautious of is the use of qualifiers, both in the question and in the passage. Qualifiers are words that change how absolute a statement is.

Qualifiers can be split into two different categories:

1. **Qualifiers of necessity.** Examples include:
    - Necessary
    - Must
    - Have to
    - Only
    - Definitely

2. **Qualifiers of possibility.** Examples include:
    - Can
    - Could
    - May
    - Should

You must understand the differences between the types of qualifiers and the effect that each qualifier has on the inferences you can draw from a statement. Qualifiers of necessity are words that are conclusive and definite, removing any doubt from the statement.

- E.g. "All cars <u>must</u> have four wheels."

Based on this statement, the reader should have no doubt that a car must have four wheels and cannot have two, three, or five wheels.

A qualifier of possibility is a word that implies probability or likelihood in a statement. However, be careful with the words "can" and "could" – while they can be used to indicate *possibility*, they can also be used to indicate *ability*. For example, here are two sentences:

- "I **can** play tennis well."
- "Tennis **can** be a great way to relieve stress."

In the first sentence, the word "can" is used to indicate ability – the speaker is able to play tennis well. However, in the second sentence, the word "can" is used to indicate possibility – tennis can possibly relieve stress, but there is no certainty to this statement, i.e. it does not definitely relieve stress. As you can see here, reading the whole sentence is imperative to understanding the context of the qualifiers used.

The *type* of qualifier used in the passage and in the question can either be the same or differ. Let us take a look at some examples.

- E.g. "Dell computers are usually black."

Dell computers are never silver.

A. True
B. False
C. Can't Tell

The answer here would have to be "Can't Tell". You can see that there is a discrepancy between the *types* of qualifiers used – "sometimes" in the passage is a qualifier of possibility, whereas "never" in the question is a qualifier of necessity. When there is a discrepancy as such, the answer is usually "Can't Tell" as there is nothing to confirm or negate the statement.

- E.g. "Dell computers are only ever black."

Dell computers are never silver.

A. True
B. False
C. Can't Tell

The answer here would be "True". The types of qualifiers used in the statement and passage are the same – qualifiers of necessity. This makes it easier to conclude whether the statement is "True" or "False".

Future Qualifiers

Another thing to bear in mind when looking at qualifiers of necessity or possibility is the tense in which they are used. Sometimes, the writer will use ***future qualifiers*** such as "would" and "will". Questions containing future qualifiers will generally be "Can't Tell", as it is difficult to predict the future with any certainty regarding a True, False, Can't Tell statement.

Let us take a look the following statement:

- E.g. "The advancement of space technology means that our goal to reach Mars is within our grasp."

Humans will soon be able to go to Mars.

A. True
B. False
C. Can't Tell

From the information we are given, we do not know enough to answer this question with any certainty. The question raises the possibility of humans being able to go to Mars, but there is no evidence to indicate that this will certainly happen, and there is no way to predict the future. The text in the question also does not directly contradict the statement, so the answer here should be "Can't Tell".

Take a look at the following passage and answer the questions based on the strategies you have learnt.

Example 6

A team of Princeton researchers reported today in the journal Cell that they have found a compound, SCH-79797, that can simultaneously puncture bacterial walls and destroy folate within their cells -- while being immune to antibiotic resistance.

Bacterial infections come in two types -- Gram-positive and Gram-negative -- named for the scientist who discovered how to distinguish them. The key difference is that Gram-negative bacteria are armored with an outer layer that shrugs off most antibiotics. In fact, no new classes of Gram-negative-killing drugs have come to market in nearly 30 years.

"This is the first antibiotic that can target Gram-positives and Gram-negatives without resistance," said Zemer Gitai, Princeton's Edwin Grant Conklin Professor of Biology and the senior author on the paper. "From a 'Why it's useful' perspective, that's the crux. But what we're most excited about as scientists is something we've discovered about how this antibiotic works -- attacking via two different mechanisms within one molecule -- that we are hoping is generalizable, leading to better antibiotics -- and new types of antibiotics -- in the future.

This poisoned arrow paradigm could revolutionize antibiotic development, said KC Huang, a professor of bioengineering and of microbiology and immunology at Stanford University who was not involved in this research.

"The thing that can't be overstated is that antibiotic research has stalled over a period of many decades," Huang said. "It's rare to find a scientific field which is so well studied and yet so in need of a jolt of new energy."

Source: https://www.sciencedaily.com/releases/2020/06/200603132541.htm

1. This new discovery will revolutionise the way in which antibiotics are developed in the future.
    A. True
    B. False
    C. Can't Tell

2. The outer layer of Gram-Negative bacteria protects it against all other antibiotics.
    A. True
    B. False
    C. Can't Tell

3. The New anti-Gram-Negative drug classes have been rare in the past 30 years.
    A. True
    B. False
    C. Can't Tell

4. The new drug's ability to attack with two mechanisms may make it more useful in fighting bacterial infection.
    A. True
    B. False
    C. Can't Tell

Answer 6

The overall strategy for this passage is to scan and read selectively.

1. The correct answer is C. The use of the future qualifier "will" means that it is difficult to prove either way, and we do not know what will happen in the future. This means that we need more information and so the answer should be "Can't Tell".
2. The correct answer is B. The word "all" is very definite here – it means that the threshold of evidence is considerably high and so you should immediately be leaning

towards "False". The evidence for this can be found in the second paragraph – "The key difference is that Gram-negative bacteria are armored with an outer layer that shrugs off most antibiotics."

3. The correct answer is B. This question is not to do with qualifiers – it is there to recap your scanning strategies. This question should have been easy to answer as there is the number "30" in the statement. Scanning for the number in the text would lead you to the sentence "In fact, no new classes of Gram-negative-killing drugs have come to market in nearly 30 years." Because the statement in the question contained the word "rare" it implied that there were still some new classes of Gram-negative-killing drugs, although the text from the passage directly states that there were none.
4. The correct answer is A. The qualifier of possibility "may", means there is a low threshold of evidence required, so you should be leaning towards "True". The evidence to back this up can be found in paragraph 3. By reading this section, it would logically follow that if an antibiotic is "better", it is more useful in fighting bacterial infection, and so the answer would be "True".

Negative Language

Sometimes, a question can use negative language, such as "none", "doesn't", or "not".

- E.g. "Which statement is not listed as a potential consequence of smoking?"

This is just a case of reading the question carefully. If you miss the word "not", you can easily be caught out and answer the opposite of what the question is asking, especially in a time-pressured exam.

You should also ensure there is not a double negative. Understand exactly what the question is asking by interpreting the "positive meaning" before you attempt to answer it.

Take a look at the following statements:

- "It is not normal to not want peace."
- "It is not impossible to write a book."

In the first example, the negative "not" is used twice, therefore, it essentially cancels itself out. The resultant positive meaning would be "It is normal to want peace."

In the second example, there are two different negatives used – "not" and "impossible". The positive meaning here is "It is possible to write a book."

Further, there may be discrepancies between the passage and the question with regards to positive and negative language. The scenarios can be as follows:

1. The statement is negative and the text in the passage is positive. This scenario is often "False."
2. The statement is positive and the text in the passage is negative. This scenario is often "False."
3. The statement is negative and the text in the passage is also negative. This scenario is often "True."

Use the following example to answer the subsequent question:

- E.g. "It is not possible to find a medication that is able to tackle every type of virus."

Scientists have not been able to invent a drug that is effective against all viruses.

a. True
b. False
c. Can't Tell

The passage says "not possible" and the question also says "not" therefore the answer is "True." Yes, the scientists have not yet been able to invent this type of drug.

Outside Knowledge

In this section, it is very important not to utilise any outside knowledge, except what you have learnt about exam technique, of course! During the course of this exam, you are only being tested on your ability to synthesise information from text and apply logic to what you are reading. You are not being tested on what you already know. However, this should not be taken the wrong way - knowledge of definitions of words is incredibly important and should be utilised.

For example, if the passage is about headphones, using the knowledge that headphones play sounds would not be considered outside knowledge – this is very general and so can be applied. However, knowledge of the intricate functioning of headphones would be considered outside knowledge, as it is more in-depth than the average person would know. The concept of definition is incredibly important here – by definition, headphones play noises into one's ears. However, the definition of headphones would not include the intricate functioning of the machine, and so would not be relevant information to use in the UCAT. It can be very easy to accidentally apply outside knowledge to a question, especially when it seems obvious.

Use the following excerpt from a passage to answer the subsequent question:

- “A volcano on Earth is a vent or fissure in the planet's crust through which lava, ash, rock and gases erupt. A volcano is also a mountain formed by the accumulation of these eruptive products.”

Volcanoes are a threat to human lives.

A. True
B. False
C. Can’t Tell

We all know that this statement is true - we’ve learnt about volcanoes since childhood. However, our knowledge is not relevant here, as a volcano, by definition, is not necessarily a threat to human lives. Therefore, this knowledge should not be used when answering the question. Nothing in the text supports this claim, so we cannot say that this is “True”. There is also nothing to refute this claim, meaning that our answer here would have to be “Can’t Tell”.

Drawing Conclusions

You can be asked in a question to identify the “best” or the “main” conclusion out of four given statements. To do this, you must understand what a conclusion is.

Identifying Premises

A premise is evidence given in support of the conclusion but is not, in itself, a conclusion.

When looking for conclusions in the text, it is important to avoid mistaking a premise for a conclusion. Take a look at the following short passage:

- Bernese Mountain Dogs shed a lot, so you shouldn’t get one. They also have a lot of fleas.

The purpose of this short passage is to highlight to the reader that they should not get a Bernese Mountain Dog. The evidences for this are as follows: Bernese Mountain Dogs shed a lot, and Bernese Mountain Dogs have a lot of fleas. Therefore, we can identify the premises which are used to support the conclusion, as follows:

- **Premise 1:** Bernese Mountain Dogs shed a lot.
- **Premise 2:** Bernese Mountain Dogs have a lot of fleas.
- **Conclusion:** You shouldn’t get a Bernese Mountain Dog.

Being able to identify premises in text is very important, as often two or three of the statements given to you in a conclusion-drawing question will just be reworded premises.

Certain words may be used before a phrase to indicate whether it is a premise or a conclusion. One sentence can include both a premise and a conclusion, but the indicating word will usually be present before its relevant portion of the sentence.

Words Indicating a Premise	Words Indicating a Conclusion
Because	Therefore
As	As such
Due to	So
For	Hence
As a result of	It follows that
Seeing that	This implies that
Owing to	For this reason
Given that	Accordingly

- E.g. "Given that my baby cries all night, it is impossible for me to get a good night's sleep."
- E.g. "My baby cries all night, hence it is impossible for me to get a good night's sleep.

Premise: My baby cries all night.
Conclusion: I cannot sleep.

Identifying the Best Conclusion

When deciphering which of four given statements is the "best conclusion", you must decide which of the statements covers all of the premises given in the passage. Statements that only address some of the premises in the passage will not be the "best" conclusion, as they are incomplete. Any statements that are off-topic or incomplete should be disregarded, regardless of how true they are. Use the following example:

Example 7

A pregnancy to a woman is perhaps one of the most determinative aspects of her life. It disrupts her body. It disrupts her education. It disrupts her employment. And it often disrupts her entire family life. And we feel that, because of the impact on the woman, this is a matter which is of such fundamental and basic concern to the woman involved that she should be allowed to make the choice as to whether to continue or to terminate her pregnancy. [Adapted from: **Roe v. Wade**, 410 U.S. 113 (1973)]

If abortion rights are denied, then a constraint is imposed on women's freedom to act in a way that is of great importance to them, both for its own sake and for the sake of their achievement of equality. [Source: http://bostonreview.net/archives/BR20.3/thomson.html]

Hint: The premises and conclusion of this passage can be identified as follows:

- ***Premise 1:*** *A pregnancy has a huge impact on the mother (with examples).*
- ***Premise 2:*** *Denying abortion rights imposes constraints on a woman's freedom.*
- ***Conclusion:*** *The mother should be given the choice to terminate the pregnancy.*

Which one of the following best expresses the conclusion drawn in the argument?

A. A pregnancy is one of the most determinative aspects of a woman's life
B. Denying the rights of a woman to terminate her pregnancy removes her freedom to choose what is best, and so a mother should be allowed to terminate her pregnancy.
C. Abortion is an inherently good idea
D. A mother should be given the choice to terminate a pregnancy in order to preserve her freedom of choice and because of the impact of a pregnancy on her and her family's lives.

Answer 7

Statement A is just a rewording of one of the premises. B is a correct conclusion but does not take all of the premises into account (premise 1 is missing), so it is incomplete. C is off topic – the text is not talking about whether or not abortion is a good thing, but is instead discussing whether mothers should have the right to abort. D is the best conclusion because it describes both premises and presents a conclusion drawn from these premises.

Assumptions

An assumption can be defined as anything that is taken to be true without proof.

It can be very easy to make assumptions when reading an extract from the passage. By definition, assumptions are a bad concept within the UCAT because everything needs evidence. If it does not come from the evidence presented to you, then it cannot be proven to be true. Assumptions can be tricky as sometimes the line between fact and assumption is unclear. Taking the definition of an object and using that to help you answer a question is not an assumption. For example, the statement "bees are able to fly" is not an assumption as, by definition, bees are insects that can fly. However, "bees are faster than wasps" would be considered an assumption if it was not backed up by clear evidence in the passage.

Have a look at this example, making sure not to use any assumptions or outside knowledge to answer the questions.

Example 8

After studying global data from the novel coronavirus (COVID-19) pandemic, researchers have discovered a strong correlation between severe vitamin D deficiency and mortality rates.
Led by Northwestern University, the research team conducted a statistical analysis of data from hospitals and clinics across China, France, Germany, Italy, Iran, South Korea, Spain, Switzerland, the United Kingdom (UK) and the United States.
The researchers noted that patients from countries with high COVID-19 mortality rates, such as Italy, Spain and the UK, had lower levels of vitamin D compared to patients in countries that were not as severely affected.
"While I think it is important for people to know that vitamin D deficiency might play a role in mortality, we don't need to push vitamin D on everybody," said Northwestern's Vadim Backman, who led the research. "This needs further study, and I hope our work will stimulate interest in this area. The data also may illuminate the mechanism of mortality, which, if proven, could lead to new therapeutic targets."
Backman and his team were inspired to examine vitamin D levels after noticing unexplained differences in COVID-19 mortality rates from country to country. Some people hypothesized that differences in healthcare quality, age distributions in population, testing rates or different strains of the coronavirus might be responsible. But Backman remained skeptical.
"None of these factors appears to play a significant role," Backman said. "The healthcare system in northern Italy is one of the best in the world. Differences in mortality exist even if one looks across the same age group. And, while the restrictions on testing do indeed vary, the disparities in mortality still exist even when we looked at countries or populations for which similar testing rates apply.
"Instead, we saw a significant correlation with vitamin D deficiency," he said.

Source: https://www.sciencedaily.com/releases/2020/05/200507121353.htm

1. According to the article, which is the best supported conclusion?
    A. Vitamin D may play a part in the way that humans respond to coronavirus
    B. Northern Italy's healthcare system is better than the UK's healthcare system
    C. Differences in healthcare quality were the main reason for the disparity in mortality rates between countries
    D. Differences in the average age of a population impacted countries' mortality rates

2. According to Vadim Backman, people should:
    A. Begin to take Vitamin D supplements
    B. Go outside more to take in more sunlight

C. Understand that a Vitamin D deficiency could play a role in coronavirus mortality
D. Get tested for a Vitamin D deficiency

3. Which of the following is not listed as an initial hypothesis for the disparity of coronavirus mortality rates?
    A. Differences in healthcare quality
    B. Differences in age distribution
    C. Differences in testing rates between countries
    D. Differences in countries' research and development capabilities

4. According to the article, why could this discovery be useful?
    A. It may help to discover the mechanism behind coronavirus mortality
    B. It will help to understand which groups of people are more at-risk
    C. It may help to find a cure for coronavirus
    D. It may help to boost vitamin D intake in the population

Answer 8

1. The correct answer is A. Whilst some of the other statements (e.g. B) are true according to some sources, they are not mentioned in this article and so the answer here would be A. This conclusion can be drawn from many different sections of the text, such as "Instead, we saw a significant correlation with vitamin D deficiency". Remember that correlation does not equal causation, but the use of the qualifier of possibility "may" in the question indicates that this statement could be true, as is it *possible* for correlation to indicate causation.
2. The correct answer is C. Again, while some of the other statements are potentially true, they aren't mentioned in the article and so would be considered as using outside information. C is backed up in the text by the sentence: "The data also may illuminate the mechanism of mortality, which, if proven, could lead to new therapeutic targets". Again, note the use of the qualifier of possibility "could".
3. The correct answer is D. While D is potentially true, it is not referenced at all in the text and so is the odd one out. To find the rest of them, it is a simple search and retrieve job – they can all be found in paragraph 5.
4. The correct answer is A. Similar to question 2, this is mentioned in the text. The rest of the options are not referenced at all in the text and so should be ignored.

Inferences

Making an inference means to draw conclusions based on the evidence and information given to you, i.e. reading between the lines.

This is different to assumptions, which are made **without** evidence. Knowing how to make inferences is essential, as this technique is used in most of the Verbal Reasoning passages. For True, False, Can't Tell questions, you will not usually need to make any inferences as these are fact-based questions that rely solely on answers found within the passage.

Let us take a look at the following statement:

- E.g. "During the weekend, I bought an iced coffee and headed to the beach with my friends."

Here are a few inferences we can draw from this statement:

1. Based on the fact that the speaker went to the beach and had a chilled drink, we can infer that the temperature was warm.
2. From this, we can infer that the most likely season is Summer.
3. The fact that the speaker is heading to the beach with friends on the weekend suggests that they had free time, which could infer that they don't work on the weekends

The point is to see what information you can take without overthinking. Sure, you could go further and suggest that they are off work because it is a bank holiday weekend, but unless stated, this is very unlikely. This kind of inference involves a degree of overthinking, because the majority of weekends in the year are not bank holiday weekends, so if there is no evidence to support this then it is not an inference that can be made.

Considering the context of the passage is very important. If the excerpt was from a passage about how the author usually spends their weekends, it would make sense to infer that they have free time on the weekend. If the text was from a passage about how people like to spend holidays from work, then we might not infer that the author is always free on a weekend, as it is more likely that this weekend is a holiday.

There will be many question types that will require you to infer bits of information from the text. Here are some examples:

- "According to the text, which is the best supported argument?"
- "Which statement can be correctly inferred from the text?"
- "What conclusion can be drawn from the text?"

Different Types of Inferences

1) The passage and the statement are directly linked.

- E.g. "Anthony was born in 1995. His parents, John and Lucy got married 6 years before his birth."
- Statement: "John married Lucy in 1989."

This is straightforward and is true as it's directly proven through the text. This answer is reached simply by reading and understanding the text. In a True, False, Can't Tell question, the answer here would be "True".

2) The statement is not directly stated in the text but can be inferred indirectly.

- E.g. "Since the early Macbooks, Apple has always been amongst the most creative and loved companies for its bespoke creation in people's eyes."
- Statement: "Apple is considered to be one of the best laptop designers in the world."

Although it is not directly stated, we can infer this to be true indirectly as the passage states, in other words, that Apple has long since been at the forefront of creativity and customer satisfaction in people's eyes. Further, this inference can be reached because the passage says that it is "among" the most creative and loved, and the statement uses similar broad terminology – "one of the best".

3) Too much inferring!

- E.g. "Since the early Macbooks, Apple has always been amongst the most creative and loved companies for its bespoke creation in people's eyes."
- Statement: "Apple is the most successful laptop designer in the world."

This statement involved too much inferring, and is therefore an assumption, rather than a logical inference. The passage infers that Apple is "among" the most successful, not that it "is". If this was a True/False/Can't Tell question, the answer would be "Can't Tell". There is a possibility that Apple could be the most successful, as the passage does not disprove this statement, nor does it confirm it.

4) Completely false inferring

- E.g. "As many footballers now enjoy playing football in England, Ronaldo followed his fellow countryman Tiago to play for Manchester United Football Club."

- Statement: "Ronaldo was the first Portuguese footballer to play for Manchester United."

This statement is disproven in the passage where "his fellow countryman" is mentioned, therefore this is not an inference that can possibly be made. The answer in a True, False, Can't Tell question would be "False."

Example 9

Liverpool Football Club is now one of the most successful football teams in the history of sport. There has been a recent injection of cash from the new owners which has funded the signing of marquee players. Liverpool Football Club has become every 11-year-old's favourite team.

1. Liverpool Football Club is one of the most prosperous teams in history.
   A. True
   B. False
   C. Can't Tell

2. Liverpool Football Club is the best football team in the world.
   A. True
   B. False
   C. Can't Tell

Answer 9

1. True. This can be directly inferred from the passage, because of the statement "...one of the most successful football teams in the history of sport."
2. Can't Tell. Is there a possibility that they are the best football team in the world? Yes, based on the passage, this is a possibility. However, is this proven in the passage? No. Therefore, we are unable to say for certain, and because there is no evidence against this statement, the answer will be "Can't Tell".

Inferring Quickly

An important skill to learn here is to not just infer, but infer quickly. As mentioned earlier, you have 21 minutes to answer 44 questions. This is not enough time to think too deeply about any particular question. By practicing your inference skills, you will be able to develop the habit of inferring naturally while reading, rather than taking everything at face value.

Here are a few steps you can take to help increase your inferencing speed:

- Just like you did with reading speed, you can read long passages such as newspaper articles to start building inferences.
- Annotate the page, as if you were in your English GCSE exams, and write down any inferences you can make from the text, underlining the evidence for your inferences.
- Once you are accustomed to annotating inferences, try to make the inferences in your head and write them down in note-form at the end of the page.

Doing this regularly will build the habit of making inferences from text naturally. This will increase the speed at which you are able to do so and will help you immensely in the UCAT.

Inferences with Numbers

It is common for the examiners to try to trick the reader with numbers. There are often situations where you need to use numbers to make logical inferences. For example, if the text states that 36% of a sample group answered "no" to a "yes or no" question, there is enough evidence to infer that 64% of the sample group answered "yes". You may also find relevant numbers distributed across the passage. For example, the start of a passage might say that 2% of the UK population suffer from a certain disease, and later in the passage you find that the UK population is 70 million. From this, you would be expected to calculate that around 1.4 million people suffer from the named disease.

Example 10

Obesity affects more than 40 percent of adults in the United States (pop. 320 million) and 13 percent of the global population (pop. 7.79 billion). With obesity comes a variety of other interconnected diseases including cardiovascular disease, diabetes, and fatty liver disease, which makes the disease one of the most difficult -- and most crucial -- to treat.

"Obesity is the biggest health problem in the United States. But, it is hard for people to lose weight and keep it off; being on a diet can be so difficult. So, a pharmacological approach, or a drug, could help out and would be beneficial for all of society," said Webster Santos, professor of chemistry and the Cliff and Agnes Lilly Faculty Fellow of Drug Discovery in the College of Science at Virginia Tech.

Santos and his colleagues have recently identified a small mitochondrial uncoupler, named BAM15, that decreases the body fat mass of mice without affecting food intake and muscle mass or increasing body temperature. Additionally, the molecule decreases insulin resistance and has beneficial effects on oxidative stress and inflammation.

The mitochondria are commonly referred to as the powerhouses of the cell. The organelle generates ATP, a molecule that serves as the energy currency of the cell, which powers body movement and other biological processes that help our body to function properly.

Source: https://www.sciencedaily.com/releases/2020/06/200608132539.htm

1. Which of the statements are best supported by the text?
    A. Obesity affects more than 160 million people in the USA
    B. Obesity affects more than 120 million people in the USA
    C. Obesity affects more than a sixth of the world population
    D. Obesity affects more than half of the American population
2. Which statement can be inferred from the text?
    A. Obesity is the most serious health issue facing the American population
    B. Obesity can't be controlled with lifestyle changes
    C. Obesity always causes cardiovascular disease in patients
    D. Obesity is the most severe global health problem
3. The new drug:
    A. Will cure obesity
    B. Decreases the body fat mass of humans without affecting food intake
    C. Works on all cells in the body
    D. Has the potential to help with the obesity problem
4. Which of the following is not listed as a complication of obesity?
    A. Diabetes
    B. Cardiovascular disease
    C. Drop in fitness levels
    D. Liver disease

Answer 10

1. The correct answer is B. 40% of 320 million is just over 120 million (320 / 10 = 32, 32 x 4 = 128) and so this would be the best supported statement. While the others may be true, we can't tell for certain from the text.
2. The correct answer is A. From the line 'Obesity is the biggest health problem in the United States', we can infer that it is the most serious health issue affecting the population. The other statements are either refuted in the text (B) or aren't backed up by the text (C, D) and so the answer here would be A
3. The correct answer is D. Note the use of the future qualifier of necessity 'will' in A, which should instantly make you wary of picking that option. D is the only one which is backed up in the text, with the other two not being mentioned.
4. The correct answer is C. A simple search-and-retrieve question.

Faulty Logic

It is important to be aware of faulty logic to avoid inferring statements without a logical basis.

Let's take a simple statement: "A lion is a mammal"

From this statement, we can conclude that any given lion would be a mammal. However, it would be false to draw the conclusion that all *mammals* are *lions*. While there is nothing in the statement to refute this idea, the statement also does not provide any evidence to suggest that this is true. Faulty logic like this can catch you out in a Verbal Reasoning question.

This can be demonstrated with the following rule:

> "If A is always B, B is not necessarily always A, unless specified."

So, when applied to the above, lion is A and mammal is B. Lions are always mammals. Mammals are not always lions, unless specified in the passage.

Correlation and Causation

This is a common topic that you should be well aware of, and that the UCAT can try to trick you with. A correlation does not always mean a causation, so be very wary of anything asking for a "cause".

- E.g. "Whenever James went to play rugby it rained."

This does not mean that James playing rugby causes it to rain. There is a correlation between James playing rugby and the clouds raining, as stated in the passage, but there is no evidence to support rugby being a cause for rain.

Do not assume a causal relationship between two things solely for the reason that they are mentioned together in the passage. Although it is possible for there to be a causal relationship where the statement indicates a correlation, there needs to be evidence to confirm this. Certain words or phrases can help identify where there is a causal relationship. Examples are as follows:

- Because
- As a result of
- Due to
- As evidenced by

Important Things to Remember

To sum up, here are 10 important things to remember when practicing for your Verbal Reasoning exam:

1. **Start early:** Giving yourself as much time as possible will allow you to fully develop core techniques such as speed reading and deduction.
2. **Speed is key:** when you are practicing any of the techniques, you should be learning to do so at an efficient speed. Without speed, you will not have enough time to answer all of the questions. Timing yourself as you do practice questions and mock papers is crucial.
3. **Learn when to discard:** There will be some styles of questions you are not as good at, or some that you find more time consuming. If you spend lots of time on a question and are still struggling for the answer, sometimes the best option is to discard that question and move on. If you are struggling on the first question out of four, it usually indicates that the other three questions are going to be of similar difficulty and that you should discard this passage and move on.
4. **Scanning vs reading:** Learning when to scan and when to read the passages given to you is one of the most important strategies in this section. When you are able to, scanning texts will save you so much time compared to reading them, allowing you to spend more time on more difficult questions.
5. **Look for similarities:** Often, the question may try to trick you with a statement phrased very similar to a sentence in the text, along with some minor changes. Reading around the section of text that you have isolated is important to make sure that it is saying exactly what the question is asking for. For example, if the sentence "All preschool children like to play outside" is in a passage, the statement "All children like to play outside" would be "Can't Tell" as they are subtly different.
6. **Subjective vs Objective:** Make sure that anything that is presented as a "fact" is backed up by evidence (unless obvious). This is important, as being able to distinguish opinions from facts will be what helps you to score highly in "best answer questions".
7. **Logic:** Make sure that any logic you are applying to a question makes sense and is viable. You can always check this in the exam by writing out your logic flow on the whiteboard. Practicing this skill while in preparation for the UCAT will also make it a lot easier in the real exam. For example, the start of a passage might say that 2% of the UK population suffer from a certain disease, and later in the passage you find that the UK population is 70 million. From this, you would be expected to calculate that around 1.4 million people suffer from the named disease. You can quickly write this out on your whiteboard.
8. **Remember to infer:** This is one of the core skills required of this section, and so making sure to read into sentences and draw logical conclusions is extremely important. This cannot be done by simply making observations or rewording the text given to you, but

equally do not overthink it – write out what comes naturally to you as a conclusion from the passage. Again, practicing this skill before starting mock questions will be very helpful.

9. **Look for qualifiers:** Remember the differences between qualifiers of necessity and possibility and look out for them in the exam. Knowing the difference between the two and immediately being able to identify them will help you answer questions more quickly and with more accuracy.
10. **There are other sections:** Spending ample time on all sections is absolutely crucial to scoring highly overall, and no university will just look at individual section scores. There is no benefit to scoring 750+ in one section at the expense of the other sections, so spending time on them all is incredibly important. That being said, remember to think about your strengths and weaknesses when coming to prepare for the UCAT to decide how much time you want to spend preparing for each section.

Verbal Reasoning Mock Test

Passage 1

When it comes to living to the ripe old age of 100, good genes help but don't tell the full story. Where you live has a significant impact on the likelihood that you will reach centenarian age, suggests a new study conducted by scientists at Washington State University's Elson S. Floyd College of Medicine.

Published in the *International Journal of Environmental Research and Public Health* and based on Washington State mortality data, the research team's findings suggest that Washingtonians who live in highly walkable, mixed-age communities may be more likely to live to their 100th birthday. They also found socioeconomic status to be correlated, and an additional analysis showed that geographic clusters where the probability of reaching centenarian age is high are located in urban areas and smaller towns with higher socioeconomic status, including the Seattle area and the region around Pullman, Wash.

"Our study adds to the growing body of evidence that social and environmental factors contribute significantly to longevity", said study author Rajan Bhardwaj, a second-year WSU medical student who took an interest in the topic after serving as a home care aide to his aging grandfather. Earlier research, he said, has estimated that heritable factors only explain about 20 to 35% of an individual's chances of reaching centenarian age.

In collaboration with co-authors Solmaz Amiri and Dedra Buchwald, Bhardwaj and Amram looked at state-provided data about the deaths of nearly 145,000 Washingtonians who died at age 75 or older between 2011 and 2015. The data included information on each person's age and place of residence at the time of death, as well as their sex, race, education level and marital status.

Bhardwaj said their findings also highlight the importance of continuing efforts to address health disparities experienced by racial minorities, such as African Americans and Native Americans. Consistent with previous research findings, for example, the data shows being white is correlated with living to 100. Looking at gender, the researchers also found that women were more likely to reach centenarian age.

Source: https://www.sciencedaily.com/releases/2020/06/200617145256.htm

1. Which statement can best be inferred from the passage?

    A. Having good genes means that you will live to at least 100 years old.
    B. People from Washington may be more likely to live to their 100th birthday.
    C. Higher socioeconomic status may influence longevity of life.
    D. Heritable factors have more of an influence than social/environmental factors on the longevity of life.

2. Which of the following is not listed as a factor in the longevity of a person's life?

    A. Their economic status.
    B. Their genetics.
    C. The environment in which they live.
    D. Their country of origin.

3. Which of the following statements is best supported by the passage?

    A. Living in different areas of a state make a minimal difference on longevity of life.
    B. 65-80% of an individual's chances of reaching 100 years old is not explained by heritable factors.
    C. Exercise doesn't contribute to an individual's longevity.
    D. Living in a mixed-age community will decrease your chances of living to 100 years old.

4. Who is Rajan Bhardwaj?

    A. A scientist at Washington State University.
    B. A participant in the study.
    C. A medical student.
    D. A resident of the Seattle region.

Passage 2

Earthquakes, also called temblors, can be so tremendously destructive, it's hard to imagine they occur by the thousands every day around the world, usually in the form of small tremors. Some 80 percent of all the planet's earthquakes occur along the rim of the Pacific Ocean, called the "Ring of Fire" because of the preponderance of volcanic activity there as well. Most earthquakes occur at fault zones, where tectonic plates—giant rock slabs that make up the Earth's upper layer—collide or slide against each other.

These impacts are usually gradual and unnoticeable on the surface; however, immense stress can build up between plates. When this stress is released quickly, it sends massive vibrations, called seismic waves, often hundreds of miles through the rock and up to the surface. Other quakes can occur far from faults zones when plates are stretched or squeezed.

Scientists assign a magnitude rating to earthquakes based on the strength and duration of their seismic waves. A quake measuring 3 to 5 is considered minor or light; 5 to 7 is moderate to strong; 7 to 8 is major; and 8 or more is great.

On average, a magnitude 8 quake strikes somewhere every year and some 10,000 people die in earthquakes annually. Collapsing buildings claim by far the majority of lives, but the destruction is often compounded by mud slides, fires, floods, or tsunamis. Smaller temblors that usually occur in the days following a large earthquake can complicate rescue efforts and cause further death and destruction.

Source: https://www.nationalgeographic.co.uk/2018/02/latest-earthquakes-and-how-earthquakes-work

5. Which statement is best supported by the passage?

    A. "Tremor" is another word for an earthquake.
    B. 80% of earthquakes occur at "fault zones".
    C. Hundreds of thousands of earthquakes occur each year.
    D. Earthquakes always cause fatalities.

6. Which is not listed as a potential consequence of an earthquake?

    A. Disease spreading
    B. Collapsing buildings
    C. Loss of lives
    D. Tsunamis

7. According to the passage, which statement is true?

    A. 10,000 people die in a magnitude 8 earthquake on average every year.
    B. An earthquake of magnitude 8 would be classified as 'Major'.
    C. Earthquakes can only occur at fault zones.
    D. Collapsing buildings are the deadliest consequence of an earthquake.

8. According to the passage, the Ring of Fire:

    A. Is an area in which 80% of all tsunamis occur.
    B. Is named after the large amount of volcanic activity that occurs there.
    C. Is the least safe place to live in the world.
    D. Gets over 5 Major earthquakes every month.

Passage 3

High school students who take music courses score significantly better on math, science and English exams than their non-musical peers, according to a new study published in the *Journal of Educational Psychology*.

School administrators needing to trim budgets often look first to music courses, because the general belief is that students who devote time to music rather than math, science and English, will underperform in those disciplines.

"Our research proved this belief wrong and found the more the students engage with music, the better they do in those subjects," said UBC education professor and the study's principal investigator, Peter Gouzouasis. "The students who learned to play a musical instrument in elementary and continued playing in high school not only score significantly higher, but were about one academic year ahead of their non-music peers with regard to their English, mathematics and science skills, as measured by their exam grades, regardless of their socioeconomic background, ethnicity, prior learning in mathematics and English, and gender."

The researchers found the predictive relationships between music education and academic achievement were more pronounced for those who took instrumental music rather than vocal music. The findings suggest skills learned in instrumental music transfer very broadly to the students' learning in school.

The researchers hope that their findings are brought to the attention of students, parents, teachers and administrative decision-makers in education, as many school districts over the years have emphasized numeracy and literacy at the cost of other areas of learning, particularly music.

"Often, resources for music education -- including the hiring of trained, specialized music educators, and band and stringed instruments -- are cut or not available in elementary and secondary schools so that they could focus on math, science and English," said Gouzouasis. "The irony is that music education -- multiple years of high-quality instrumental learning and playing in a band or orchestra or singing in a choir at an advanced level -- can be the very thing that improves all-around academic achievement and an ideal way to have students learn more holistically in schools."

Source: https://www.sciencedaily.com/releases/2019/06/190624111504.htm

9. Which statement can be best inferred from the passage?

   A. Music is commonly undervalued by school administrators.
   B. Students that can play a musical instrument will do better in science exams than those who cannot.
   C. Students who devote time to music rather than math, science and English will underperform in those disciplines.
   D. Singing is linked more heavily to better grades than playing the piano.

10. Which factor is not listed as something that does not impact this study?

   A. Socioeconomic Background
   B. Ethnicity
   C. Type of musical instrument played
   D. Gender

11. Which statement is true, according to the text?

   A. Skills learned in instrumental music transfer well to academic subjects.
   B. Learning to sing will have a negative impact on a student's academic grades.

C. Peter Gouzouasis believes that the more students engage with music, the less time they have to spend on their academics and so the worse they perform in these subjects.
D. School administrators should look to academic courses when their budgets need cutting down.

12. Which of the following would be a viable future step?

A. Reducing funding for math, English and science courses.
B. Increasing access to music classes in elementary school.
C. Increasing access to music classes in high school.
D. Restricting the number of students that can take music classes, so as to only allow brighter students to study music.

Passage 4

In the second century, Origen wrote, "For those who are adorned with religion use physicians as servants of God, knowing that He himself gave medical knowledge to men, just as He himself assigned both herbs and other things to grow on the earth."
The practice of medicine in the Middle Ages was rooted in the Greek tradition. Hippocrates, considered the "father of Medicine," described the body as made up of four humors—yellow bile, phlegm, black bile, and blood—and controlled by the four elements—fire, water, earth, and air. The body could be purged of excess by bleeding, cupping, and leeching—medical practices that continued throughout the Middle Ages.
In 65 A.D., Dioscorides, a Greek, wrote his *Materia Medica* . This was a practical text dealing with the medicinal use of more than 600 plants. In the second century, Galen synthesized much of what has been attributed to Hippocrates. To further his understanding of bodily functions, he performed animal and even human dissections and was able to demonstrate that the arteries carried blood rather than air. Galenic theories had great longevity, prevailing in western Europe until the sixteenth century.
The Arabs were the great translators and synthesizers of medical texts. Many Greek texts were translated first into Arabic and then into Hebrew. Consequently, Arabs and Jews were renowned for the practice of medicine, and Arabic and Jewish doctors were often employed by kings (for example, James II of Aragon [died 1327]).

Source: https://www.metmuseum.org/toah/hd/medm/hd_medm.htm

13. Kings only hired Arabic and Jewish doctors

A. True
B. False
C. Can't Tell

14. Origen was active in the same century as Galen

A. True
B. False
C. Can't Tell

15. Hippocrates proved that arteries carried blood rather than air

A. True
B. False
C. Can't Tell

16. James II of Aragon died in the 13th century

A. True
B. False
C. Can't Tell

Passage 5

Ever heard of a seed bank? The basic idea is this: When the apocalypse is over and the forests are nothing but smoking ruins and the fields barren of grain, fear not! We can reboot the world thanks to our banked seeds stored in bunkers strategically located from here to eternity. The Svalbard International Seed Vault in Norway, for instance, currently holds more than 880,000 seeds and has the capacity to hold 2.5 billion seeds.

Seeds are amazing that way; all you need to do is dry them out and freeze them solid and they can last for years. It's a comforting thought — an ace up civilization's sleeve in the less-and-less-unlikely scenario that we self-destruct. The U.N.'s Global Strategy for Plant Conservation plans to bank 75 percent of all plant species by 2020.

But hold the comforting thought. According to a study from researchers at the Royal Botanic Gardens, Kew, there's a significant catch. Researchers discovered that a whole whack of plant seeds just can't be banked — including avocado, cacao and mango. Their findings, which were published in the Nov. 2, 2018, issue of the journal Nature Plants, detail how a full 33 percent of tree species alone are on this list, including oak and chestnut trees. Worse still, 36 percent of our "critically endangered" species are also unbankable. That's not even counting 27 percent of the plain old "endangered" plants, or 35 percent of the "vulnerable" ones.

Why can't these seeds be banked? Apparently, not all seeds like the drying out process. And for this, they're labelled "recalcitrant seeds," which seems a little unfair.

"Ex-situ conservation of plants is more critical than ever, with many threats to plant populations including climate change, habitat conversion and plant pathogens, we need to make sure we're doing all we can to conserve the most important and threatened species," John Dickie, head of Seed & Lab-based Collections at Kew's Millennium Seed Bank and an author of the paper, said in a statement. "As successful as seed banking is for some species, it is not suitable for all seed plants and we need to invest in other ways to safeguard recalcitrant seeds.

Source: https://science.howstuffworks.com/environmental/green-science/worlds-rarest-seeds-cant-be-banked.htm

17. According to the text, what is the main advantage of having seed banks?

    A. To hold expensive seeds so that they don't get stolen.
    B. To boost tourism.
    C. To re-plant seeds that go extinct.
    D. So that the U.N. can control all plant growth.

18. According to the text, what is the main disadvantage of seed banks?

    A. They are expensive to run.
    B. A lot of endangered seeds cannot be stored in the seed banks.
    C. They are subject to theft.
    D. The Svalbard International seed bank is running out of space.

19. Which of the following seed types can be stored in seed banks?

    A. Chestnut
    B. Cacao
    C. Barley
    D. Mango

20. Which statement about the Svalbard International Seed Vault is correct?

    A. It can be found in international waters.
    B. Its capacity is 20% full.
    C. It has the capacity to hold 2.5 billion seeds.
    D. Every country in the world has contributed to its seed collection.

Passage 6

Elephants are the largest mammals living on land these days. Today's African elephants comprise two species (originally considered a single species, but confirmed as distinct in 2010) and the Asian elephant. But their closest current relative is probably the hyrax, a small, furry rodent-like mammal. However, not all their relatives have been so teensy — some extinct elephant relatives were larger even than the modern behemoths.

A new study analyzing genetic data and published in the journal eLife finds that this XXL ancestral elephant is more closely related to one of today's African elephants than it is the modern Asian elephant. This is surprising, because the ancient straight-tusked giant

Palaeoloxodon antiquus actually lived in Eurasia between 1.5 million and 100,000 years ago. The elephant that grew to around 13 feet (four meters) tall and weighed in at about 13 tons (11.8 metric tons) — basically twice as big as modern elephants.

The research team examined the mitochondrial DNA (passed only from mother to offspring) and nuclear DNA (which includes information about the father) of African and Asian elephant species, and compared them to DNA extracted from the fossilized bones of 16 wooly mammoths collected from permafrost in cold climates, and four from *P. antiquus* bones collected in Germany. This is the first time such a good genetic sample has been taken and successfully sequenced from fossils from such a warm climate.

Using this new data, the researchers pieced together a new phylogenetic tree for elephants. They found the ancestor shared by *P. antiquus* and today's African forest elephant (*Loxodonta cyclotis*) lived between 1.5 million and 3.5 million years ago, while its shared ancestor with the African bush elephant (*Loxodonta africana*) lived between 3.9 and 7 million years ago. *P. antiquus* also moves further from the Asian elephant (*Elephas maximus*). So, while African elephants are sometimes managed and protected under the assumption they are all the same species, this study proves they are not.

Source: https://animals.howstuffworks.com/mammals/elephant-family-tree-dna-analysis-species.htm

21. What is the main conclusion in the text?

    A. Elephants are the largest mammals living on land.
    B. Mitochondrial DNA is passed from mother to offspring.
    C. African elephants are not all the same species.
    D. African and Asian elephants are different species.

22. P. Antiquus:

    A. Was 3x bigger than a normal elephant.
    B. Lived in Africa between 1.5 million and 100000 years ago.
    C. Was the largest land animal.
    D. Grew up to 4m tall.

23. Which of the statements is true?

    A. Mitochondrial DNA is passed down matrilineally.
    B. African elephants consist of +10 different species.
    C. The four DNA samples from P. Antiquus bones were collected from Asia.
    D. The Hyrax is the second largest land animal, after the elephant.

24. Which of the following is not given as an example of a relative to modern African Bush elephants:

    A. Hyrax
    B. P. Antiquus

C. Loxodonta cyclotis
D. Elephas Maximus

Passage 7

The term "aphantasia" comes from the Greek words *a*, which means "without," and *phantasia*, meaning "a capacity to form mental images." The phenomenon was first described by psychologist Francis Galton – one of the pioneers in the science of eugenics – in 1880. The term, which denotes the lack of a "mind's eye," or inability to visualize in the mind, was coined to describe the phenomenon in 2015 by neurologist and University of Exeter Medical School professor Adam Zeman.

While Zeman believes that heredity and environment both are likely to be relevant causes, the exact cause of aphantasia is still unknown. Aphantasia could potentially occur in different ways in different people. Neuroimaging has shown that mental imagery is definitely associated with the left temporal lobe and requires an extensive series of pathways in the brain to occur. Scientists are still studying why these pathways might work in different ways in different people. Zeman theorizes that, while people with a functional ability to see things in the mind's eye use visual circuitry, some people use non-visual paths to process visual data. Research does suggest, however that people with aphantasia are more likely to pursue STEM – science, technology, engineering or math – careers. In fact, Zeman's University of Exeter study polled 2,000 people with aphantasia and discovered that 20 percent of those with little or no visual imagery selected careers in mathematics, computing or science. This, compared with people who experience hyperphantasia (exceptionally vivid mental imagery), 25 percent of whom opt for careers in creative industries such as arts, entertainment or design. Still, Zeman insists that these numbers are no more than "statistical trends," so people shouldn't limit themselves based on the ability of their mind's eye.

While aphantasics typically don't experience any deficits due to it, there are some potential, albeit rare, problems. "Aphantasia is associated with face recognition difficulties, impoverishment of autobiographical memory and – probably – autistic spectrum disorder. But each of these associations occurs in only a minority of people with aphantasia," Zeman notes.

Source: https://health.howstuffworks.com/human-body/systems/nervous-system/aphantasia.htm

25. Which statement is best supported by the text?

A. Aphantasia was discovered in 2015.
B. Aphantasia is caused by environmental factors only.
C. People with aphantasia can only do STEM-related jobs.
D. Mental imagery is definitely associated with the left temporal lobe region of the brain.

26. Which statement best defines aphantasia?

A. A condition which makes people less skilled at creative tasks.
B. A term to describe people without the capacity to visualize objects in their mind.
C. A term to describe a condition which causes the patient to have an inability to visualize objects in their mind.
D. A term to describe a condition which causes a patient to have exceptionally vivid mental imagery.

27. Which statement can be best inferred from the text?

A. 500 people with hyperphantasia opted for a career in creative industries.
B. 400 out of 2000 people in a study with aphantasia pursued a career in mathematics, computing or science.
C. Hereditary factors have a bigger influence than environmental factors on aphantasia.
D. 25% of people in a creative field of work have hyperphantasia.

28. Francis Galton:

A. Was a founder of modern psychological science.
B. Didn't believe in aphantasia.
C. Was a pioneer in the field of eugenics.
D. Worked at the University of Exeter.

Passage 8

A Newcastle University study involving thousands of families is helping prospective parents work out whether they are likely to have sons or daughters.

The work by Corry Gellatly, a research scientist at the university, has shown that men inherit a tendency to have more sons or more daughters from their parents. This means that a man with many brothers is more likely to have sons, while a man with many sisters is more likely to have daughters.

The research involved a study of 927 family trees containing information on 556,387 people from North America and Europe going back to 1600.

"The family tree study showed that whether you're likely to have a boy or a girl is inherited. We now know that men are more likely to have sons if they have more brothers but are more likely to have daughters if they have more sisters. However, in women, you just can't predict it," Mr Gellatly explains.

The Newcastle University study suggests that an as-yet undiscovered gene controls whether a man's sperm contains more X or more Y chromosomes, which affects the sex of his children.

On a larger scale, the number of men with more X sperm compared to the number of men with more Y sperm affects the sex ratio of children born each year.

"The gene that is passed on from both parents, which causes some men to have more sons and some to have more daughters, may explain why we see the number of men and women roughly balanced in a population. If there are too many males in the population, for example, females will more easily find a mate, so men who have more daughters will pass on more of their genes, causing more females to be born in later generations," says Newcastle University researcher Mr Gellatly.

Adapted from: https://www.sciencedaily.com/releases/2008/12/081211121835.htm

29. Which of the statements below is best supported by the text?

    A. A woman with many brothers is more likely to have a son than a daughter.
    B. A man with many brothers is more likely to have a daughter than a son.
    C. A man with many sisters is more likely to have a daughter than a son.
    D. A woman with many sisters is more likely to have a son than a daughter.

30. Which of the statements can be inferred from the text?

    A. Attempting to predict the gender of a child based on the mother's genes would be pointless at this stage.
    B. The number of men is equal to the number of women born every year.
    C. The presence of certain genes in the father will definitively control the gender of the baby.
    D. The family trees researched went back to the 16th century.

31. Which of the statements is true?

    A. There is a gene that controls whether a man's sperm contains more X or more Y chromosomes.
    B. The likelihood of a father having a boy or a girl is inherited.
    C. This discovery will lead to people being able to 'decide' what gender their child is through genetic engineering.
    D. The research involved over 500,000 families.

32. Which of the following could be a viable next step in the research?

    A. Isolating the suggested gene.
    B. Restricting the study to look at fewer families, making it easier and cheaper.
    C. Attempting to find a way to "switch off" this gene.
    D. No more research needed.

Passage 9

Following the fast spread of COVID-19 across Europe and North America in March 2020, many people began stockpiling commodities including toilet paper. Some companies reported an increase of up to 700 percent in toilet paper sales, despite calls from the government to refrain from "panic buying."

In the new study, researchers surveyed 1,029 adults from 35 countries who were recruited through social media. Between 23 and 29 March 2020, participants completed the Brief HEXACO Inventory -- which ranks six broad personality domains -- and shared information on their demographics, perceived threat level of COVID-19, quarantine behaviors, and toilet paper consumption in recent weeks.

The most robust predictor of toilet paper stockpiling was the perceived threat posed by the pandemic; people who felt more threatened tended to stockpile more toilet paper. Around 20 percent of this effect was also based on the personality factor of emotionality -- people who generally tend to worry a lot and feel anxious are most likely to feel threatened and stockpile toilet paper. The personality domain of conscientiousness -- which includes traits of organization, diligence, perfectionism and prudence -- was also a predictor of stockpiling.

Other observations were that older people stockpiled more toilet paper than younger people and that Americans stockpiled more than Europeans. The researchers pointed out that the variables studied explained only twelve percent of the variability in toilet paper stockpiling, which suggests that some psychological explanations and situational factors likely remain unaccounted for. "Subjective threat of COVID-19 seems to be an important trigger for toilet paper stockpiling. However, we are still far away from understanding this phenomenon comprehensively," concludes Theo Toppe, co-author of the study.

Adapted from https://www.sciencedaily.com/releases/2020/06/200612172227.htm

33. Sales of toilet paper increased by over 700% for some companies.

    A. True
    B. False
    C. Can't Tell

34. The subjective threat of COVID-19 was the key factor found by the researchers for influencing the stockpiling of toilet paper.

    A. True
    B. False
    C. Can't Tell

35. Older Americans were more likely to stockpile than younger Europeans.

    A. True
    B. False

C. Can't Tell

36. Certain traits, such as prudence and perfectionism, could lead to a higher likelihood of stockpiling.

    A. True
    B. False
    C. Can't Tell

Passage 10

The amount of time teenagers spend on social networking sites has risen 62.5 percent since 2012 and continues to grow. Just last year, the average time teenagers spent on social media was estimated as 2.6 hours per day. Critics have claimed that more screen time is increasing depression and anxiety in teenagers.

However, new research led by Sarah Coyne, a professor of family life at Brigham Young University, found that the amount of time spent on social media is not directly increasing anxiety or depression in teenagers.

"We spent eight years trying to really understand the relationship between time spent on social media and depression for developing teenagers," Coyne said about her study published in Computers in Human Behavior. "If they increased their social media time, would it make them more depressed? Also, if they decreased their social media time, were they less depressed? The answer is no. We found that time spent on social media was not what was impacting anxiety or depression."

Mental health is a multi-process syndrome where no one stressor is likely the cause of depression or anxiety. This study shows that it is not merely the amount of time spent on social media that's leading to an increase in depression or anxiety among adolescents.

"It's not just the amount of time that is important for most kids. For example, two teenagers could use social media for exactly the same amount of time but may have vastly different outcomes as a result of the way they are using it," Coyne said.

The goal of this study is to help society as a whole move beyond the screen time debate and instead to examine the context and content surrounding social media use. Coyne has three suggestions to use social media in healthier ways:

- Be an active user instead of a passive user. Instead of just scrolling, actively comment, post and like other content.
- Limit social media use at least an hour before falling asleep. Getting enough sleep is one of the most protective factors for mental health.
- Be intentional. Look at your motivations for engaging with social media in the first place.

Source: https://www.sciencedaily.com/releases/2019/10/191022174406.htm

37. Which of the following statements best describes the conclusion of the passage?
    A. More screen time directly leads to depression and anxiety in teenagers.
    B. Time spent on social media doesn't directly impact anxiety or depression.
    C. The amount of time that teenagers spend on social media is more influential to their mental health than what they are using the media for.
    D. If teenagers decrease the time spent on social media, they will become less depressed.

38. Which of the following statements was not listed as a way to use social media more healthily?
    A. Actively engaging with content on social media, rather than just observing.
    B. Use filters to block harmful content.
    C. Think about your motivations for engaging with social media.
    D. Don't use social media within the hour before you go to sleep.

39. According to the passage, which of the following statements is true?
    A. Teenagers spend at least 2.6 hours a day on social media.
    B. Teenagers tend to stop using social media as they get older.
    C. This study was conducted over 12 years.
    D. Sarah Coyne's specialty is Family Life.

40. The goal of the study was:
    A. To find an answer to the screen time debate.
    B. To highlight the negative impacts of social media use.
    C. To discover what caused depression in youth.
    D. To learn more about the processes behind mental health disorders.

Passage 11

Adolescents are disproportionately affected by HIV worldwide, and yet are rarely specifically prioritized in national HIV-plans and programming efforts. In 2016, 260 000 adolescents between 15 and 24 years were infected with HIV, with 44% more infections amongst young women than their male counterparts.

Within the larger at-risk population of adolescents, there are specific concentrated groups that are particularly vulnerable. Young women outside of the school system are isolated and unsupported by the networks and structures that could contribute to healthy development and reduce their vulnerability. Their vulnerabilities often stem from family economic imperatives, teenage pregnancy or a lower social priority to keep young women in school. In addition, young key populations throughout the world carry a high burden of HIV and increased risk. These key populations include young MSM, transgender youth, young people who inject drugs as well as young people who find themselves on the wrong side of the law. Although large-scale interventions are needed when combating a generalized epidemic, a targeted and focused approach that caters to these key populations is required to efficiently and successfully prevent new infections.

HIV prevention for adolescents is particularly critical in a world where the youth population is rapidly expanding. Over half the population of the world is currently under the age of 30 and the majority of these young people reside in developing countries; it is predicted that this proportion of youth will increase markedly in the next 20–30 years. Beyond HIV, almost 35% of the global burden of disease has its roots in adolescence. Adolescence is a critical transition period for adolescents, as well as a critical investment period, where rewards of prevention efforts can be significantly multiplied across health and sociostructural domains. Described as the triple dividend, meaningful investment in prevention in this age group is likely to impact both the immediate and longer-term horizons.

Source: Pettifor, Audrey et al. "Adolescent lives matter: preventing HIV in adolescents."

41. What is the main conclusion that can be drawn from the passage?
    A. People living in poorer areas are disproportionately affected by HIV.
    B. 260,000 adolescents between 15 and 24 years were infected with HIV in 2016.
    C. There needs to be better HIV prevention for adolescents.
    D. Over half of the world's population is under the age of 30.

42. Which of the following groups is not vulnerable to HIV infection?
    A. Young women outside of the education system.
    B. People who inject drugs.
    C. People living in places with poorer sanitation and healthcare.
    D. Transgender youth.

43. Which of the following statements is true?
    A. Young men are more likely to contract HIV than young women.
    B. There were over 260,000 new infections in people aged 16-25 in 2016.
    C. The world's population distribution is going to change, with younger people taking up less of the global population as a proportion.
    D. A targeted approach would be less effective at preventing the spread of HIV in youth than a large-scale intervention.

44. It is important to target HIV in youth because:
    A. Young people are more likely to die of HIV than adults.
    B. This issue is currently overlooked in most healthcare systems.
    C. There are other problems to target in older population groups.
    D. 35% of all HIV cases are found in youth.

Verbal Reasoning Answers

Passage 1

1. The correct answer is C. "...where the probability of reaching centenarian age is high are located in urban areas and smaller towns with higher socioeconomic status, including the Seattle area and the region around Pullman, Wash". Be careful of the use of the future qualifier of necessity "will" in statement A. C is the only statement supported by the text.
2. The correct answer is D. A simple search and retrieve question; the other three factors can all be found in the second paragraph.
3. The correct answer is B. A and D are directly contradicted by the text, C is not supported, and B is merely the inverse of the statement "Earlier research, he said, has estimated that heritable factors only explain about 20 to 35% of an individual's chances of reaching centenarian age."
4. The correct answer is C. Make sure to completely read around the section which mentions his name. If you just read "study author" you may be tempted to choose the answer "scientist", but reading later into the section would show you that he is first and foremost a medical student.

Strategies

This is a typical statement-based question, so you should read the entire passage before attempting the questions. When looking at individual statements, you may scan to find the relevant section but having a good understanding of the text will be very useful in making inferences. Some of the vocabulary in the passage is specific to scientific text, so if you are unsure of a word, try to read around it to gain a better understanding.

Passage 2

5. The correct answer is C. This can be inferred from the line "it's hard to imagine they occur by the thousands every day around the world." "Thousands" multiplied by 365 days would equal a minimum of 365,000. The other statements are either refuted by the text or not mentioned.
6. The correct answer is A. Whilst Geography GCSE would have taught you that this is true, it is not mentioned anywhere in the text and so would be the correct answer.
7. The correct answer is D. This is supported by the statement "Collapsing buildings claim by far the majority of lives." If this is the consequence that claims the most fatalities, then it is the deadliest.

8. The correct answer is B. None of the other options are mentioned anywhere in the text. Remember the importance of reading every statement carefully when looking for its supporting text. In this question, excerpts from the passage may look similar to some of the statements, but if read carefully, you will find the statements to be incorrect.

Strategies

This text is quite short, and the subject matter is not overly complex, so you should follow the normal route of reading the entire passage for statement-based questions. Something to bear in mind with this text is that because the subject matter is relatively easy, it is important not to bring outside information and assumptions into the picture when answering these questions. Stick to what is stated in the text.

Passage 3

9. The correct answer is A. C and D are both refuted by the text and the use of the future qualifier of necessity "will" in B means that this option should be discarded, as it is difficult to predict the future. Statement A is supported by the text and therefore is the correct answer.
10. The correct answer is C. The text states that the results are regardless of ethnicity, socioeconomic background and gender, meaning that by process of elimination the answer must be C
11. The correct answer is A. As you go down the list of statements, this one should immediately be clear. There is no need to look at the others, as this can quickly be confirmed by scanning the text. The correct section of text is: "The students who learned to play a musical instrument in elementary and continued playing in high school not only score significantly higher, but were about one academic year ahead of their non-music peers with regard to their English, mathematics and science skills"
12. The correct answer is B. The two clear answers here are B and C, but it states in the text "The students who learned to play music in elementary and continued playing in high school...", indicating that B is a better answer.

Strategies

The text is written more in the style of a science paper, and so the level of reading will be more complex. Scanning may not give you the full picture, and so you should be reading this text. Make sure that you read the statements carefully: a lot of them are worded similarly but mean completely different things and so it is important to have a clear understanding of what you're looking for in the text.

Passage 4

13. The correct answer is B – False. The use of the qualifier of necessity "only" compared the text in the passage which says "often" means that this statement would be false. When qualifiers of necessity are used, the answer is very rarely "Can't Tell", as the statement is a strict "yes" or "no" without any ambiguity.
14. The correct answer is A – True. In the first sentence of the passage, Origen is said to have been active in the second century. Later, the passage says, "In the second century, Galen synthesized much of what has been attributed to Hippocrates."
15. The correct answer is B – False. This discovery is credited to Galen, but if that section is not read carefully it would be easy to only see the name Hippocrates. The relevant section of text is: "In the second century, Galen synthesized much of what has been attributed to Hippocrates. To further his understanding of bodily functions, he performed animal and even human dissections and was able to demonstrate that the arteries carried blood rather than air." Whilst this statement may have been attributed to Hippocrates, it is clear from the passage that it was Galen who discovered it.
16. The correct answer is B – False. "James II of Aragon (died 1372)" means that he died in the 14th century.

Strategies

In this passage, you should understand the use of qualifiers and make sure that you are comfortable reading dates – often, students can be caught out with working out what century a particular year is in. To clarify: The years 0-99 are in the 1st century, the years 100-199 are in the 2nd century, and so on. Therefore, the year 1372 is in the 14th century.

Passage 5

17. The correct answer is C. This would be made clear by reading the first paragraph. None of the other options are mentioned. The relevant section of text is "When the apocalypse is over and the forests are nothing but smoking ruins and the fields barren of grain, fear not! We can reboot the world thanks to our banked seeds."
18. The correct answer is B. Similar to the first question, this would be made clear by reading the third paragraph. Again, none of the other options are mentioned. "Researchers discovered that a whole whack of plant seeds just can't be banked" is the important sentence here.
19. The correct answer is C. By process of elimination, we can work out that A, B and D cannot be stored in a seed bank (mentioned in the 3rd paragraph) and so the answer

must be C. The relevant section of text is the same as the last question - "including avocado, cacao and mango."

20. The correct answer is C. This is mentioned in the first paragraph. The word "international" may lean you towards A or D, but reading the text will show you that these options are not mentioned.

Strategies

The first question is not an inference question, and so you can assume that the rest will be of a similar difficulty. The questions are relatively easy in this passage, as they are each very short, and the answer options are sometimes a single word. Therefore, scanning would be your best bet here as it will save you lots of time to then use on the more difficult questions.

Passage 6

21. The correct answer is C. Conclusions are usually prefixed with words like "so", "therefore", etc. The relevant sentence is, "So, while African elephants are sometimes managed and protected under the assumption they are all the same species, this study proves they're not.", meaning that the correct answer would be C.
22. The correct answer is D. You can see immediately that A and C are incorrect. B appears correct because of the dates, but looking closely would show you that the statement says "Africa" and the text states "Eurasia". Therefore, the correct answer is C.
23. The correct answer is A. Do not let the unusual word "matrilineally" catch you out (it means down the mother's genetic line). Checking the other statements and ruling them out would have helped you reach the answer, even if you did not understand the statement.
24. The correct answer is C. Loxodonta Cyclotis is actually the name of the African Bush elephant mentioned in the question, and so it cannot be a relative to itself.

Strategies

The text is complex and contains unfamiliar words, and so reading the text would be the best strategy to go with here. Reading around the relevant sections carefully once identified is very important, as the use of unfamiliar words can create some confusion. Understanding the concept of conclusion-drawing and making sure that your chosen conclusion is, indeed, a conclusion rather than a fact or premise will help you.

Passage 7

25. The correct answer is D. Be careful of similarities between some of these statements and the text. A is incorrect as the condition was named in 2015, but discovered earlier. B is incorrect as it is stated that a mixture of hereditary and environmental factors can

contribute to aphantasia. C is incorrect, as the text suggests that STEM is the area of choice for some people with aphantasia and does not mention a restriction at all.

26. The correct answer is C. B and C are very similar, but the key here is that aphantasia describes the condition rather than the patient. Reading the first paragraph would help you to infer this. . The text also uses the phrase "people with aphantasia" multiple times, indicating that the term 'aphantasia' is used to describe the condition rather than the patient.
27. The correct answer is B. 20% of 2000 is 400. This is referred to in the following sentence: "Zeman's University of Exeter study polled 2,000 people with aphantasia and discovered that 20 percent of those with little or no visual imagery selected careers in mathematics, computing or science."
28. The correct answer is C. Similar to previous questions, this is a search-and-retrieve style question. C is the only possible answer and can be found in the first paragraph: "... psychologist Francis Galton – one of the pioneers in the science of eugenics – in 1880." The other three options are not mentioned.

Strategies

Again, the text subject is complex and so requires reading. The key with these questions is to look out for similarities, especially in 1 and 2. Understanding the statements and then making sure that your chosen section of the passage matches up with your understanding of the statements is essential.

Passage 8

29. The correct answer is C. All of the statements are similar and so it is important to read them all carefully. Finding and understanding the relevant section of the passage (paragraph 2) will give you this answer. Simplifying the logic in each statement here and writing it down may be helpful in determining exactly what each statement is saying. For example, you can use the whiteboard to take a quick note of each option using initials, such as "W+B=S" for "woman+brother=son".
30. The correct answer is A. The text states, "In women, you just can't predict it", implying that with our current scientific knowledge, it would be pointless to try to use data gathered from the mother to predict the gender of a child.
31. The correct answer is B. A sounds correct, but it is too definite. The text suggests the possibility of such a gene existing, but statement A says that this gene definitely exists. Thus, the answer would be B as it is the only one out of the remaining 3 that can be drawn from the text.
32. The correct answer is A. This question is more logic-based. Having a reasonable understanding of science would suggest that A is the correct answer. B and D are illogical. Although C would be a potential step in research, it is not the best "next step"

as trying to switch off the gene could only be useful in a potentially long-term study comparing the results in groups with and without this gene. This is far too complex and would not be expected from you in the UCAT. Therefore, it is not the logical next step in research.

Strategies

The style of the text is scientific and factual, and so the best strategy would be to read the whole text as it could be very complex. The first question is difficult – all of the statements are very similar and so it is important to carefully understand and differentiate each one.

Passage 9

33. The correct answer is B – False. The text states, "up to 700%", meaning that anything over 700% would be false
34. The correct answer is A – True. This is backed up twice in the text – "The most robust predictor of toilet paper stocking was the perceived threat of the pandemic" and "Subjective threat of COVID-19 seems to be an important trigger.."
35. The correct answer is A – True. The text says that older people tended to stockpile more than younger people and Americans tended to stockpile more than Europeans. It would be logical to suggest that older Americans may be more likely to stockpile than younger Europeans.
36. The correct answer is A – True. This is referenced in the third paragraph – "The personality domain of conscientiousness -- which includes traits of organization, diligence, perfectionism and prudence -- was also a predictor of stockpiling."

Strategies

As it is A True, False, Can't Tell question, the best strategy is to scan the text. As the text subject is complex, you may need to read around your isolated sections a bit more than usual to grasp the relevant concepts.

Passage 10

37. The correct answer is B. All of the other statements are refuted by the passage. Note that A and D are fundamentally saying the same thing with different wording – they follow the same flow of logic. If more screen time leads to more instances of depression, then it follows that less screen time would lead to a lower number of instances of depression. However, this is not what the text is saying – it argues the converse.
38. The correct answer is B. While this may be true, it is not mentioned in the article. You can find the other statements in the three bullet points given in the text.

39. The correct answer is D. All of the other statements may have references in the passage, but upon looking closely, none of them could be true and so D is the answer here. Be careful with statement A – it is a generalisation and is not said in the text. The text says that on average, teenagers spend 2.6 hours on social media a day, but statement A generalises and says that teenagers spend 2.6 hours on social media every day.
40. The correct answer is A. Again, whilst all of these may be true, A is the only one referenced by the text and so is the correct answer. The supporting text can be found in the sixth paragraph: "The goal of this study is to help society as a whole move beyond the screen time debate."

Strategies

Reading is your best bet here to understand fully what the text is saying. The first question asks for the main conclusion of the text, and so it is important to have that better understanding. Again, it is important not to bring any outside information or assumptions into the question when reading the text: the answers should be purely based off the text's contents.

Passage 11

41. The correct answer is C. All four statements are mentioned in the text, but only one of them is a conclusion. The other three are merely statements or facts presented in the text. The conclusion draws from these facts.
42. The correct answer is C. This may be true, but it is not mentioned in the text. The other three points can be found together in the second paragraph: "Young women outside of the school system are isolated... transgender youth, young people who inject drugs."
43. The correct answer is B. All of the other statements are directly contradicted by the text, and so B is the correct answer. It is referenced nearly word-for-word in the first paragraph - "In 2016, 260 000 adolescents between 15 and 24 years were infected with HIV"
44. The correct answer is B. D may also seem correct, but looking closely at the section of text which mentions the 35% would show you that this figure is actually referring to disease as a whole rather than HIV, and so the correct answer is B.

Strategies

This text is considerably harder than the others, as it is taken from a science journal. Therefore, you would need to read the text fully to understand the contents. When you get to the questions, making sure that you understand what a conclusion is and read the statements carefully to help you answer the questions. Again, be careful not to bring any outside knowledge into your answers.

SECTION 2

Decision Making

INTRODUCTION

Decision Making is the second section of the UCAT. It consists of 29 questions to be solved in 31 minutes, giving you approximately a minute per question. In 2020, this section had the second-lowest overall average – 625.This section aims to assess you on your ability to analyse and deduce information from complex sources of data, interpret and decipher crucial details, and extrapolate inferred information to derive conclusions. The data within the questions is given in the form of passages, graphs, charts, visual diagrams, and text. Some questions have key concepts taken from Verbal Reasoning and Quantitative Reasoning. It is worth revising some Critical Thinking material to aid your learning in this section.

In this section of the book, you will learn how to answer questions involving Venn diagrams, syllogisms, drawing conclusions, shape equations, and more! The best time-saving strategies are explained in detail to help you understand each question. There are various examples throughout that you can try under timed conditions, and a mock test towards the end.

Types of Questions

There are various different types of questions listed in the table below. Some questions will take long, while some should be completed in a shorter amount of time. You can refer back to this table once you familiarise yourself with the types of questions. A large portion of questions will require use of your whiteboard, and some will require you to use the on-screen calculator.

Category	Question Types	Time Needed	Number of Questions
Statistical & Figural Reasoning	• Venn Diagrams • Probabilistic Reasoning	• 40-60 seconds	• Approximately 8-9 Questions
Deductive Reasoning	• Syllogisms • Logical Puzzles • Shape Equations	• 60-80 seconds • 20-30 seconds for shape equations	• Approximately 9-11 Questions
Evaluating Arguments	• Justifying Assumptions • Drawing Conclusions	• 20-40 seconds	• Approximately 10-11 Questions

Question Format and Scoring

There are two formats of questions in this section.

1. Multiple choice questions: you are given a choice of 4 possible answers where you must select one. Each of these is worth a single mark.
2. 5 statement questions: there are 5 statements and you must assign either "Yes" or "No" to each statement.

    5 correct = 2 marks

    4 correct = 1 mark

    $\leq$ 3 correct = 0 marks

Probabilistic Reasoning

Probabilistic reasoning is unlike the probability questions that present in Quantitative Reasoning. Some questions will require calculations, while others will simply require you to justify and apply the correct reasoning to a scenario regarding probability. Aside from explaining the strategies for these types of questions, this section focusses on the use of tree diagrams to work out probability. No formulae will be given, as they can be found in Quantitative Reasoning, but you can focus on the basic "and/or rule".

- To work out the probability of an event *and* another event, multiply each individual probability.
- To work out the probability of an event *or* another event, add the individual probabilities.

Let us use the following scenario to understand the creation and use of tree diagrams.

Natalia tosses an unbiased 2-sided coin.

1. What is the probability that it lands on heads?
2. If she tosses it twice, what is the probability that it will land on heads both times?
3. If she tosses it twice, what is the probability of landing on both heads and tails, in any order?

Let us construct the tree diagram for tossing a two-sided unbiased coin twice. The two possible outcomes in the first throw are heads and tails. This can be drawn as follows:

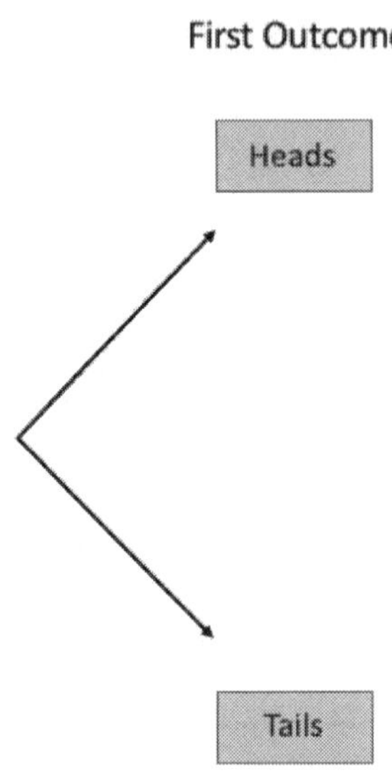

We should now outline the probability of each outcome occurring. The probability of landing on heads is ½ and the probability of landing on tails is ½. This can be drawn as follows:

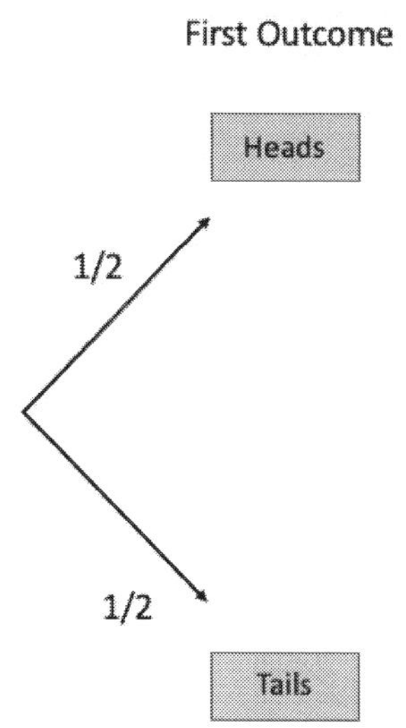

We must now define the possible outcomes in the second toss. If the first outcome is heads, the second outcome can be either heads or tails. If the first outcome is tails, the second outcome can also be either heads or tails. This can be demonstrated as follows:

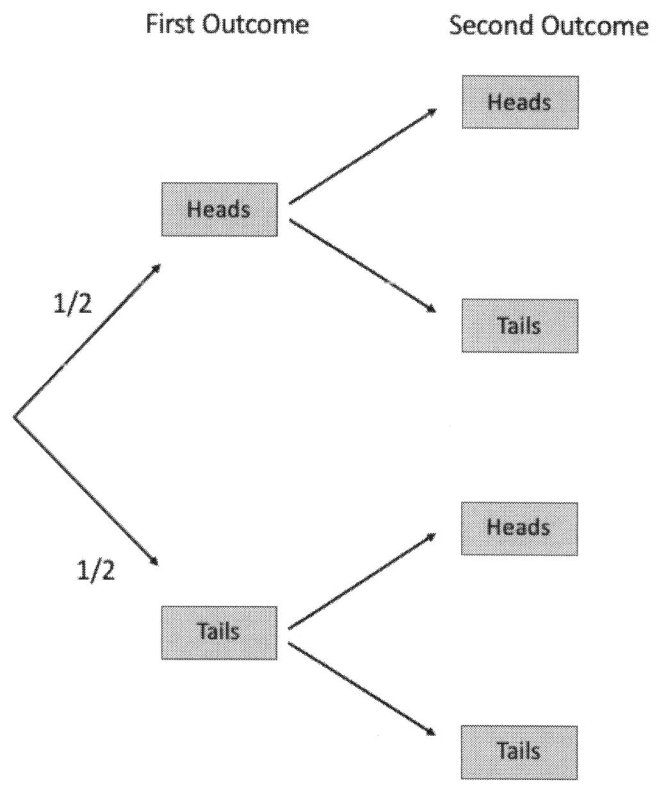

You must now specify the probability of each of the possible second outcomes. The probability of landing on heads or tails will remain the same no matter how many times a coin is flipped, as the second outcome is not dependent on the first. Therefore, each of these probabilities will also be ½, as follows:

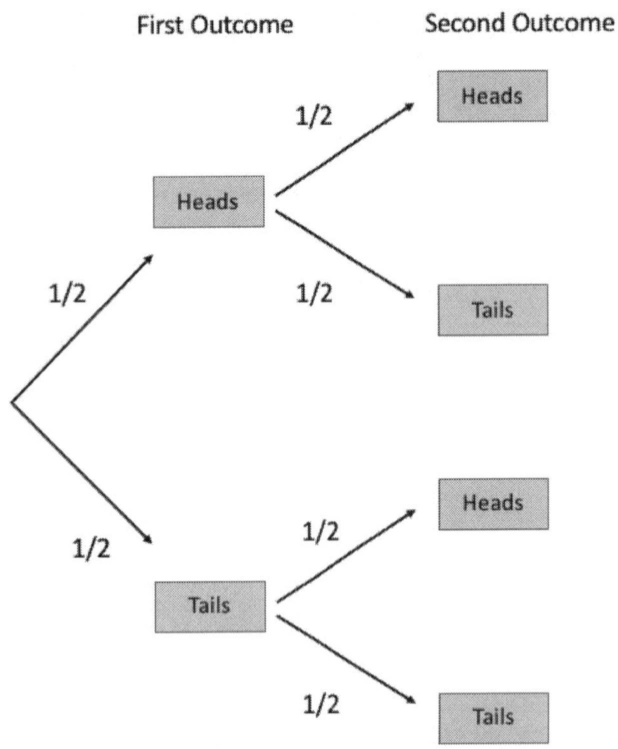

Using this tree diagram, let us now attempt to answer the questions.

1. What is the probability that it lands on heads?

This refers to the first outcome only. The probability of landing on heads is ½.

2. If she tosses it twice, what is the probability that it will land on heads both times?

The first outcome must be heads and the second outcome must be heads. The two probabilities you must consider are as follows:

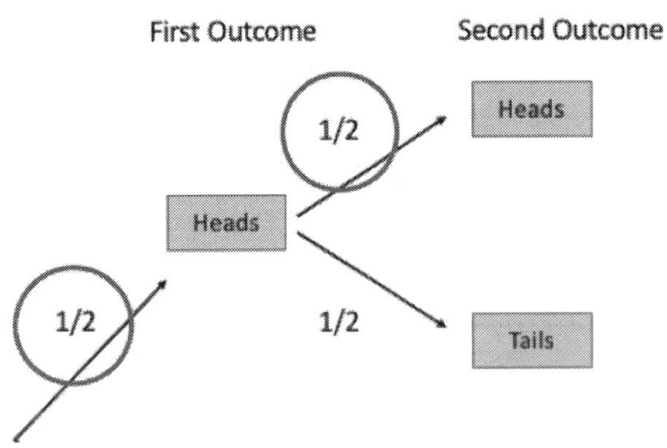

The probability of *both* of the above outcomes occurring can be found by multiplying their individual probabilities. The formula for this is further explained in Quantitative Reasoning, or you can refer to the "and/or rule" to recognise the need to multiply.

$$\frac{1}{2} \times \frac{1}{2} = \frac{1}{4}$$

3. If she tosses it twice, what is the probability of landing on both heads and tails, in any order?

This time the question is slightly different. Natalia could land on either heads first, then tails, or tails first, then heads. These possible combinations are demonstrated by the tree diagram below:

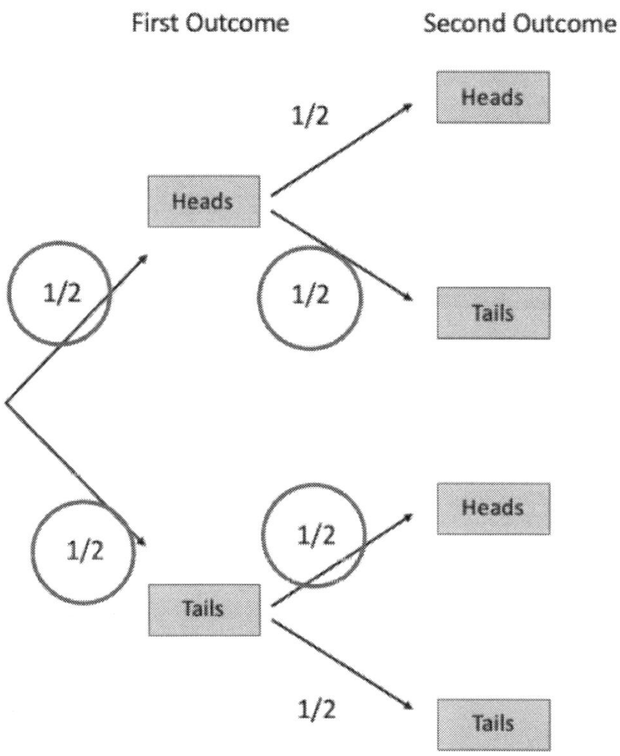

The probability of landing on heads first, then tails, can be calculated by multiplying the individual probabilities of both outcomes, as follows:

$$\frac{1}{2} \times \frac{1}{2} = \frac{1}{4}$$

The same can be done to calculate the probability of landing on tails first, then heads:

$$\frac{1}{2} \times \frac{1}{2} = \frac{1}{4}$$

Because there are two ways that this combination of outcomes can occur, the two individual probabilities for each *combination* need to be added up. Therefore, the probability of landing on heads *and* tails, in any order (i.e. the first combination *or* the second combination) is:

$$\frac{1}{4} + \frac{1}{4} = \frac{1}{2}$$

Hopefully, this demonstration has given you a good overview of how to construct and use a tree diagram to answer probability questions. In this case, each of the individual probabilities are identical. However, this is not always the case. Tree diagrams are especially useful for dependent events, as they allow you to visualise the change in probability from one outcome to the next. An example of this can be seen on page 56 of Quantitative Reasoning.

Example 1

Jasmine is tossing an unbiased coin repeatedly and noting down the outcomes. She is currently on her 50th throw. So far, she has landed on heads 48 times and tails once.

The probability of her obtaining heads on her fiftieth throw is more than that of her obtaining tails.

A. Yes, because the previous outcomes strongly support this statement.
B. Yes, because the outcomes of her previous throws influence her next one.
C. No, because the coin is unbiased.
D. No, this data cannot be concluded.

Answer 1

The correct answer is C.

This is a simple, yet common type of question. You are required to calculate the probability of Jasmine obtaining heads or tails in her 50th throw and use this value to answer the question. Once you have your value, which you should know is 0.5, you must determine which option correctly justifies this. This is where the questions are different to Quantitative Reasoning – you are not simply calculating an answer, but further justifying the answer with a correct statement.

Option C notes that the coin is unbiased, therefore, the probability of landing on heads or tails is identical. This requires a sufficient understanding of probability. It may appear strange that Jasmine continues to obtain heads, and the probability of 48 heads in 50 throws is very low, but is not 0. Likewise, the individual probability of heads or tails is 50% regardless of previous throws.

Make a mental note of the important terms here. The word unbiased is in fact the most important word, as the word means that the coin has a 50/50 chance of landing on either heads or tails. This means that the coin has an equal probability of landing either a head or tail, and is definitely not influenced by previous outcomes; hence the answer is (c).

These questions involve the mathematical concept of probability; however, the questions of this type also require candidates to select the option which justifies the answer correctly. Hence, both the answer, and the justification provided have to be correct for the candidate to be awarded with full credit.

Example 2

Jacob has two urns – a big one and a small one. Both the urns contain balls which are either red or blue. The big urn contains 15 balls of which 10 are blue. The small urn contains 2 red balls and a total of 10 balls. Jacob asks Hasan to pick up one ball from each urn.

What is the probability of Hasan picking one red and one blue ball in any order?

A. 1/3
B. 2/5
C. 1/5
D. 8/15

Answer 2

The correct answer is B.

You must understand the question and process the information given. This is most easily done by constructing a tree diagram. There are 10 blue balls and 15 balls in total, so there must be 5 red balls. If the first ball is selected from the large urn, the probability of it being blue is 10/15, and the probability of it being red is 5/15. This is demonstrated as follows:

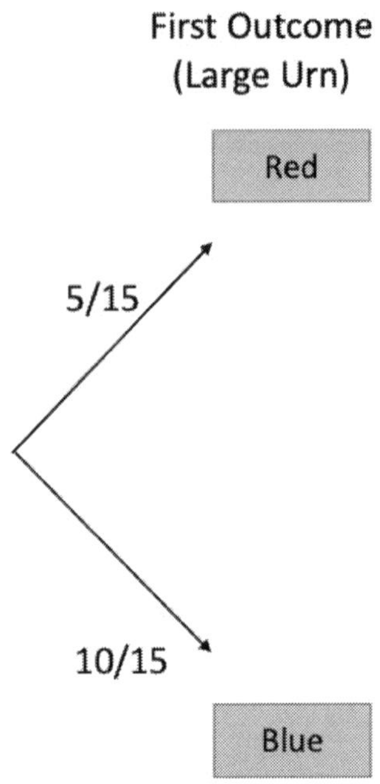

The second outcome, picking a ball from the small urn, can then be shown as following on from each of the first possible outcomes. There are a total of 10 balls: 2 red balls and 8 blue balls. This can be demonstrated as follows:

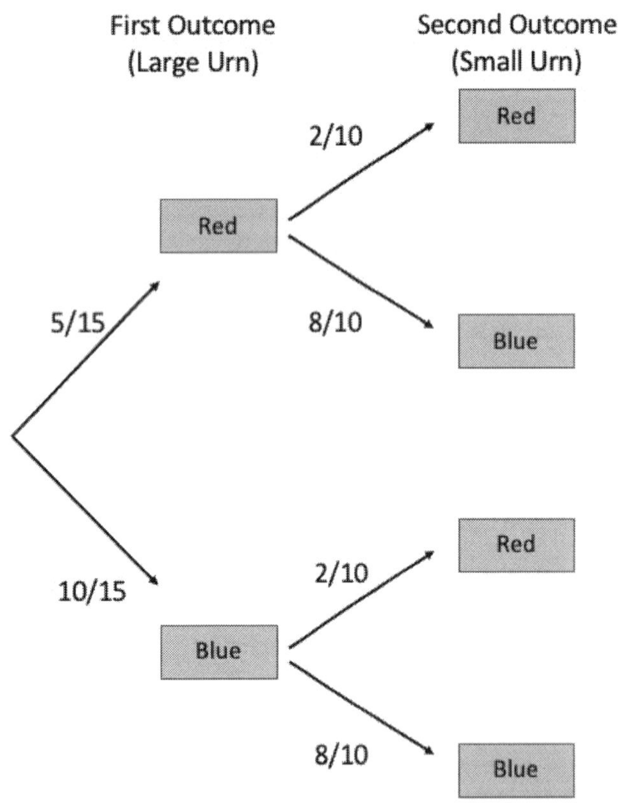

In the above question, if Hasan picks a red ball from the large urn *and* blue ball from the small urn, the probability would be:

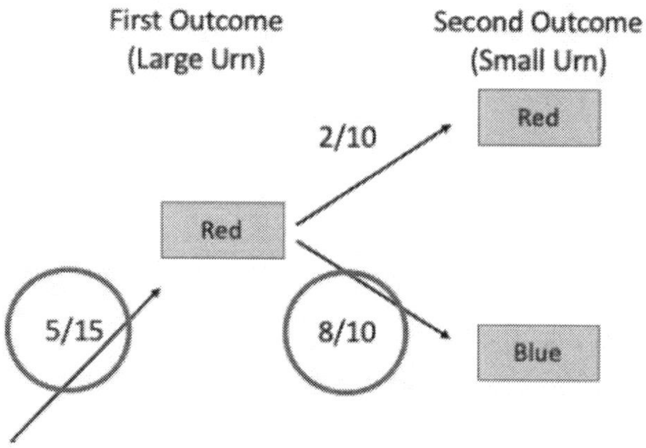

$$\frac{5}{15} \times \frac{8}{10} = \frac{40}{150}$$

Remember the "and/or" rule – you multiply the probabilities in this case.

Similarly, if Hasan picks up a blue ball from the large urn and red ball from the small urn, the probability would be:

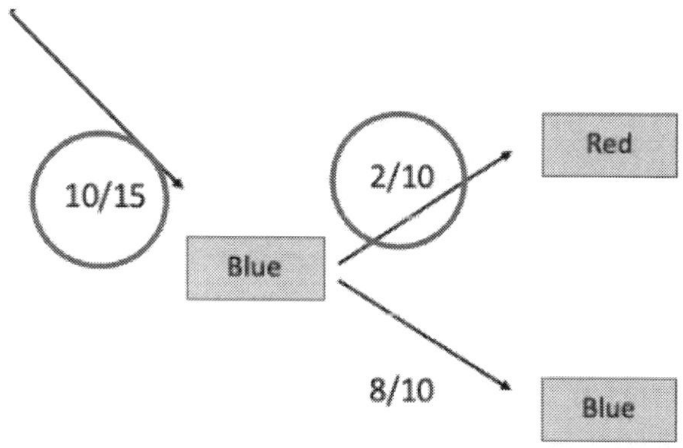

$$\frac{10}{15} \times \frac{2}{10} = \frac{20}{150}$$

The question asks you to find the probability of Hasan selecting a blue ball *and* a red ball *in any order*. The probabilities of the two possible combinations of events that will result in him selecting a blue ball and a red ball are 40/150 and 20/150, as calculated above. These two probabilities must be added together to find the probability of this sequence of events occurring in any order.

$$\frac{40}{150} + \frac{20}{150} = \frac{60}{150}$$

60/150 can be further simplified to 2/5.

Example 3

Ally is taking part in a game, and the rules are as follows:
She has to initially select one of two decks, deck A or deck B.
Deck A has 10 Red, 15 Blue, 6 Green, and 8 Black Cards.
Deck B has one more Blue & Black Cards than Deck A
Deck A has 4 less Red Cards and 3 less Green Cards than Deck B.

The probability of Ally choosing a blue card from either deck is greater than the probability of choosing a green card from either deck.

A. Yes, because Deck B has 48 cards and a greater number of blue cards.
B. Yes, because the difference in probability between the two is greater than 0.1.
C. No, because there are two decks of cards and hence probability cannot be calculated.
D. No, because the probability of choosing a blue card from the first deck is less than choosing a blue card from the second deck.

Answer 3

The correct answer is B.

Without even working out the answer, you can eliminate all of the incorrect or irrelevant choices.

A. Although it is true that Deck B has 48 cards and it also has a greater number of blue cards than Deck A, this is not sufficient justification to answer the question. It does not explain why the probability of selecting a blue card is greater than the probability of selecting a green card. Moreover, it makes no comparison at all to green cards, thereby overlooking the primary goal of the question. Watch out for options that provide the correct answer but have an incorrect or irrelevant justification.
C. This is simply incorrect. Probability can be calculated even though there are two decks of cards. If the information was incomplete, perhaps you would not be able to calculate the probability, but there is no reason here why it cannot be done.
D. This is not relevant to the question, just like option A. It does not involve green cards at all, therefore, it can be eliminated based on irrelevant justification. Further, if you actually calculate it, the probability of choosing a blue card from Deck A is 0.384 whereas the probability of choosing a blue card from Deck B is 0.333. Therefore, this answer is not only irrelevant, but is incorrect.

You may have been able to answer this question by eliminating all of the incorrect and irrelevant answer choices. Alternatively, you can work out the probability, which may take longer than the elimination method above. To construct a tree diagram, remember the steps taking place and account for each of them:

- Select a deck – A or B
- Select a card – Blue or green

You must also work out the probabilities of each of the possible choices.

- Deck A has 39 cards in total. 15 are blue and 6 are green.
- Deck B has 48 cards in total. 16 are blue and 9 are green.

You do not need to include the probabilities of each of the cards that are irrelevant to our question. Using this information, you can construct a tree diagram as follows:

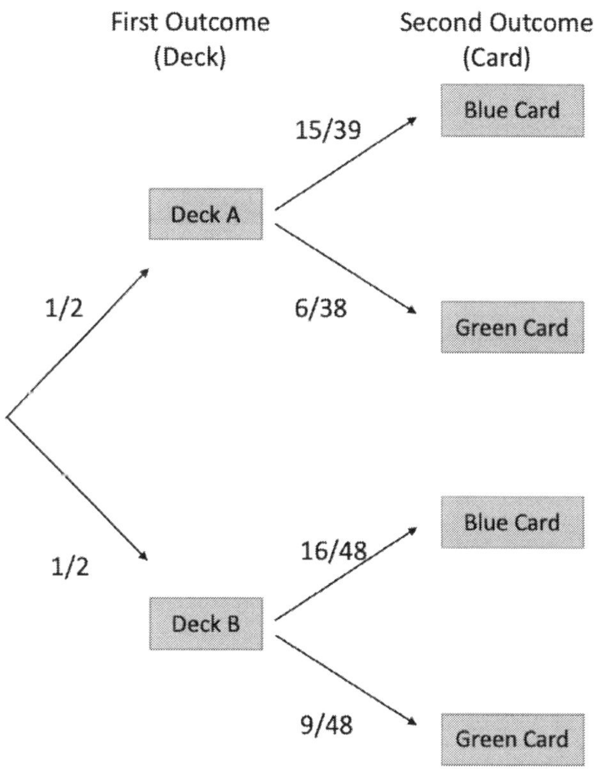

Using this tree diagram, you can calculate the total probability of selecting a blue card, i.e. from Deck A *or* from Deck B. *Hint: add them together!*

Deck A: $\frac{1}{2} \times \frac{15}{39} = \frac{15}{78} = 0.192$

Deck B: $\frac{1}{2} \times \frac{16}{48} = \frac{16}{96} = 0.166$

$0.192 + 0.166 = 0.358$

The total probability of selecting a green card from any deck can be calculated as follows:

Deck A: $\frac{1}{2} \times \frac{6}{39} = \frac{6}{78} = 0.077$

Deck B: $\frac{1}{2} \times \frac{9}{48} = \frac{9}{96} = 0.094$

$0.077 + 0.094 = 0.171$

Hence, the difference in probability = ~0.188, which is greater than 0.1.

You can see that this calculation would have taken much longer than simply answering the question through a process of elimination. Ensure that you practice eliminating answers to increase your speed, and do not feel the necessary urge to calculate every probabilistic reasoning question.

Shape Equations

Each question has four rows of shapes, each with two sides, connected by an equals sign. The final row has a missing shape, which you need to decipher. This form of maths is not commonly practiced, so although the equations are generally simple, they can be very challenging to understand. Your whiteboard or scratchpad will be of essential use. Many students like to replace the shapes with letters and solve each question algebraically, while others prefer to work with shapes. It takes far less time to solve equations using letters, but you can use whichever method you find easiest.

Strategy

We will call the first three rows "equations 1-3" and the final row "equation 4".

1. Start with the equation with the missing shape – equation 4.
2. Look through equations 1-3. Determine whether any equation can be substituted into equation 4 to **reduce the number of shapes** in equation 4. Sometimes there will be multiple equations that you can substitute, and sometimes there will be none. Conduct as many substitutions as possible before moving on to the next step.
3. If there are no possible substitutions, or if you have completed all of the possible substitutions and have not yet solved the equation, start substituting equations 1-3

within themselves to form your own equations that can be substituted into equation 4. To do this, find an equation that contains the same shapes as equation 4, and remove any extra shapes that do not exist in equation 4 through substitution.

4. Once you have removed any extra shapes, substitute your new equation into equation 4. If you have not yet solved the question, repeat step 3.

Tips

1. After making some substitutions to equation 4, you will often find that you are left with a question mark on one side, which represents a single missing shape, and the other side looks exactly like one of the sides present in equations 1-3. You can use that equation to deduce the shape that is represented by the question mark.
2. There are many ways to solve an equation. You need to find the fastest and most effective way to do so. During your Decision Making practice, if you find that a question has taken you many, many steps to solve, try it again. Find a faster way, as there must be one. This will help you to quickly solve future questions that may have a similar pattern of equations.
3. Any equation with a shape that exists nowhere else in all of the equations should be discarded immediately. That equation is there to waste your time. You can rearrange and substitute as much as you like, but you will always have that single shape that you cannot make use of.
4. Try not to substitute any shape into equation 4 that does not already exist there. Sometimes, it will be necessary to do so, as you may need to completely replace one of the shapes in equation 4 with another one in order to solve the equation. However, unless you recognise an absolute need to add an extra shape, do not do this!

These strategies and tips will be demonstrated to you through two different examples.

Example 4

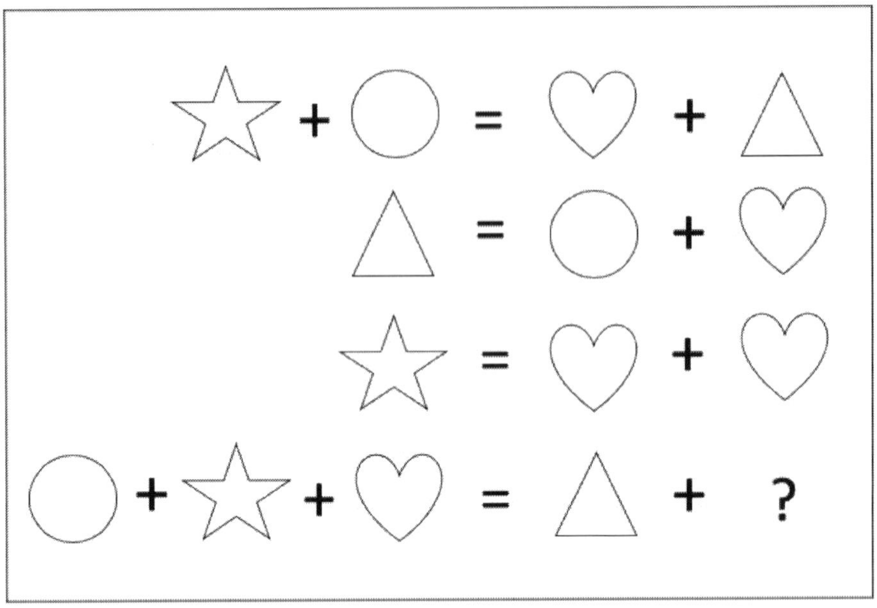

Which of the following makes the last equation true?

A. Triangle
B. Circle
C. Heart
D. Star

Answer 4

The correct answer is D. A solution will be demonstrated below using shapes, then a better and quicker solution will be demonstrated using letter replacements for the shapes. Remember, the first three rows are equations 1, 2 and 3 respectively, while the final row is equation 4.

Solving with shapes

Start with the equation that has a missing variable – equation 4. There are four different shapes, so we must try to reduce the number of shapes in order to solve the equation. If any of equations 1-3 can easily replace one of the shapes in equation 4, they should be substituted now.

1. Equation 3 is simple: 1 star = 2 hearts. Substitute the star in equation 4 for two hearts. This will reduce the number of shapes in equation 4 from four to three.

Working Out	Previous Step for Reference
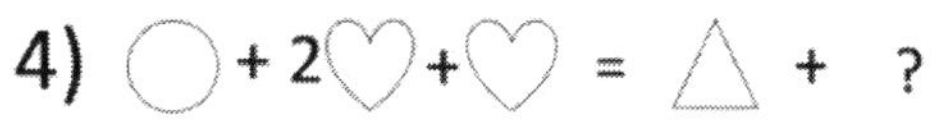 **Now simplify.** 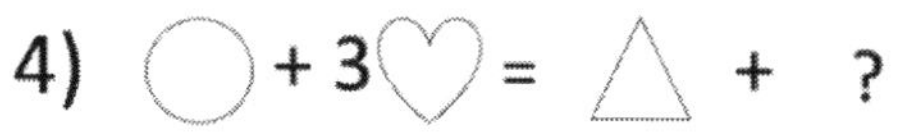	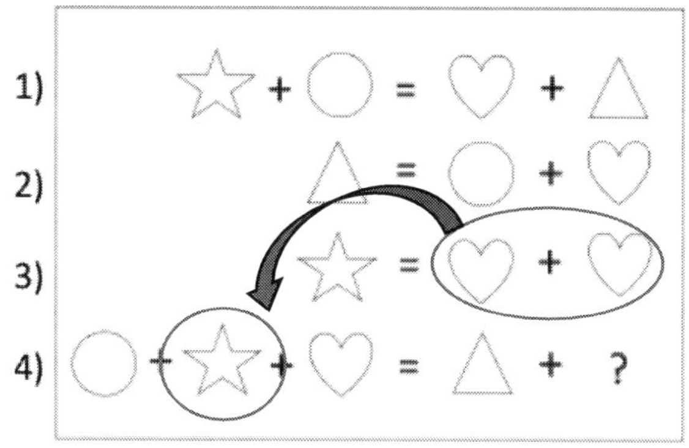

2. You can now go back to equations 1-3 to find anything else that can be substituted into equation 4. The triangle in equation 2 is equal to 1 circle and 1 heart. We can remove the triangle in equation 4 by substituting it for a circle and a heart. It may feel pointless to substitute one shape for two, but you will notice that equation 4 consists of only circles, hearts and triangles. The goal is to reduce the number of shapes in the equation, and by replacing the triangle for a circle and heart, there will only be two different shapes in the equation, rather than three.

Working Out	Previous Step for Reference
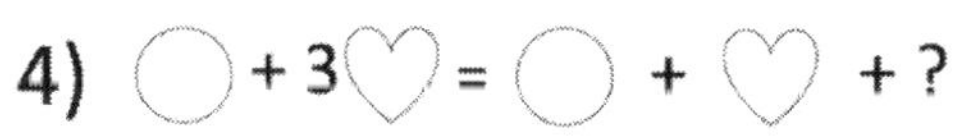	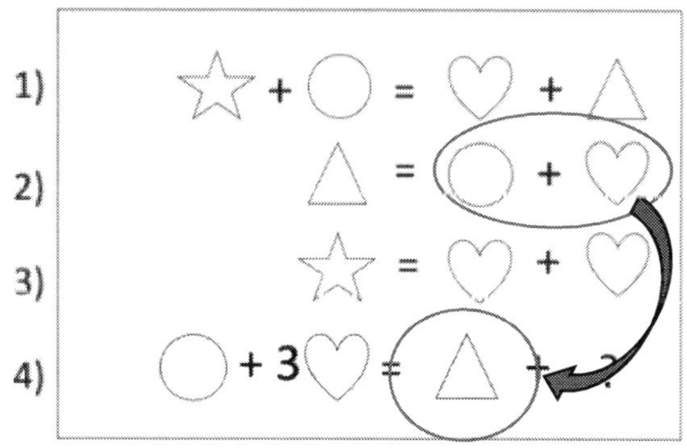

3. You can now rearrange the equation. A circle on each side of the equals sign cancels out, and a heart on the right side can be subtracted on the left side to give two hearts on the left.

Working Out	Previous Step for Reference
	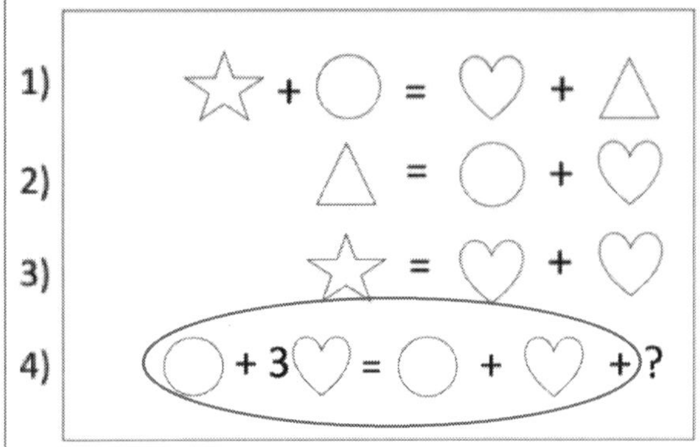

4. We know from equation 3 that 1 star = 2 hearts. Therefore, 2 hearts = 1 star. The missing shape is a star.

Solving with letters

Note: This is a different technique to the one shown above and is much quicker. The demonstration is using letters, rather than shapes.

If you choose to solve the equation with letter replacements, a star shape can be replaced with the letter "s", a triangle can be replaced with the letter "t", a circle can be replaced with the letter "c", and a heart with the letter "h". The equations would then become:

1) 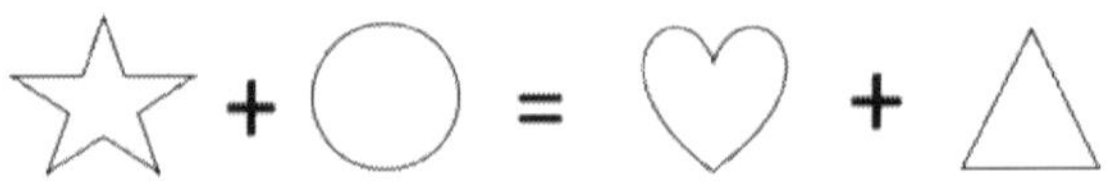	1) s + c = h + t
2) 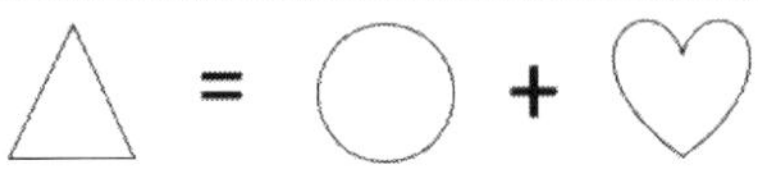	2) t = c + h
3) 	3) s = h + h
4) 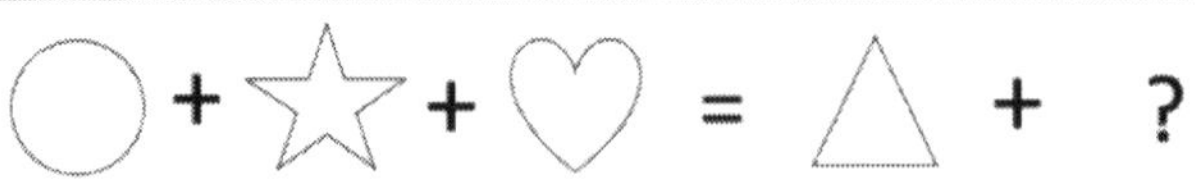	4) c + s + h = t + ?

1. Start with the equation with a missing variable:

   c + s + h = t + ?
2. Reduce the number of letters in the equation via substitution. Substitute either equation 2 or 3 into the equation. Even though it appears less simple to begin with, we will start with equation 2. Equation 4 has a circle and a heart that are separated by

a star to make their connection more difficult to see. You will notice from equation 2 that a circle and heart can be replaced with a single triangle. This removes two shapes in one step.

c + s + h = t + ?

Substitute the coloured letters above for the coloured letter below:

s + t = t + ?

3. Without even cancelling out the triangle on either side, you should recognise that the right side is missing a star. If s + t = t + ?, then the ? = s.

You can see that this method was far easier. This demonstrates that the simplest substitution that first appears to you may not be the quickest substitution! It is best to substitute multiple shapes at once from equation 4, if possible, rather than trying to substitute one shape at a time. Further, you should always look for any tricks, such as the placement of a star between the circle and heart in equation 4 in an attempt to hide their relationship.

Either of the above methods will provide you with the correct answer, but it is best to find the quickest way to save you time. This may mean spending a few more seconds analysing the equations to decide which one you should begin with. This would be more efficient than starting with the wrong equation and wasting time doing long, multi-step substitutions where they are unnecessary.

Example 5

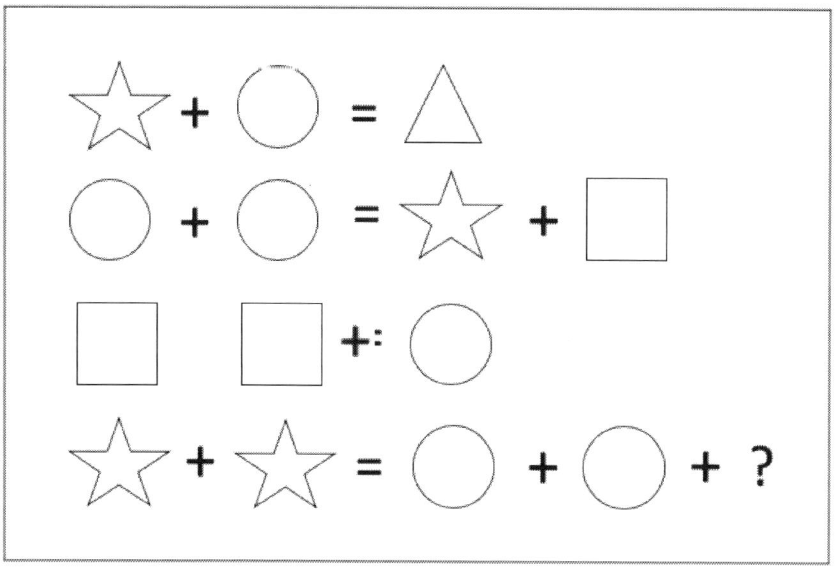

Which of the following makes the last equation true?

A. Triangle
B. Circle

C. Square
D. Star

Answer 5

The correct answer is B.

This question is different to the previous one, as equation 4 only consists of 2 shapes, rather than a large variety. Therefore, there is not much we can directly substitute into equation 4. Instead, we will need to work with equations 1-3, making our own equations that can be used to solve equation 4. This can be done as follows:

1. Firstly, as in the previous example, check equations 1-3 to find anything that can possibly be substituted into equation 4. There is nothing that would reduce the number of shapes, therefore, none of the equations are suitable for substitution in their current states.
2. Secondly, identify any equation that contains the same shapes as equation 4. If there are extra shapes, determine a way to remove the extra shapes.
    a. Equation 1 has a circle and a star, but it also contains a triangle. There is no other triangle in all of the equations. Therefore, this equation can immediately be discarded, as there is no way for us to make use of the triangle within it.
    b. Equation 2 has both circles and stars, but it also contains a square. Therefore, it would be useful to remove the square. However, you should not substitute the square for another shape that does not *already exist* in the equation, as this will not be beneficial. For example, if possible, substituting the square for a triangle would be pointless, as the equation would then have a triangle that requires removal.
3. To remove the square, we should substitute it for a shape, or shapes, that already exist in equation 2. Equation 3 has squares and a circle. If we find the value of a single square, we can substitute it into equation 2 to remove the square and replace it with circle(s). This is seen below. *Note:* When forming equations, do not be afraid of decimals and fractions!

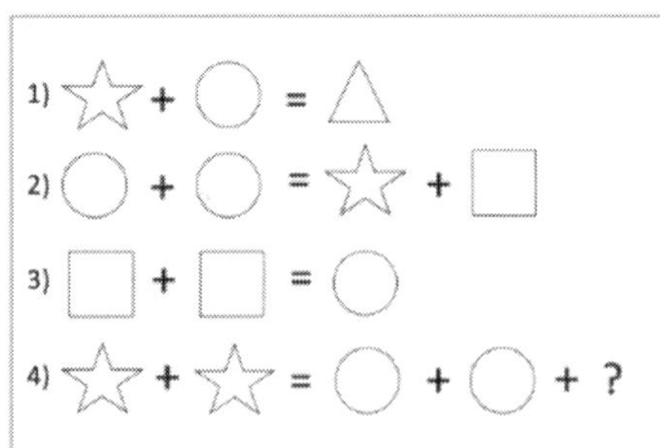

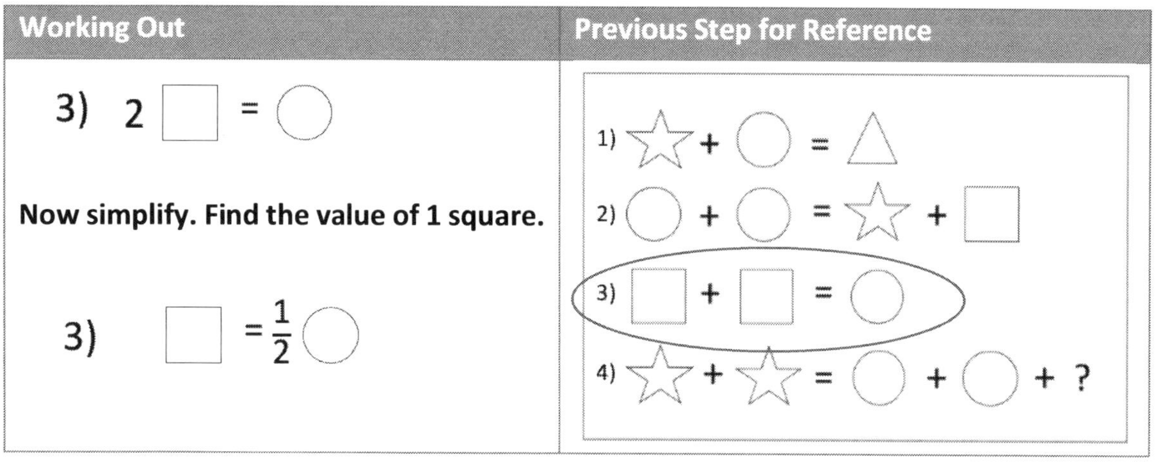

4. We can now substitute equation 3 into equation 2 to reduce the number of shapes in equation 2. We must replace the square with $\frac{1}{2}$ circle.

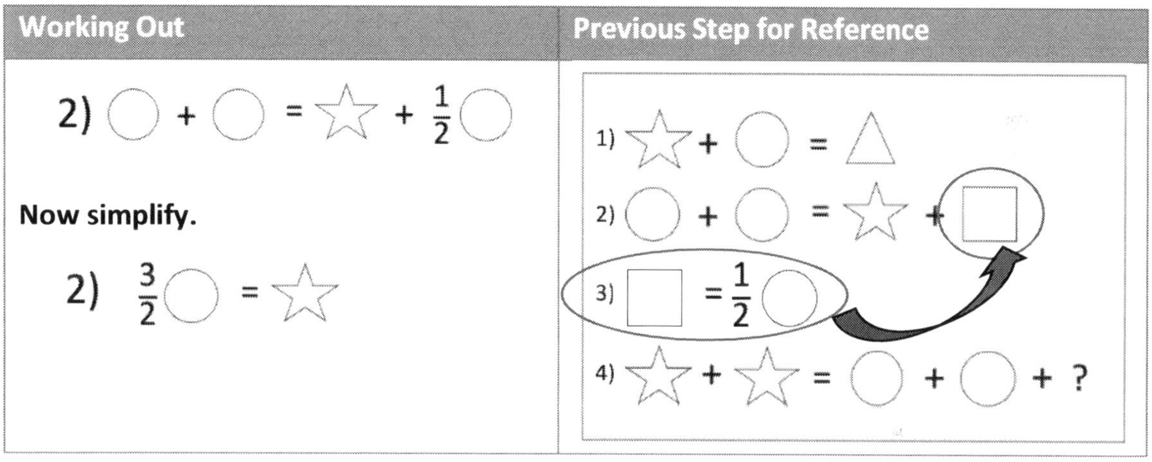

5. We now have an equation that has only circles and stars – the sole shapes that exist in equation 4. Substitute the simplified equation 2 into equation 4 by replacing each of the stars with $\frac{3}{2}$ circle.

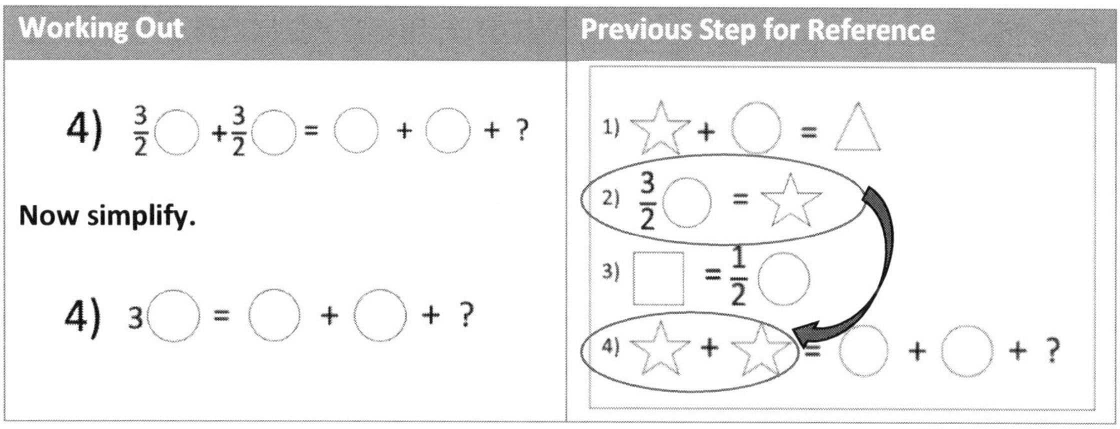

6. One more circle is needed to complete equation 4. It is clear now that the answer is B.

Hopefully, you can see the difference in strategy between the two examples. Example 5 had a missing shape in an equation that consisted of four different shapes. Therefore, the aim was to replace the shapes as much as possible and reduce their variety. Equations 1-3 did not really need to be altered, as they were already in states that were easily substituted directly into equation 4. However, example 5 required a lot more work. Rather than simply substituting existing equations into the question, we had to rearrange and create our own equations. This was conducted by identifying the equation that consisted of the same shapes as the question, then removing any additional shapes it contained. After forming our own equation through this process, we substituted our equation into equation 4, allowing us to solve the question.

You will come across questions that are a mixture of these two formats, so you should be able to use the strategies from each to solve those questions. *Always substitute for any existing equations before creating new equations.*

Evaluating Arguments

An argument is a set of reasons that address a problem or an idea, either given in support of or against it. It is made up of premise(s) and a conclusion, with the premise(s) acting as evidence for the conclusion. More information on premises and conclusions can be found in the Verbal Reasoning section of this book.

Factors That Strengthen an Argument	Factors That Weaken an Argument
The premises are based on facts/research/studies	The premises are based on opinion or subjectivity
The premises are directly linked to the subject of the argument	There is no clear link between the premise and the subject of the argument
The conclusion logically follows from the premises	The premises do not cover all of the points of the argument
No assumptions are made	Assumptions are made
No external knowledge is used	External knowledge is used

It is also important to ensure that no bias is present in your thought process when evaluating an argument. The questions will commonly contain themes that are of general knowledge, so many students may have their own opinions on the idea in question. Further, when it is worded as "Should X occur?" it is easy to use your own biases when deciding the correct answer. However, you must ensure that you use only the knowledge presented to you and evaluate the argument based on facts and relevance to the subject matter.

E.g. Should America host a cricket world cup?

A. Yes, of course they should.
B. No, the American cricket team has no star players.

Both of the above arguments are weak.

A. "Yes, of course they should." There is not a single piece of evidence given here to support the conclusion of "Yes". Without evidence, or a premise, an argument is weak.
B. "No, the American cricket team has no star players." This is a subjective statement which is not backed up by any factual evidence. Further, it does not directly link to the topic of the question. To host a world cup, you would need stadiums, staff, security, and so on. Having "no star players" in the team is not an ideal reason for concluding that America should not host a cricket world cup.

A better argument might be: "Yes, because they have a great infrastructure and many state-of-the-art stadiums." This addresses the main question and provides a valid and logical premise to support the argument that they should host the world cup.

Idea

Should America host a cricket world cup?

Yes, they should host the world cup because they have a great infrastructure and many state-of-the-art stadiums

Conclusion

Premise

Argument

Strategy

1. Understand the subject matter in the idea and identify key points. What exactly is being asked? Is the idea universal or does it refer to a specific group?
2. Read the arguments (all of the answer options). You cannot choose a conclusion (Yes/No) without reading the full argument, as the correct conclusion must be paired with the correct premises to support it. There are likely to be options that have the correct conclusion (Yes/No) but have illogical or irrelevant reasoning.

3. Eliminate any arguments that are weak due to assumptions, bias, irrelevance, or subjectivity.
4. Evaluate the remaining arguments, separating them into premises and conclusions. Identify whether the premises specifically address each of the key points in the idea. Eliminate any argument that misses out a key point.
5. Select the strongest argument. This should be relevant to the topic, evidence-based, and address all of the key points in the idea. You may not find the *best* argument to support or reject the idea, but it should be the best out of all of the options presented.

Detailed Evaluation of Arguments

E.g. In order to reduce pollution, should all manufacturing industries be required to adhere to emission control norms issued by the government?

The idea here is "All manufacturing industries should be required to adhere to emission control norms". There is no justification for why this should occur. Therefore, a strong and valid argument is necessary in support of this idea.

Argument 1

"Yes, as following the rules issued by the state will ensure that hefty fines will be imposed on violators, thereby ensuring a reduction in air pollution and emission of harmful gases."

- Premise 1: The rules issued by the state will ensure that hefty fines will be imposed on violators.
- Premise 2: This will ensure a reduction in air pollution and emission of harmful gases. *Note:* Both of these premises act as supporting evidence for *why* the idea should occur.
- Conclusion: Yes, all manufacturing industries should be required to adhere to emission control norms issued by the government in order to reduce pollution.

The idea refers to reducing *pollution*. Pollution can take many forms, and while imposing hefty fines might help reduce air pollution, this argument does not address land, water, or other areas of pollution. Further, this argument relies on the assumption that fines will lead to this reduction, but does not provide any evidence for this. These premises are not strong enough to back up the conclusion, and thus this argument is weak.

Argument 2

"No, as emission control laws only address air pollution and are found to have no impact on land or water pollution, hence this is not a sufficient method of reducing pollution."

- Premise: Emission control laws only address air pollution and are found to have no impact on land or water pollution.
- Conclusion: No, all manufacturing industries should not be required to adhere to emission control norms issued by the government in order to reduce pollution.

The premise is based on facts, rather than opinions or assumptions. The word "found" shows that evidence is being used. This directly links to the idea which talks about pollution in general, and clarifies that the general pollution mentioned in the idea will not be solved through this measure. The conclusion logically follows from the premise – it is clear that if there is no impact on many areas of pollution, this is not an ideal measure. This argument is strong.

Argument 3

"Yes, but air pollution is mostly caused by cars."

- Premise: Air pollution is mostly caused by cars.
- Conclusion: Yes, all manufacturing industries should be required to adhere to emission control norms issued by the government in order to reduce pollution.

The premise has no relevance to the subject matter (idea). The question discusses pollution emitted from manufacturing industries while the argument shifts the attention to cars. It gives no evidence to support the conclusion that this idea should occur, but rather, it seems to go against it by suggesting that manufacturing industries do not cause much pollution at all. This is a weak argument.

Argument 4

"Yes, because all industries will follow the laws issued and allow for a reduction in the overall pollution within that country."

- Premise 1: All industries will follow the laws.
- Premise 2: This will allow for a reduction in the overall pollution within that country.
- Conclusion: Yes, all manufacturing industries should be required to adhere to emission control norms issued by the government in order to reduce pollution.

This argument does well to address overall pollution, as is specified in the idea. However, it is based on the assumption that all industries will follow the laws, but no evidence is provided to support this. Therefore, it is a weak argument.

Example 6

Should the legal driving age be reduced to 15 to overcome the issue of illegal driving?

Select the strongest argument from the statements below.

A. Yes, if younger people can drive, they will be happier citizens and abide by the laws.
B. Yes, by reducing the driving age you will reduce the number of young people smoking cannabis on the street.
C. No, because 15-year-olds are not mature enough to drive, so they may cause more car accidents.
D. No, because studies have shown that there is no association between age and likelihood of illegal driving.

Answer 6

The correct answer is D.

A. "Yes, if younger people can drive, they will be happier citizens and abide by the laws." This is a subjective statement that is irrelevant as it is not directly addressing the subject matter. Although "abiding by the law" can refer to the avoidance of illegal driving, it is not directly clear, and there is no evidence provided. Therefore, this is a weak argument.
B. "Yes, by reducing the driving age you will reduce the number of young people smoking cannabis on the street." This is irrelevant as it is making its own argument, providing a different outcome of a reduced driving age. There is also no evidence provided to suggest that the number of young people smoking cannabis on the street will be reduced by simply reducing the driving age. Therefore, it is a weak argument.
C. "No, because 15-year-olds are not mature enough to drive, so they may cause more car accidents." This is another subjective statement and it does not address the issue of illegal driving. It addresses a separate issue which is unrelated to the subject matter. Therefore, it is a weak argument.
D. "No, because studies have shown that there is no association between age and likelihood of illegal driving." This directly addresses the subject matter, providing a factual basis, therefore, it is a strong argument. Because there is no association between age and likelihood of legal driving, there is no need to reduce the legal driving age in an attempt to decrease illegal driving.

Venn Diagrams

A Venn diagram is used to represent relationships between different elements, with overlaps suggesting a common factor, and the non-overlapping areas suggesting something unique to the set in question. Venn diagrams can come in different shapes, sizes, and combinations.

There are four types of Venn diagram questions:

1. Interpreting Venn diagrams: Understand and interpret information given in the form of a Venn diagram, then use this information to answer a question.
2. Creating Venn diagrams: Construct your own Venn diagram to better understand the text, then use this to answer a question.
3. Choosing Venn diagrams: Select one of four Venn diagrams which represents the given text.
4. Euler diagrams: Similar to Venn diagrams, but they only show real-life scenarios.

Below is a common form of Venn diagram.

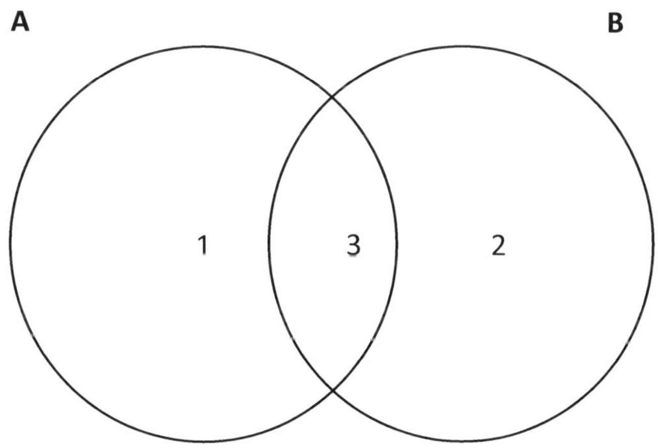

In this simple Venn diagram, region 1 represents the elements that belong to only set A (the first circle) and region 2 represents the elements belonging to only set B (the second circle). Region 3, on the other hand, represents elements belonging to *both* set A and set B.

Venn diagrams can further be complicated by adding another set of data, such as set C shown below:

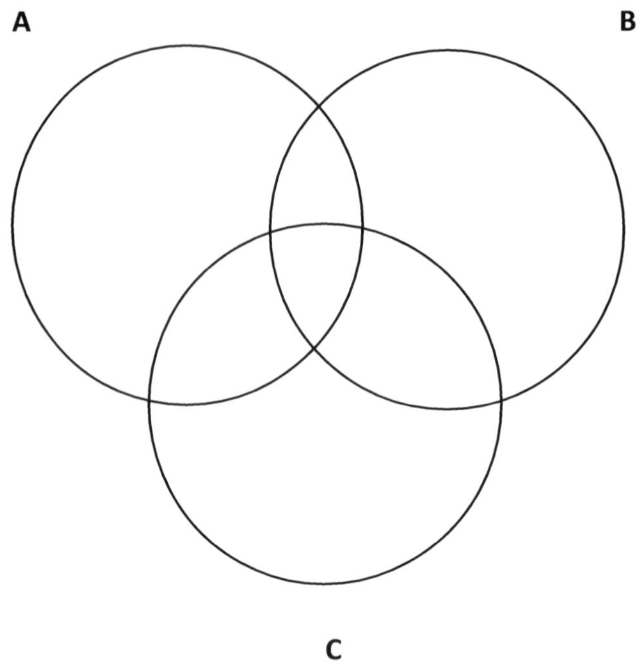

Compared to the three previously shown relations between the data in sets A and B, this Venn diagram now has seven possible relations:

1. Only A
2. Only B
3. Only C
4. Both A and B
5. Both B and C
6. Both A and C
7. A, B and C

1. Interpreting Venn diagrams

You are given a Venn diagram which you must interpret in order to answer the follow-up question. You should read the question *before* attempting to interpret the Venn diagram, as this will help you focus your interpretation in the correct area.

Example 7

The Venn diagram below represents the number of employees working in various departments in a company.

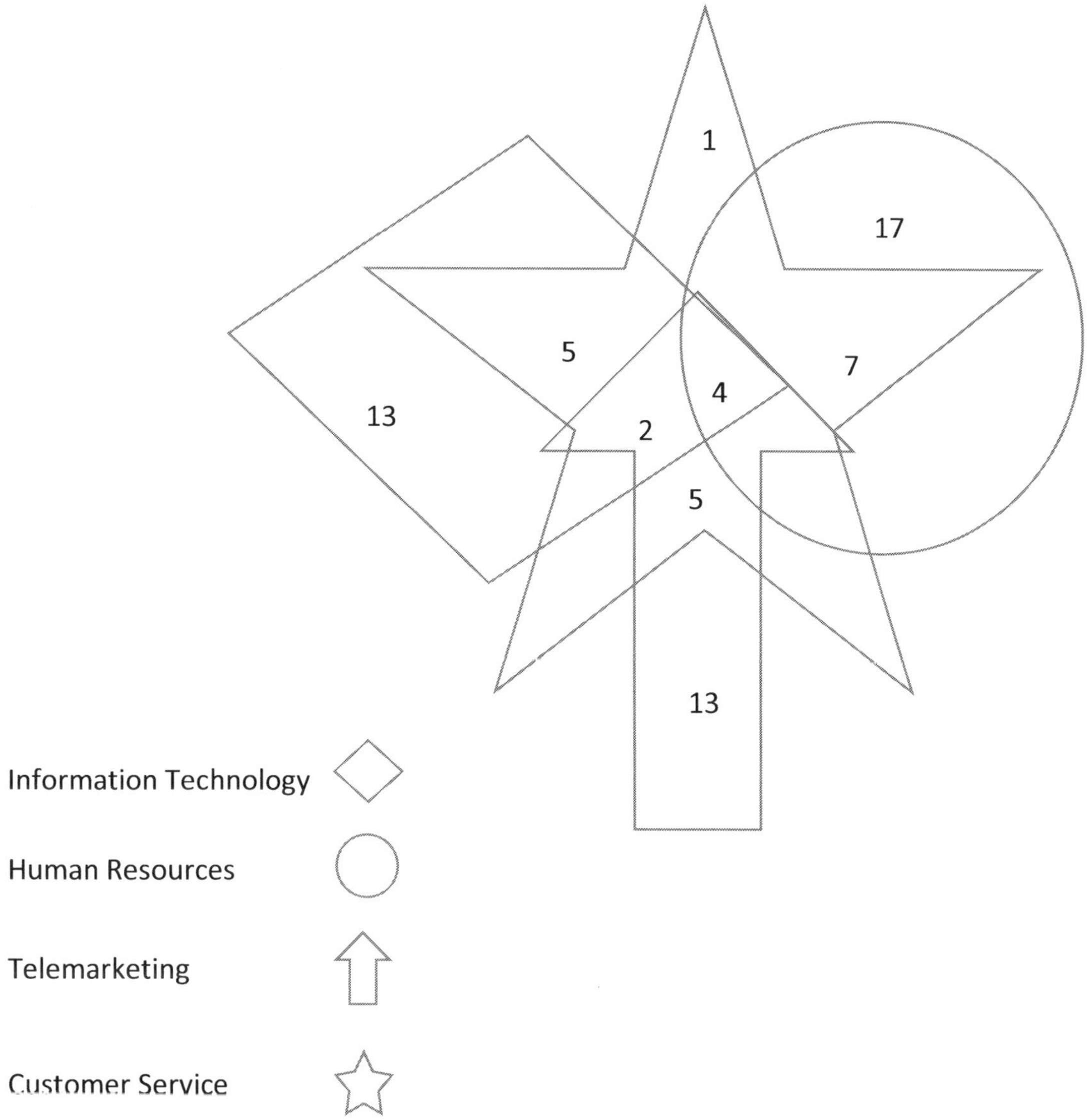

In a particular financial year, only those employees working in exactly one department are eligible for two weeks of paid leave.

Based on the above diagram, how many employees are not eligible for two weeks of paid leave?

A. 44
B. 17
C. 16
D. 23

Answer 7

The correct answer is D. This is a very simple example of a Venn diagram question that requires a level of interpretation. The number of employees **not** eligible for two weeks of paid leave will be the number of employees that work in more than one department, i.e. all of the numbers that are part of the overlapping sectors. This can be calculated as follows:

7 + 5 + 4 + 2 + 5 = 23

Although this example may seem fairly simple, it is easy to make errors in interpretation, especially as there are a number of different shapes and overlaps. You must ensure that you count the correct numbers in the overlapping areas and exclude any number that is not part of these areas.

Example 8

The diagram below depicts the result of a survey conducted on USA citizens that travelled to Italy, France and Greece in the last year. Tourists from USA require a visa to enter any country in the west of Europe. Greece belongs to the east of Europe and the other countries in the survey belong to the west. Those who visited France spent a minimum of $3500, whereas those who visited Italy spent a maximum of $5000, and those who visited Greece spent a minimum of $2500 on souvenirs. Obtaining a visa costs an additional fee of $300.

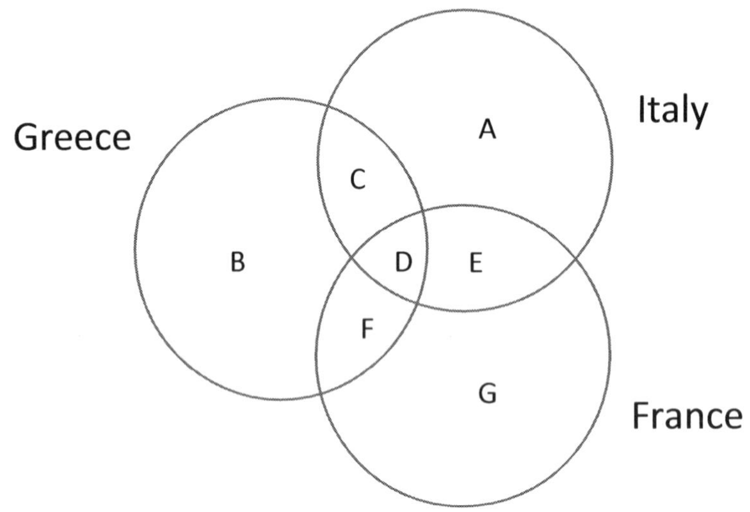

Which of the following statements is true about the tourists?

A. Those belonging to category D spent a maximum of $6000.
B. Those who belong to category G required a visa and spent a maximum of $7000.
C. Those who belong to category D spent a minimum of $300 more than those who belong to category F.
D. Those who belong to category C spent a maximum of $7800.

Answer 8

The correct answer is C.

Simplify the data before reading the questions, as they will be much easier to understand once you understand the data. This can be done as follows:

Country	Visa (Yes = $300 extra) (No = $0 extra)	Expenditure
France	Yes	>$3500
Italy	Yes	<$5000
Greece	No	>$2500

Note: On your whiteboard or scratchpad, this can be simplified much further. Try using initials to represent countries, "Y" and "N" or a check and cross rather than "Yes" or "No", and omitting the column headers. After interpreting the data, eliminate options by focussing on the ones that are most easily calculable.

A. Category D represents tourists who visited all three countries. You must add up the total expenditures: 2 visas ($600) + minimum $2500 (Greece) + minimum $3500 (France) = a minimum of $6600. The expenditure in Italy is given as a maximum, but it is possible for the number to be 0, so we will not include any value here. We know that the minimum expenditure *must* be $6600, so it is not possible for the maximum to be $6000.
B. Category G represents those travelling to only France. There is no maximum expenditure in France, so this option can easily be eliminated.
C. Category D has a minimum expenditure of $6600, which we already calculated for option A. Category F represents those who travelled to France and Greece, where the minimum expenditure is $300 (visa for France).+ $3500 (France) + $2500 (Greece) = $6300. Therefore, those belonging to category D spent at least $300 more than those in category F, as they had one extra visa to pay for. Remember, these are minimum values and they may have spent much more than this.
D. Category C represents those who travelled to Greece and Italy. Although Italy has a maximum spending limit, Greece does not. Therefore, it is not possible that there was a maximum spending limit between the two, as they could have spent as much as they wanted in Greece. This option can be eliminated.

Time saving tips

You will have noticed that some options were easily eliminated on the basis of their wording – sometimes it is just not possible to select an answer, and therefore, you should not waste your time trying to calculate it. If you worked out options A and B, then realised that option

C required a longer calculation, you could have skipped to D to determine whether it was any simpler. D was found to be incorrect, thus the calculations for C would not be necessary as it would be correct on the basis of elimination.

2. Selecting A Venn Diagram

Example 9

11 of the students in St James' Academy study English at A level. 8 of those who study English also study Maths. A total of 19 students in the Academy study Maths, out of which 10 also study Physics. A total of 15 students study Physics, and 3 study all three of the mentioned subjects.

A.

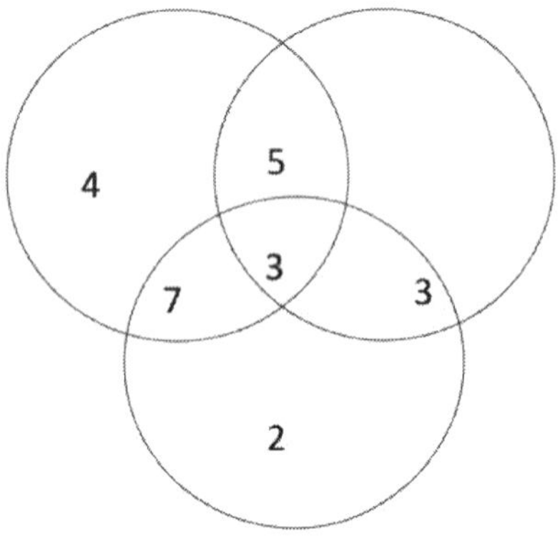

B.

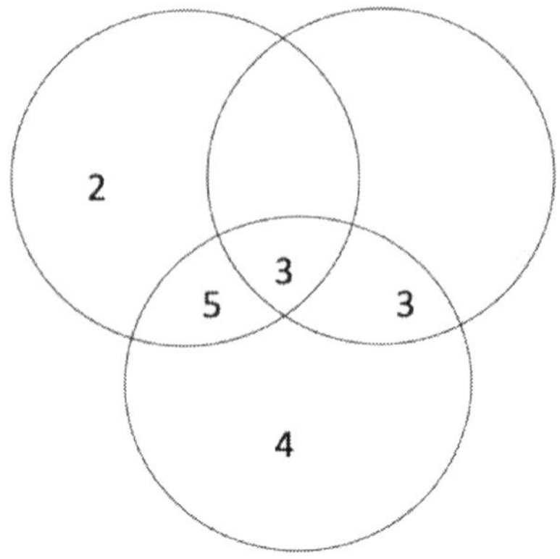

C.

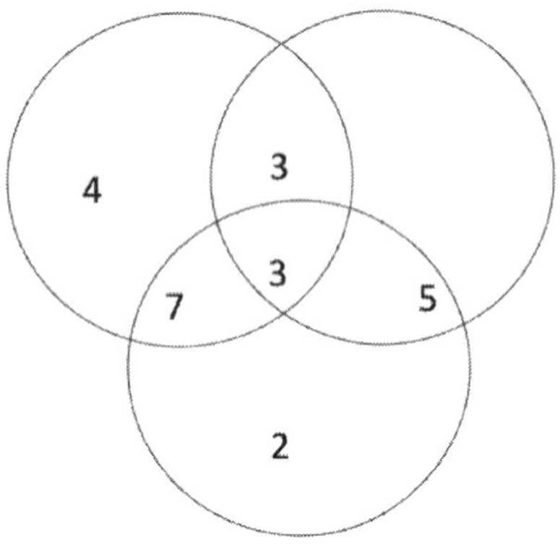

D.

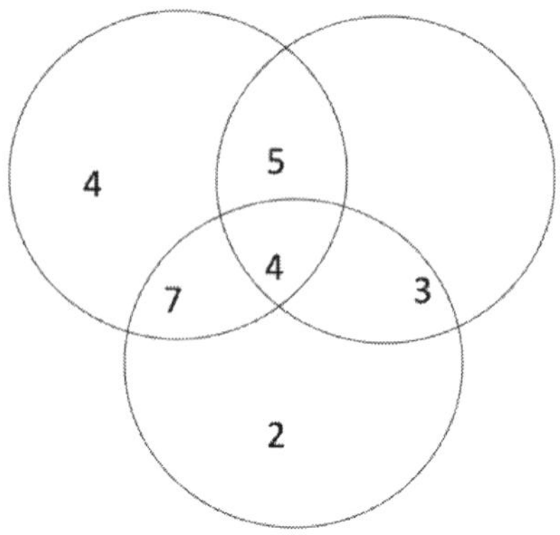

Answer 9

These questions, like many others in the UCAT, can be particularly confusing as there is a lot of information to understand. You can either create your own Venn diagram and find a matching option, or analyse the options to find the correct answer. Creating your own Venn diagram may take longer, depending on your own speed and skills at analysing and interpreting such data. Selecting from the given options can be done in a shorter amount of time, as you are able to eliminate options and guess the answer.

In this case, we will use the second option, as it can save a lot of time.

1. Read the whole passage and eliminate what you are able to. The final thing we read was that 3 students study all three subjects, so we can eliminate option D, as it has a 4 in the area that is an overlap of all three circles.
2. You can then re-read the passage, eliminating one step at a time based on what you read. The first sentence states that 11 students study English at A-level. We do not know which of these circles represents English, but we know that one circle out of the three must have 11 students. We can count the numbers in each circle from A to C. This needs to be done quickly using mental maths. You will find that option B has no circle with 11 students, so it can be eliminated.
3. The next sentence states that the overlap between English and Maths must be 8 students. Both A and C have an overlap of 8 students, so this sentence did not help much, except to determine which of the circles in the respective options might represent Maths.
4. The next sentence states that the total number of students studying Maths is 19. If you count the number of students in the Maths circle which you discovered in the last step, you will find that 19 study Maths in option A, whereas 17 study Maths in option C. Therefore, C can be eliminated. Hence, A is the correct answer.

This clearly takes a bit of time, so you must go through all of the steps speedily, ensuring that you take note of what you have already discovered about each option (which circle represents English, which represents Maths, etc.). If you are running out of time, you can guess an answer after eliminating some options, as your chances of guessing the correct answer improve after each elimination. You may find it quicker to draw your own Venn diagram, but generally, this can take much longer as you need to continually account for each of the values added in each overlap of a circle, subtracting it from the total. Also, you do not need to go in the order of the paragraph, but can choose any sentence and eliminate in a way that works for you. However, if you have a routine of following the order of the paragraph, this may save you time as your brain is accustomed to answering the question in a specific way.

3. Euler Diagrams

Euler diagrams look very similar to Venn diagrams and both show relationships between sets. However, the relationships in a Venn diagram do not need to be true in the real world, whereas the relationships in a Euler diagram must be true in the real world. Therefore, Venn diagrams may show relationships that do not make sense e.g. some fish are humans. A Euler diagram would show such an impossible relationship as follows:

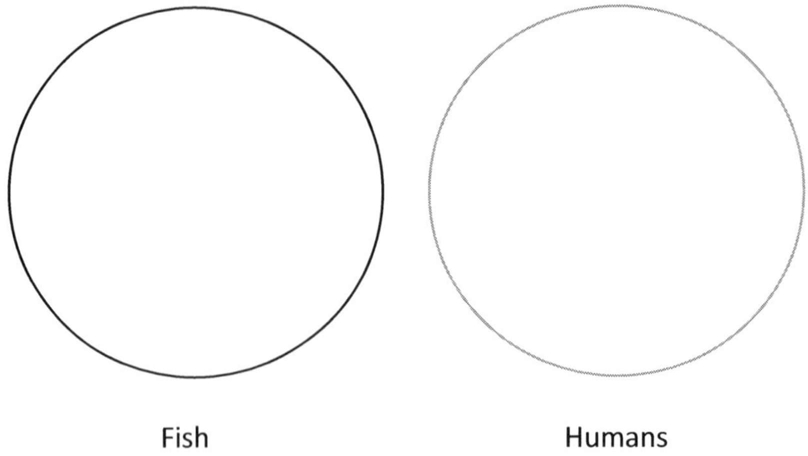

A Venn diagram would show the relationship as follows:

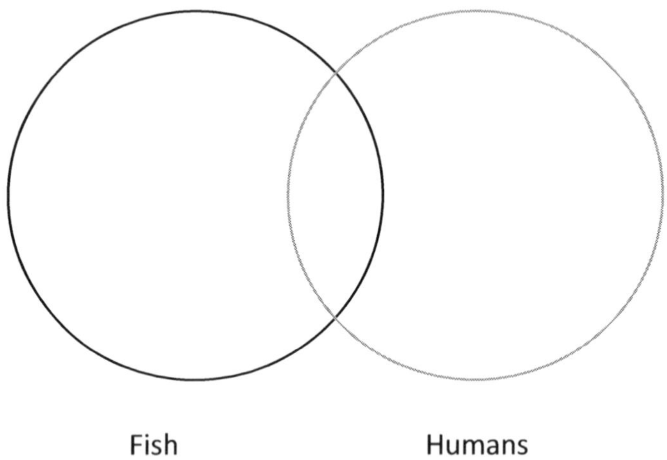

You can see the clear difference between the two. A Euler diagram will not accept this impossible relationship, and will completely separate the two circles that represent each set.

Example 10

Which of the following diagrams most accurately shows the relationship between pens, stationary, cars, vehicles and rats?

A.

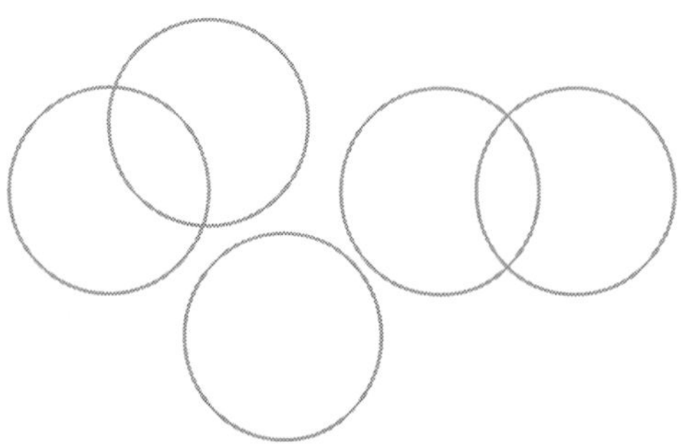

B.

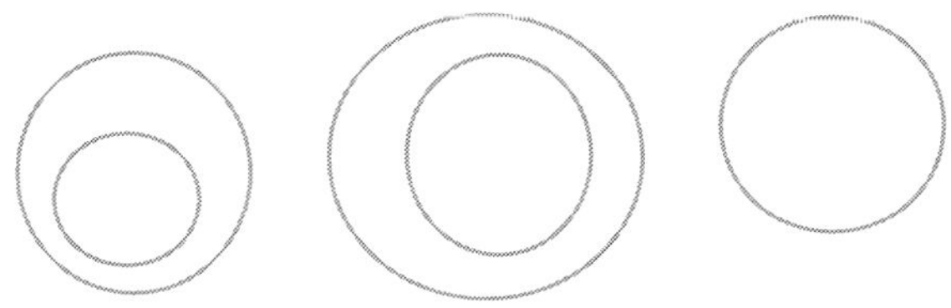

C.

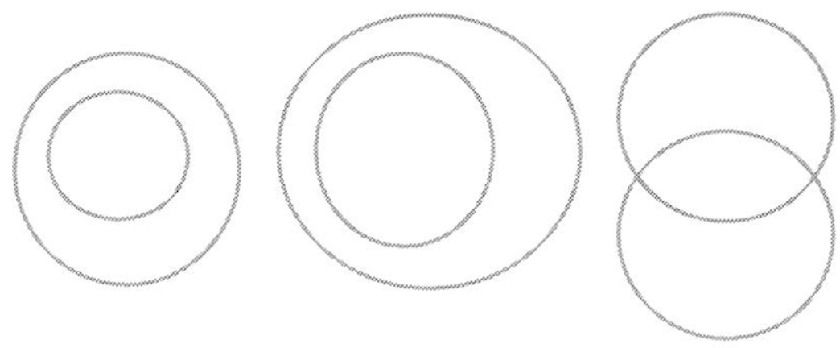

D.

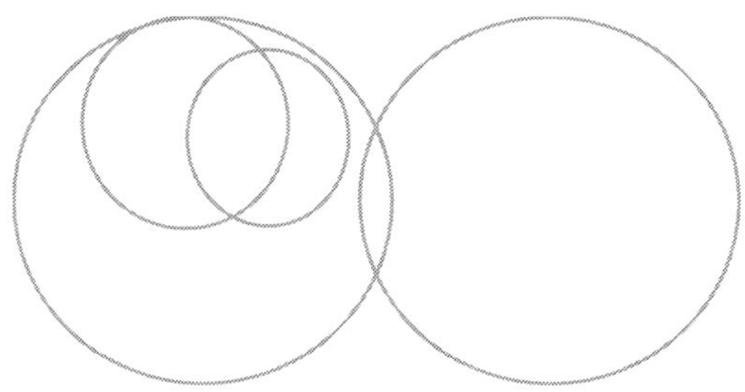

Answer 10

The correct answer is B.

This is the only diagram which shows the real-life relationship between pens, stationary, cars, vehicles and rats. We know that all pens are a subtype of stationary, thus must be contained within the circle representing stationary, rather than overlapping it. These two terms have no relationship with the rest of the terms in real life, so they are separated from the rest of the diagram. We also know that all cars are vehicles, thus the circle representing cars must be contained within the circle representing vehicles. Finally, rats have no association with anything on the list so they must be represented by a standalone circle.

4. Create Your Own Venn Diagram

You will be given information in text format which is easiest to process by drawing a Venn diagram. This type of question can be time consuming, so you should ensure that you are comfortable drawing Venn diagrams.

Example 11

Layla, a medical student, conducted a survey at her GP practice to determine how many patients there are with diagnoses of diabetes or hypertension. 75 patients volunteered to participate in the survey. 25 patients had diabetes whilst 16 said they had hypertension. 13 said they had both diabetes and hypertension.

What is the probability that a patient picked at random from the survey has diabetes but not hypertension?

A. 12/28
B. 25/75
C. 12/75
D. 25/28

Answer 11

The correct answer is C

This is a very simple example that should demonstrate how a Venn diagram can be constructed. There will be more complicated examples in the mock test, but the principles used are the same.

If there are 25 patients with diabetes and 13 with both diabetes and hypertension, the number of patients with diabetes alone is:

$$25 - 13 = 12$$

We also know that the number of patients with hypertension is 16. However, 13 patients have hypertension *and* diabetes. So the number of patients with hypertension alone is:

$$16 - 13 = 3$$

We can now complete our Venn diagram.

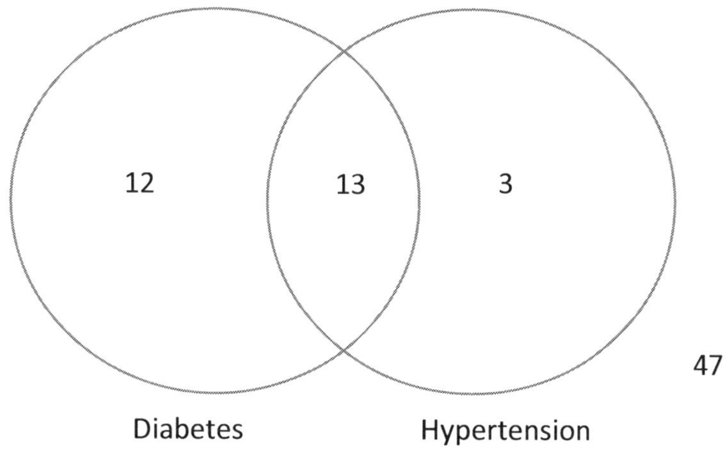

There are 75 patients in total, but only 28 have stated that they have at least one of the diseases in question. Therefore, 47 people have neither disease (75 - 28 = 47). It is not essential to calculate this for the question given, but it is essential to remember that the total number of patients in the survey is 75, *not* 28.

Syllogisms

A syllogism is a method of logical reasoning use to derive a conclusion from two or more premises. Although the statements and conclusions may not make sense in reality, they will logically follow from the information provided. This can be demonstrated through the following example:

> Based on the statements below, is the conclusion true or false?
>
> Statement 1: All dogs are animals.
> Statement 2: All animals have four legs.
> Conclusion: All dogs have four legs.

The conclusion is true. We can see from this statement that the conclusion logically follows. If all dogs are animals, and all animals have four legs, we can logically conclude that all dogs have four legs. We have used statement 1 and statement 2 to come to a logical conclusion. This is a simple example of a syllogism question where you must use the conditions given in a question to arrive at a conclusion.

Sometimes the information provided may not be logical in real life. This can be demonstrated through the following example:

> All dogs are animals.
> All animals are human.

Thus, all dogs are human.

These statements are clearly untrue in real life. However, from the information provided, the conclusion logically follows. It is essential that you use the information provided to derive conclusions, disregarding any outside knowledge.

Question Format

Questions will contain information followed by a series of conclusions. You must decide whether or not each conclusion can be drawn from the information provided. Questions are in a drag-and-drop format, where you must drag the "Yes" and "No" buttons, dropping them next to each conclusion they belong to.

A typical question would appear as such:

All scholars at the conference who study Biology also study Philosophy. All the scholars in the conference were students at the ABC university. None of the scholars studied Mathematics; and a few of them liked environmental studies. All the scholars present had a strong inclination to believe that global warming is impacting the ecology adversely.

Place "Yes" if the conclusion does follow. Place "No" if the conclusion does not follow.

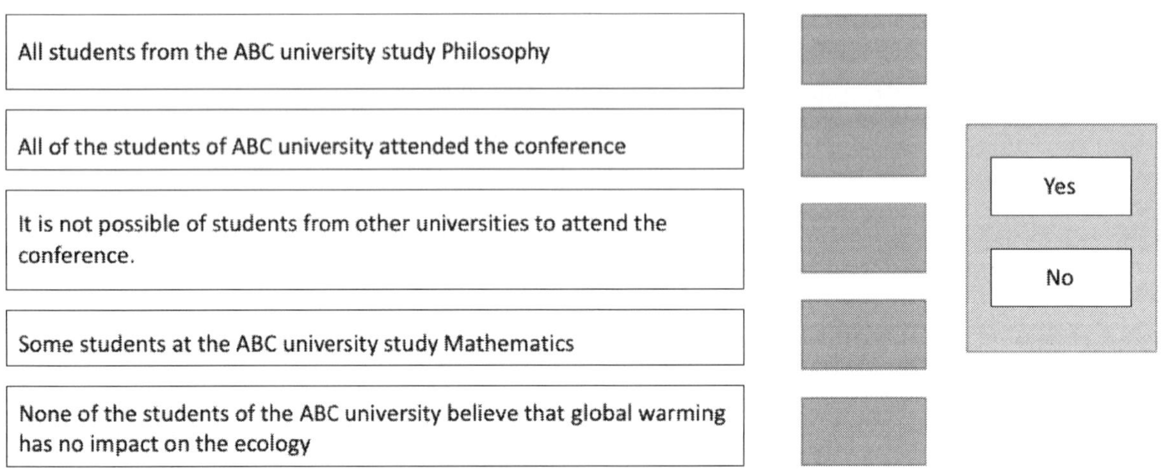

Note: The above represents the official UCAT version of syllogism questions, whereby you must drag and drop the "Yes" and "No" from the right side into the dark grey boxes next to each conclusion. The questions in this book will be in plain text format.

You must understand the following definitions to answer these questions:

- **Yes:** From the information given in the text, this statement logically follows. The answer is only "Yes" if you are certain that the given conclusion can be made.

- **No:** From the information given in the text, this statement does not logically follow. There is not a 100% logical conclusion that can be made. Even with a small amount of doubt, the answer will be "No".

Your analysis of the information provided in each question must be very clear in order to answer the question with certainty. Let us try the following example. Practice summarising the information as you read the example.

Example 12

All those who are thirsty are hungry. Motorcyclists are always hungry, but they are not always thirsty. All those who are intelligent are not always thirsty, but they are always hungry.

Place "Yes" if the conclusion does follow. Place "No" if the conclusion does not follow.

A. All those who are hungry are intelligent.
B. Someone who is hungry will not be a thirsty motorcyclist.
C. An intelligent person cannot be hungry.
D. Some intelligent people will not be motorcyclists.
E. More intelligent people are hungry than thirsty.

Answer 12

We can work this out by quickly writing the information in an easy-to-understand model. Let us represent Thirsty with "T", Hungry with "H", Motorcyclists with "M" and Intelligent with "I". Going through the written passage above, we can deduce that:

All T → H
All M → H
Some M → T (they are not all thirsty, so some must be thirsty)
Some I → T
All I → H

Now, let us assess each of the options.

A. All those who are hungry are intelligent

We know that all I → H, but this does not mean all H → I. Thus, this statement does not logically follow, and the answer is no. It is important to understand that a sentence of logic usually only flows in one direction, so do not mix up the order as the logic does not flow both ways.

For example: "All dentists learn how to drill". This can be broken up into:

A= Dentists
B= Learning how to drill
We can therefore say A → B
However, we cannot say that everyone who learns how to drill is a dentist. This would not follow from the above statement as logic flows in one direction.

B. Someone who is hungry will not be a thirsty motorcyclist.

We know that:
Some M → T
All M → H

If all motorcyclists are hungry, and some motorcyclists are thirsty, we can logically conclude that a thirsty motorcyclist will be hungry.

C. An intelligent person cannot be hungry.

No, because the information we are given tells us that all intelligent people are hungry.
All I → H

D. Some intelligent people will not be motorcyclists.

No, as there is no logical relationship we can conclude with certainty about intelligent people and motorcyclists.

E. More intelligent people are hungry than thirsty.

Yes, as All I → H whereas only some I →T. We can logically conclude that there are more intelligent people who are hungry than thirsty.

Seven HeaVenns

Around a third of syllogism questions can be solved using Venn diagrams. There are seven Venn diagrams that we have named the "Seven HeaVenns". Going through these Seven HeaVenns, you will learn to appreciate how Venn diagrams can be used to clarify the relationships between different objects in a syllogism. Thus, you will be able to quickly and accurately draw logical conclusions from the given text.

1st HeaVenn: No X are Y

We can express this visually by using the following Venn diagram. The orange outlined shape is X and the black outlined shape is Y.

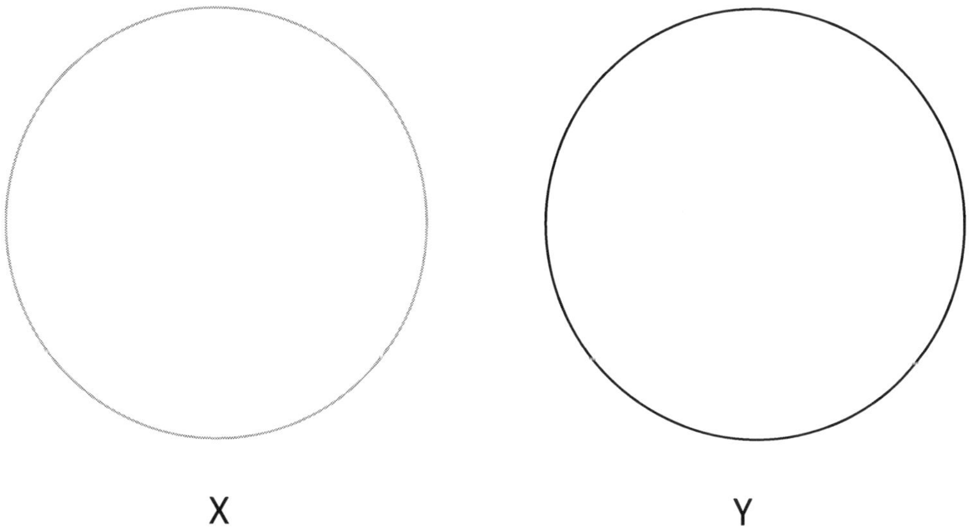

As per the above image, it is evident that No X are Y. We can also deduce from the statement that No Y are X. This is reinforced by the image.

Let us now replace "X" and "Y" with nouns.
Rather than "No X are Y", if the statement was "No shoes are boots," we could logically conclude from the statement, with the help of the Venn diagram, that no boots are shoes.

2nd HeaVenn: Some X are Y

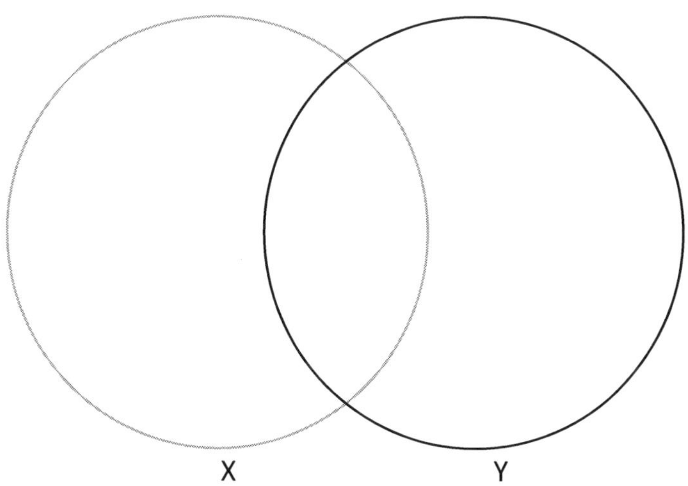

The statement above has been manipulated into a Venn diagram. This now makes it easier for us to make further logical conclusions. We already know that "Some X are Y". We can now say that the following conclusions also logically follow:

1. Some Y are X
2. Some X are not Y
3. Some Y are not X

If we replaced X and Y with nouns and the statement was "some lions are mammals", we could draw the following Venn diagram:

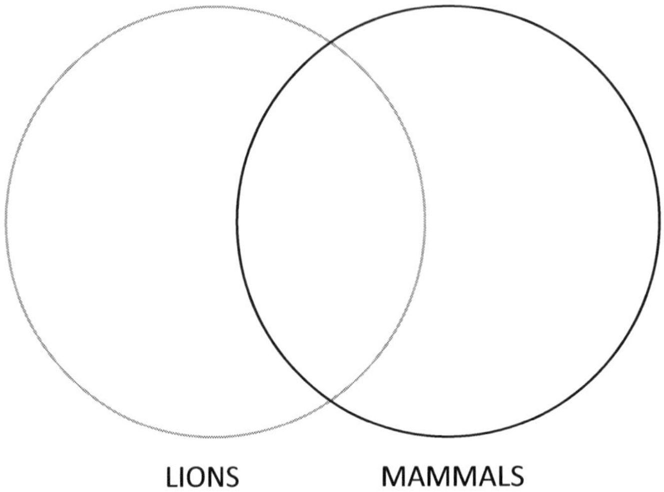

We can easily deduce that some lions are mammals, some mammals are lions, some lions are not mammals and some mammals are not lions. All of the statements mentioned are logical conclusions that can be made. Although we know from our outside knowledge that all lions are in fact mammals, this statement does not logically follow from the information provided. You must not use any outside knowledge when interpreting syllogisms.

3rd HeaVenn: All X are Y

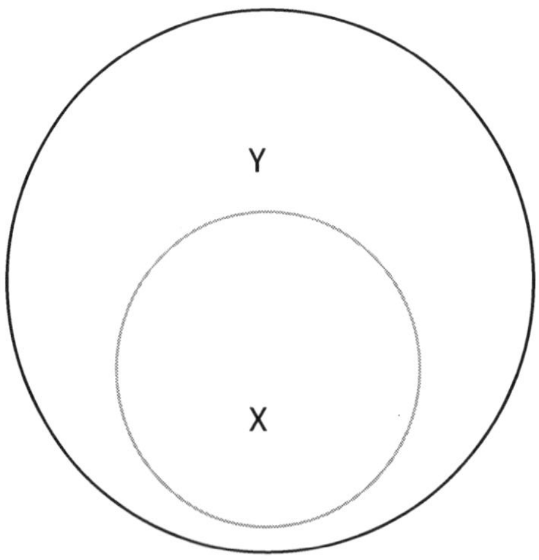

By forming the statement into a Venn diagram, it is easier to see all possible conclusions that we can derive. If all X are Y, we can also say:

1. some X are Y (if all X are Y, then *some* X must definitely be Y)
2. some Y are X

Let us replace "X" and "Y" with "pigeons" and "birds". The statement would then be "all pigeons are birds". Using this statement and the Venn diagram above, you will deduce correctly that:

1. Some pigeons are birds (if all pigeons are birds, some of them must definitely be birds).
2. Some birds are not pigeons.

4th HeaVenn: Some X are Y and some Y are Z

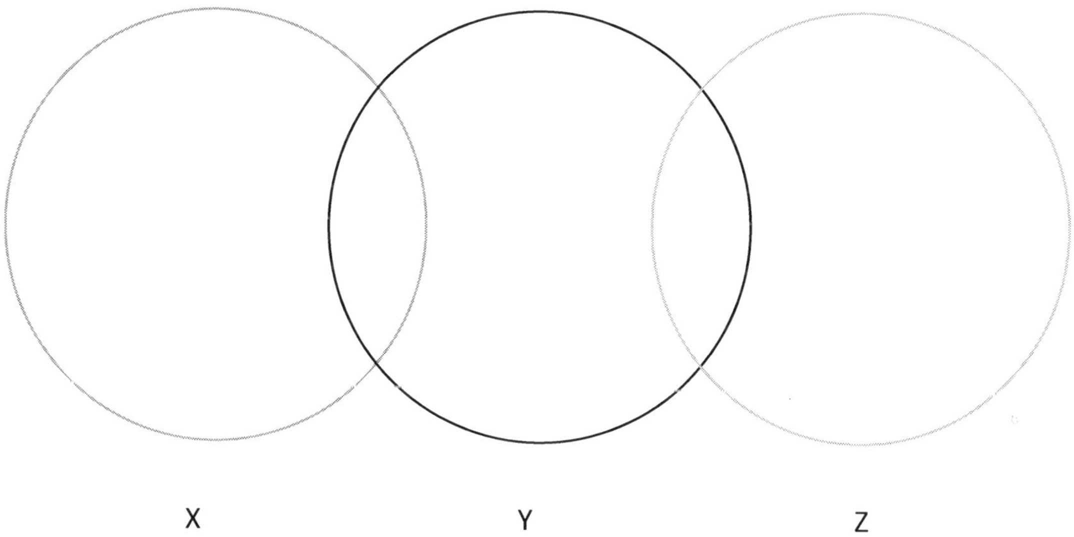

By drawing a Venn diagram, we can now see that certain conclusions can be drawn from the above statement. The following conclusions logically follow from "Some X are Y and some Y are Z":

1. Some Y are X
2. Some Z are Y
3. Some X are not Y
4. Some Y are not X
5. Some Z are not Y
6. Some Y are not Z

It is important to note that in the above example, no conclusions can be made about the relationship between X and Z. We can assume or speculate whether there is a relationship, but we cannot logically show this, as no information has been given in this regard. Whenever there is an unknown element to a relationship the answer is always "No".

Let us look at another similar statement: "Some cars are trucks and some trucks are lorries." Try drawing out the Venn diagram and listing each conclusion that can be made.

We can logically conclude the following from the statement as shown by the above Venn diagram:

1. Some trucks are cars
2. Some lorries are trucks
3. Some cars are not trucks
4. Some trucks are not cars
5. Some trucks are not lorries
6. Some lorries are not trucks

We cannot logically conclude anything about the relationship between cars and lorries from the information given.

5th HeaVenn: Some X are Y, and all Y are Z

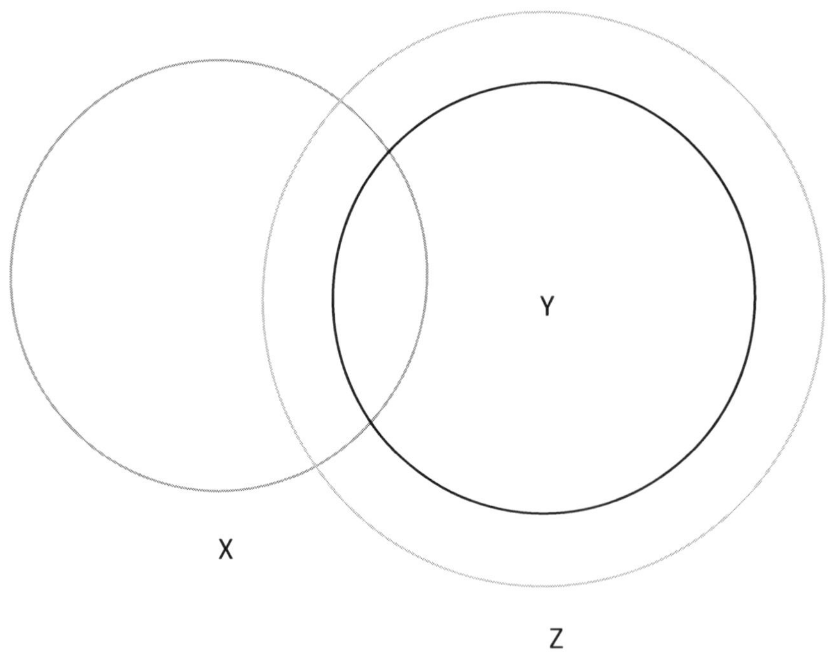

By converting the statement into the above Venn diagram, it is much easier to deduce conclusions. We can now logically conclude that:

1. Some Y are X
2. Some X are not Y and some Y are not X
3. Some Y are Z (If all Y are Z then *some* Y must definitely be Z)
4. Some X are Z
5. Some Z are X

Note: It is important to recognise that in this statement, the relationship between X and Z *can* be proven logically. This is further confirmed by the Venn diagram.

If oranges are X, fruits are Y, and flowers are Z, we can turn this statement into: "Some oranges are fruits and all fruits are flowers." Try to draw out the Venn diagram that represents this statement and write down each conclusion that can be made.

Along with what is obvious from the statement, we can also deduce that:

1. Some fruits are oranges
2. Some oranges are not fruits and some fruits are not oranges
3. Some fruits are flowers (if all fruits are flowers, some fruits must be flowers)
4. Some oranges are flowers
5. Some flowers are oranges

6th HeaVenn: All Y are X and all Z are X

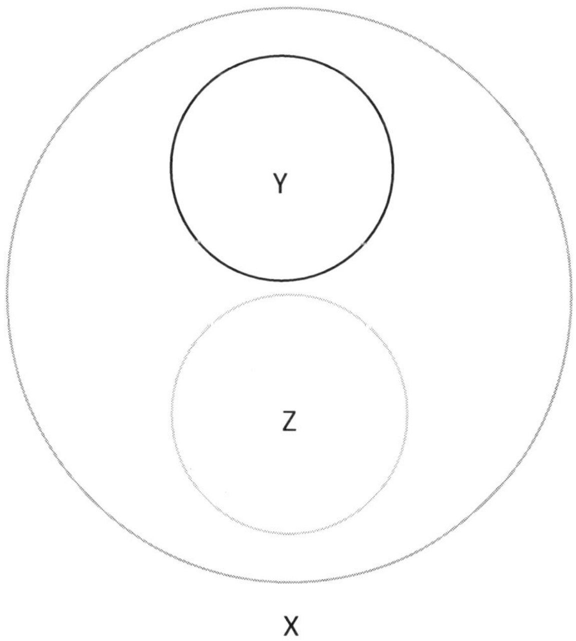

We can deduce the following conclusions from the above statements:

1. Some Y are X
2. Some Z are X
3. Some X are Y, some X are not Y
4. Some X are Z, some X are not Z

Note: We cannot conclude a relationship between Y and Z with the given information.

Let us use an example to further understand the above. Using the following statement, what conclusions logically follow?

"All cats are pets and all dogs are pets."

Along with what is obvious from the statement, we can also deduce that:

1. Some cats are pets
2. Some dogs are pets
3. Some pets are cats and some pets are not cats
4. Some pets are dogs and some pets are not dogs.

We cannot comment on the relationship between cats and dogs as there is no logical conclusion that follows in their regard.

7th HeaVenn: All X are Y and no Y are Z

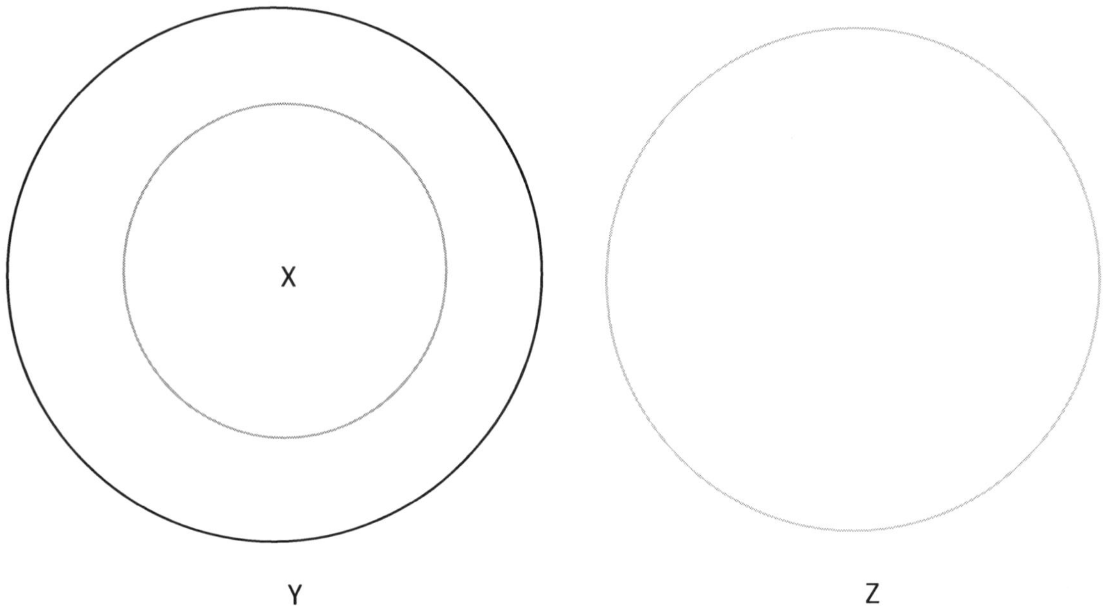

We can make the following additional conclusions from the above statement as depicted by the Venn diagram:

1. Some X are Y
2. Some Y are X
3. No X are Z
4. No Z are X
5. Some X are not Z
6. Some Z are not X
7. No Z are Y
8. Some Y are not Z (if all Y are not Z, some Y are definitely not Z)

9. Some Z are not Y (if all Z are not Y, some Z are definitely not Y)

Let's use an example to further understand the above. Using the following statement, what conclusions logically follow?

"All hens are chicken and no chickens are roosters."

Along with what is obvious from the statement, we can also deduce that:

1. Some hens are chickens
2. Some chickens are hens
3. No hens are roosters
4. No roosters are chickens
5. Some hens are not chickens
6. Some chickens are not roosters
7. No roosters are chickens
8. Some chickens are not roosters
9. Some roosters are not chickens.

Example 13

Some bananas are fruits. All fruits are herbs. Apples are all herbs.

Place "Yes" if the conclusion does follow. Place "No" if the conclusion does not follow.

A. All fruits are bananas.
B. All herbs are apples
C. Some fruits are not bananas
D. Some apples are herbs
E. Some bananas are apples

Answer 13

We can answer this very quickly by drawing a Venn diagram based on the information provided. If some bananas are fruits, their respective circles should overlap. All fruits are herbs, so the circle for herbs should be fully contained within the circle for fruits. All apples are herbs, so the circle for apples should be fully contained within the circle for herbs. The Venn diagram should appear as follows:

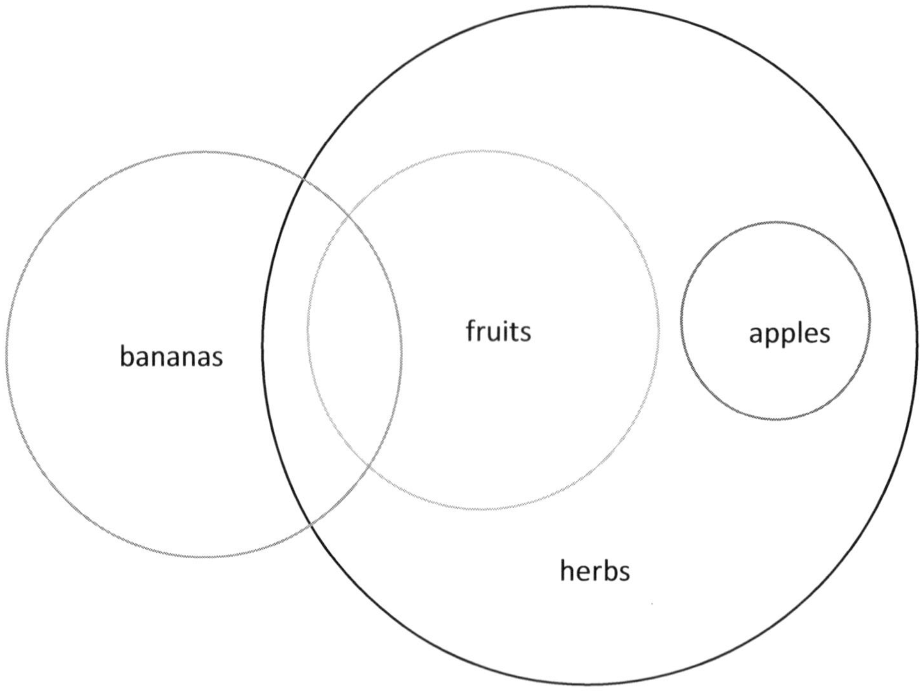

Based on this information, we can deduce the following:

A.	All fruits are bananas.	NO
B.	All herbs are apples	NO
C.	Some fruits are not bananas	YES
D.	Some apples are herbs	YES
E.	Some bananas are apples	NO

Although the statements do not make sense in real life, we can use Venn diagrams to summarise the information and quickly deduce whether or not a statement logically follows based on the information provided.

Drawing Conclusions

Conclusion drawing questions consist of information provided in the form of text, diagrams, tables, charts, and graphs. You must interpret the information and decide whether a proposed conclusion can be made from the information given. Similar to syllogisms, the questions are usually in a drag-and-drop format.

Does it Hold True?

It is vital to develop your ability to decipher whether or not a conclusion holds true. A conclusion can only hold true when, based on the information provided, it necessarily follows.

If a conclusion *may* follow, or is *likely* correct, but not necessarily, it cannot hold true. Remember some key points from Verbal Reasoning:

- Pay attention to key words
- Do not use outside knowledge
- Do not make any assumptions
- Watch out for faulty logic

E.g. 1) Stephanie has 3 pets – a dog, a cat and another mammal. Hamsters are mammals.

Place "Yes" if the conclusion does follow. Place "No" if the conclusion does not follow.

A. Stephanie's third pet is a hamster.

The correct answer is "No". Her third pet is a mammal, and simultaneously, hamsters are mammals, but there is no condition given that her third pet is necessarily a hamster. It is definitely possible, but cannot be said for certain. If it said "Only hamsters are mammals" then this would be true, as it would not be possible for Stephanie to have any other mammal as a pet if no other mammals exist. However, based on the information, she may have any other mammal as a pet, therefore, this conclusion cannot hold true.

B. It is a possibility that Stephanie's third pet is a hamster.

The correct answer is "Yes". Pay attention to the word "possibility". This completely changes the meaning of the conclusion being drawn. As hamsters are mammals, and her third pet is a mammal, there is definitely a possibility that that her third pet is a hamster. Therefore, this conclusion holds true.

C. The dog is a mammal.

The correct answer is "No". It says that her third pet is "another mammal" but this does not necessarily mean that the first two are mammals. Alternatively, it could mean that the cat is a mammal, and the third pet is "another mammal". It does not mention anywhere that the dog is a mammal, therefore, you cannot assume this. In real life, dogs are mammals, but you cannot use outside knowledge to draw conclusions. You must base your conclusion solely on the information given, so this conclusion cannot hold true.

E.g. 2) All adults in a room are wearing black tops. James is wearing a black top.

Place "Yes" if the conclusion does follow. Place "No" if the conclusion does not follow.

A. James is an adult.

The correct answer is "No". You cannot use faulty logic or assumptions to draw a conclusion. James may be a child, a baby, an animal, or anything else. All adults are wearing black tops, but it does not say "only adults are wearing black tops". There are no restrictions on who or what else is able to wear a black top. Therefore, you cannot conclude that James is an adult based on the fact that he is wearing a black top.

Example 14

All employees of a specific firm are eligible for yearly bonuses provided they have worked for 3 consecutive years in the company. Some employees are eligible for other bonuses as well. Staff who have received an "exceptional rating" are eligible for an additional £3500 add-on to their yearly salary, and staff who helped design project "Alpha" are eligible for an additional two weeks of paid leave. Any employee with a yearly salary of £30,000 or more is not eligible for any kind of bonus.

Place "Yes" if the conclusion does follow. Place "No" if the conclusion does not follow.

A. David has worked for 5 years in this company, and has received an "exceptional rating", so he is eligible for a minimum of two bonuses.
B. Maxine receives a salary of £29,000, but due to her "exceptional rating" she gains another £3500. Therefore, she is not eligible for any other bonus.
C. David is part of project "Alpha" so he is definitely eligible for an additional two weeks of paid leave.
D. Emily's salary is double that of David, while Maxine's salary is twice as much as Emily. If Maxine earns £140,000, David is not eligible for any kind of bonus.
E. Emily earned £12,000 in the month of August, so her yearly salary will make her unqualified for any kind of bonus.

Answer 14

This question has a lot of information, so it would be useful to use your whiteboard or scratchpad to note down your interpretations and any key points.

A. The correct answer is "No". David worked for 5 years, but it is not evident from this information that he definitely worked for a minimum of 3 *consecutive* years. It is possible that he may have taken breaks, or left and re-joined the company in that period of time. Hence, he may not be eligible for the yearly bonus which requires 3 consecutive years of work. His salary is also not given, so it is possible that he has a yearly salary of £30,000 or more. In that case, he would not get any bonus at all.

B. The correct answer is "No". This question changes the rules that are applied in the scenario. The information in the passage states that the £3500 add-on is a bonus in itself. If an employee earns a yearly salary of £30,000 or more, they will be eligible for no bonuses at all. £30,000 most likely refers to the salary *prior* to any bonuses paid, as it says "... they are not eligible for any kind of bonus". If this £30,000 limit included bonuses, it would say "... they are not eligible for any *additional* bonus." Additionally, it is clear that Maxine is already getting a bonus, so it would not make sense to apply this rule to her.
C. The correct answer is "No". The keyword is "definitely". The text states that those who helped design this project will get an additional two weeks of paid leave. Although it is possible that David helped design it, given that he is "part of" the project, it is not certain. Therefore, this conclusion cannot hold true.
D. The correct answer is "Yes". This is a simple maths question. If Maxine earns £140,000 which is double Emily's salary, Emily will earn half of that, which is £70,000. Further, David will earn half of what Emily earns, which is £35,000. The text states that anyone with a salary over £30,000 will not be eligible for any kind of bonus.
E. The correct answer is "No". This is based on the assumption that Emily will definitely earn more than £30,000 in a year if she earned £12,000 in one month. She may have a variable pay every month, or only work for one or two months in a year, so this cannot be assumed.

Example 15

The graph below shows the speed of 3 sprinters in the first 30 seconds of their race. Haseeb wore purple trainers, Jared wore green and Obafemi wore orange.

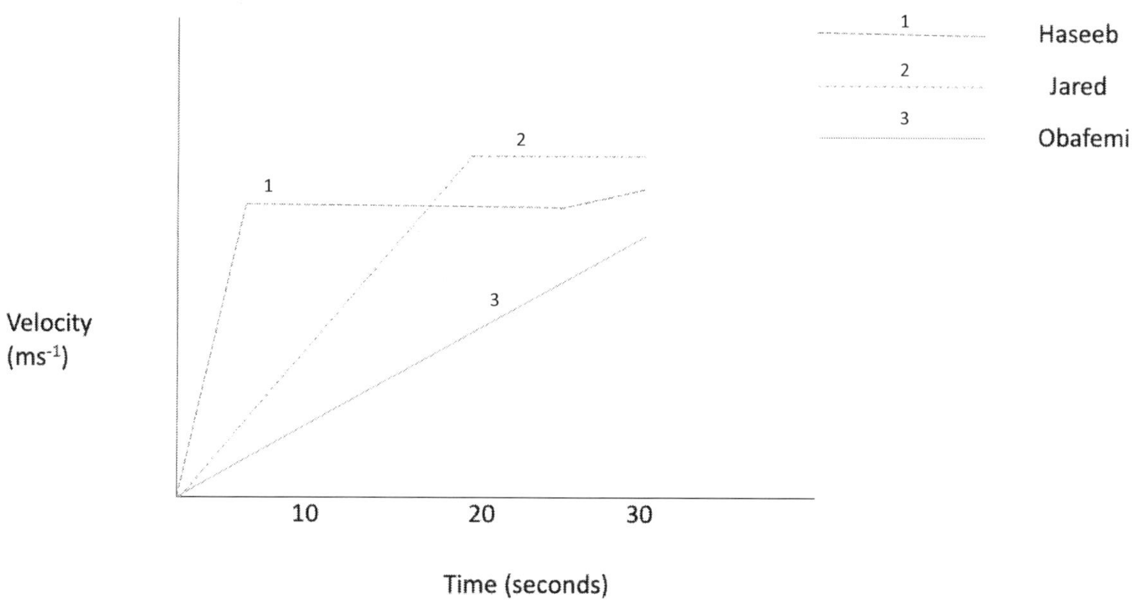

Place "Yes" if the conclusion does follow. Place "No" if the conclusion does not follow.

A. Obafemi was always behind Haseeb.
B. Haseeb seems to have covered the most distance in 30 seconds.
C. Jared's initial acceleration was greater than Haseeb's.
D. Orange trainers decrease the speed of the runner.
E. The fitness of the sprinters was the deciding factor in the race.

Answer 15

This question requires you to understand velocity-time graphs and their associated formulae.

A. The correct answer is "Yes". Distance is represented by the area of the space under the line in a velocity-time graph. The space under the line representing Obafemi has a far smaller area than that of Haseeb's line, thus it is clear that the distance he covered was far less.
B. The correct answer is "Yes". The area under Haseeb's line appears largest. Without values to calculate, it may be uncertain, but the conclusion says that he "seems to", rather than a qualifier of necessity like "definitely", therefore this conclusion does hold true.
C. The correct answer is "No". Haseeb had a greater acceleration, as acceleration=velocity/time. Thus, a steeper curve shows a greater acceleration.
D. The correct answer is "No". This conclusion is assuming that correlation equals causation. We know that it does not, therefore, this conclusion cannot hold true.
E. The correct answer is "No". There is no mention about the fitness of the sprinters, so this conclusion relies on an assumption. Thus, it cannot hold true.

Logical Puzzles

Scenarios involve a large number of details which you must interpret in a format that is reasonable for yourself to understand. They can be nearly impossible to solve without using a whiteboard to simplify the information. Logical puzzles may appear as a drag-and-drop format, but are generally in the form of option selection.

Example 16

Daniel, Mohammed, Adrian, Aaron, Stephanie and Rachel went shopping together and bought trousers. These trousers were either short, medium or long in length and black, red or grey in colour.

- Only one of the friends had medium length trousers.

- Daniel's trousers were long and were not black in colour.
- There was one more pair of long trousers than short trousers.
- Mohammed and Rachel bought the exact same trouser length and colour combination.
- The length of Daniel's trousers was exactly the same as Rachel's.
- The number of black trousers was equal to the number of long ones.
- There was only one pair of red trousers and they belonged to Daniel.
- Rachel's trousers were grey in colour.

Which of the following combinations of trouser length and colour is possible?

A. Adrian's trousers were medium and black.
B. Rachel's trousers were short and grey.
C. Aaron's trousers were medium and grey.
D. Daniel's trousers were short and red.

Answer 16

The amount of information given is very difficult to comprehend, thus it is advisable to create a table of the various domains in the question. This would appear as follows:

	Length	**Colour**
Daniel		
Mohammed		
Adrian		
Aaron		
Stephanie		
Rachel		

In a time-pressured exam, you would not have the time to create a table with the gridlines and each word spelled out completely. You would, instead, use initials for each name, or the first two letters when there are multiple names starting with the same initial. On your whiteboard, it would more likely appear as follows:

	L	**C**
D		
M		
Ad		
Aa		
S		
R		

For the purposes of clarity, we will demonstrate the step-by-step method of filling in this table using the full names and words, rather than initials.

Once you have created your table, read the passage again, adding any information that you are able to. Some points will not allow you to add anything to the table immediately, so you can skip those points and come back to them at the end. Let us go through all of the points, stopping at each one that allows us to write something in the table.

- Only one of the friends had medium length trousers.
  You cannot yet write anything using this information.
- Daniel's trousers were long and were not black in colour.

Daniel	Long	Not black

- There was one more pair of long trousers than short trousers.
  You cannot yet write anything using this information, as we do not know how many short trousers there are.
- Mohammed and Rachel bought the exact same trouser length and colour combination.
  Their trouser length is unknown. You could either write "Mohammed" in Rachel's boxes, and "Rachel" in Mohammed's boxes, or leave them blank and see if more information will come up.
- The length of Daniel's trousers was exactly the same as Rachel's.
  We previously found out that Daniel bought long trousers. We now know that Daniel, Mohammed, and Rachel all have long trousers.

	Length	**Colour**
Daniel	Long	Not black
Mohammed	Long	
Adrian		
Aaron		
Stephanie		
Rachel	Long	

- The number of black trousers was equal to the number of long ones.
  You cannot yet write anything using this information.
- There was only one pair of red trousers and they belonged to Daniel.
  Replace "not black" with "red".
- Rachel's trousers were grey in colour.
  We know that Mohammed bought the same colour of trousers as Rachel.

	Length	**Colour**
Daniel	Long	Red
Mohammed	Long	Grey
Adrian		
Aaron		
Stephanie		
Rachel	Long	Grey

Now, you can go back and check each of the points again to see if there is anything that you missed.

- Only one of the friends had medium length trousers.
  We still do not know who these belong to, but it will be either Adrian, Aaron, or Stephanie.
- There was one more pair of long trousers than short trousers.
  There are 3 long trousers, so there must be 2 pairs of short trousers.
- The number of black trousers was equal to the number of long ones.
  There are 3 long trousers, so there must be 3 black trousers. There are 3 empty boxes for "colour", so they must all be black. We can fill this in below.

Daniel	Long	Red
Mohammed	Long	Grey
Adrian		Black
Aaron		Black
Stephanie		Black
Rachel	Long	Grey

This is all of the information we are able to fill in. We also know that out of Adrian, Aaron, and Stephanie, two will have short trousers and one will have medium length. We do not have any more information than this.

Using the table we have constructed, we can now answer the question.

Which of the following combinations of trouser length and colour is possible?

A. Adrian's trousers were medium and black.
B. Rachel's trousers were short and grey.
C. Aaron's trousers were medium and grey.
D. Daniel's trousers were short and red.

It is clear from the table that options B, C and D cannot be true. Rachel's trousers are long, Aaron's trousers are black, and Daniel's trousers are long. The question asks what is *possible*. Adrian's trousers must be black, and they are either short or medium length. Thus, it is possible that they are medium length.

Example 17

There are 6 houses in a lane, belonging to each of Arav, Barbara, Chang, Derek, Eric and Fatima. Barbara and Fatima are women, whereas the remaining are men. One of the houses on either end belongs to a woman. Arav's house is next to Fatima's house, and is 5th in the sequence of houses. Derek's house is adjacent to Barbara's house, and Derek has only one neighbour. The remaining houses chronologically belong to the remaining owners based on their names in alphabetical order.
(Assume the houses are numbered 1, 2, 3, 4, 5, 6 starting from left to the right.)

Who is the owner of the fourth house from the left?

A. Eric
B. Fatima
C. Chang
D. Derek

Answer 17

The correct answer is A.

As in the previous example, you need to summarise the data in a way that will make sense to you. You should first read the passage to understand the context of the question, then create a quick sketch to represent the 6 houses. You can read the passage for a second time, adding on information to the sketch as you read.

- One of the houses on either end belongs to a woman.
  You cannot yet write anything using this information.
- Arav house is 5th in the sequence of houses.

____ ____ ____ ____ A ____

- Fatimah's house is next to Arav's *(could mean left or right).*

____ ____ ____ F A F

- Derek has only one neighbour.
  This means that Derek must own one of the end houses.
- Derek's house is adjacent to Barbara's house.

This means that Derek must own the first house, as he cannot have the 6th house and also have Barbara as a neighbour (Arav would be his neighbour in that case).

D B ___ F A F

- If we go back to the earlier point that one of the end houses must belong to a woman, we know that Fatimah must own house 6, as the first house has been taken by David. Therefore, we can remove her from house 4, as that is not her house.

D B ___ ___ A F

- The remaining houses chronologically belong to the remaining owners based on their names in alphabetical order.
  Only Chang and Eric remain. If we arrange these names alphabetically, Chang will come first, then Eric.

D B C E A F

Therefore, the owner of the fourth house from the left is Eric.

Decision Making Mock Test

Question 1

A car manufacturer has only 4 types of vehicles in her showroom: SUVs, sedans, hatchbacks, and pickups. On a particular day, she decides to put 15 of the vehicles in her showroom for sale.

6 of the vehicles put up on sale have a 2L engine.
None of the hatchbacks have a 2L engine.
There were equal number of SUVs and pickups put on sale.
The number of sedans put on sale was 1 more than the number of hatchbacks put on sale.
Only SUVs and pickups have a 2L engine.

Place "Yes" if the conclusion follows. Place "No" if it does not follow.

A. There were more SUVs than sedans put up for sale. YES/NO
B. The difference in the number of sedans and pickups put up for sale was half of the number of hatchbacks up for sale. YES/NO
C. The number of hatchbacks put for sale was less than the number of pickups put up for sale. YES/NO
D. There are more sedans than SUVs in the showroom. YES/NO
E. It is possible for the car manufacturer to put up more types of vehicles for sale, given that the number of vehicles put up do not change. YES/NO

Question 2

At a fun fair, you approach a stall that allows you to win money, provided that you play a game and win. The game consists of a dice and a deck of cards. The conditions of the game are as follows:
If you are able to draw a club, and then roll a 5, the organiser will give you £50.
If the organiser draws a spade, and then rolls a 4, you have to give the organiser £40.

The game takes place in turns: you start first, then the organiser plays her turn. You carry on taking turns until someone wins.

Should you take part in the game?

A. No, because the probability of either person winning is numerically equal.

B. No, because there could be other biased reasons allowing the organiser to win easily, hence you are at greater risk of losing money.
C. Yes, because you will win more money than you will lose.
D. Yes, because given the fact that you are starting first, you have a greater chance of winning.

Question 3

Should all countries be forced to adapt to newer and more renewable sources of energy in order to increase sustainability and promote environmental harmony?

A. Yes, because our current dependence on non-renewable fossil fuels will not serve us in the long run.
B. Yes, because the burning of fossil fuels is slowly and steadily harming the environment.
C. No, because studies show that many countries are not economically developed and do not have the infrastructure to shift into a system that only relies on renewable sources of energy for survival.
D. No, because all European countries are economically developed and switching over to renewable sources of energy may not help reduce global warming.

Question 4

Choose the correct relation which represents the following fact: All frogs are amphibians, all toads are amphibians, and no frog is a toad. Some cells are reptiles, frogs or toads.

A.

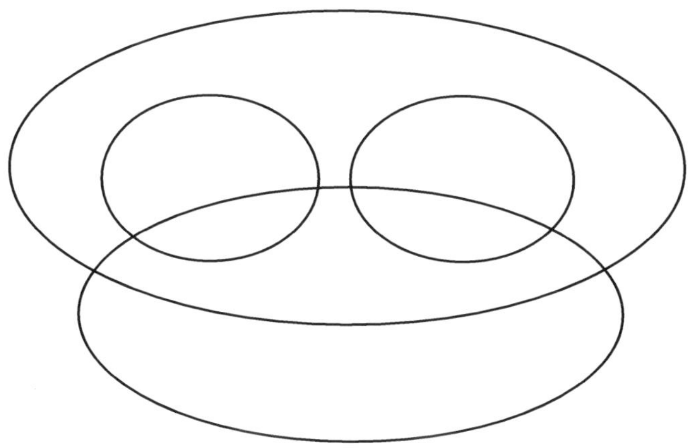

B.

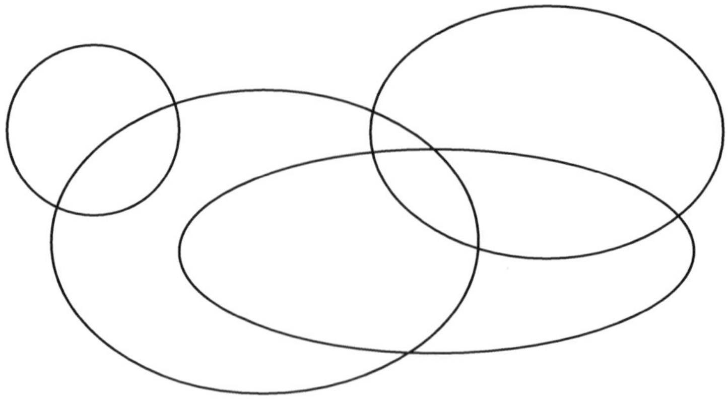

C.

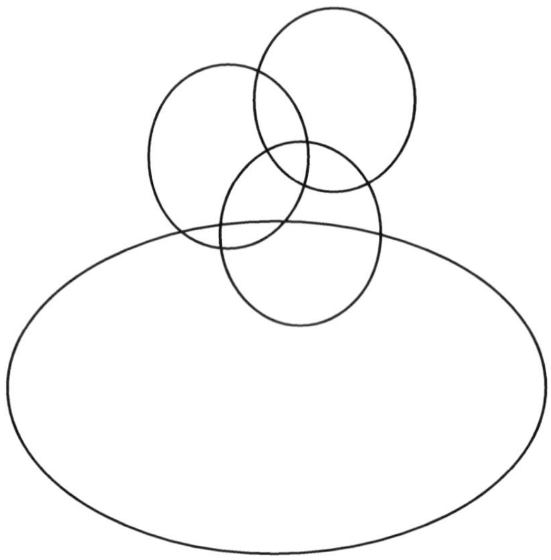

D.

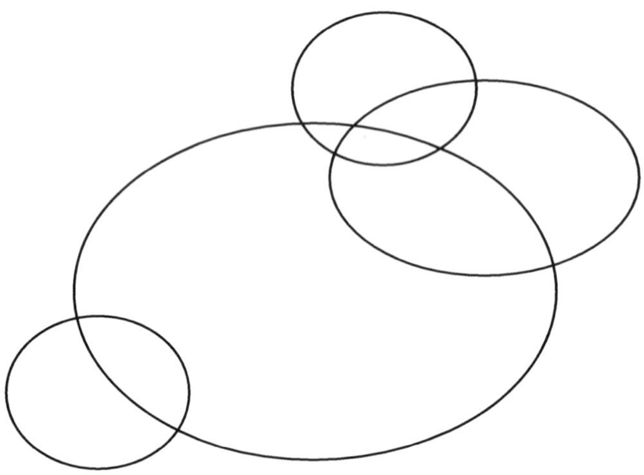

Question 5

Out of all the Mathematics graduates from university, some of them go on to do further jobs in data analysis. However, those who studied only analytical mathematics do not work in data analysis.

Place "Yes" if the conclusion follows. Place "No" if the conclusion does not follow.

A. Only mathematics graduates can work in data analysis. YES/NO

B. Analytical mathematics graduates are not eligible for a career in data analysis. YES/NO

YES/NO

C. Some of the graduates of this university are employed. YES/NO

D. David studied analytical mathematics, therefore he cannot be working in data analysis. YES/NO

E. Some mathematics students did not graduate from university

Question 6

The following diagram depicts the number of students studying different subjects at university.

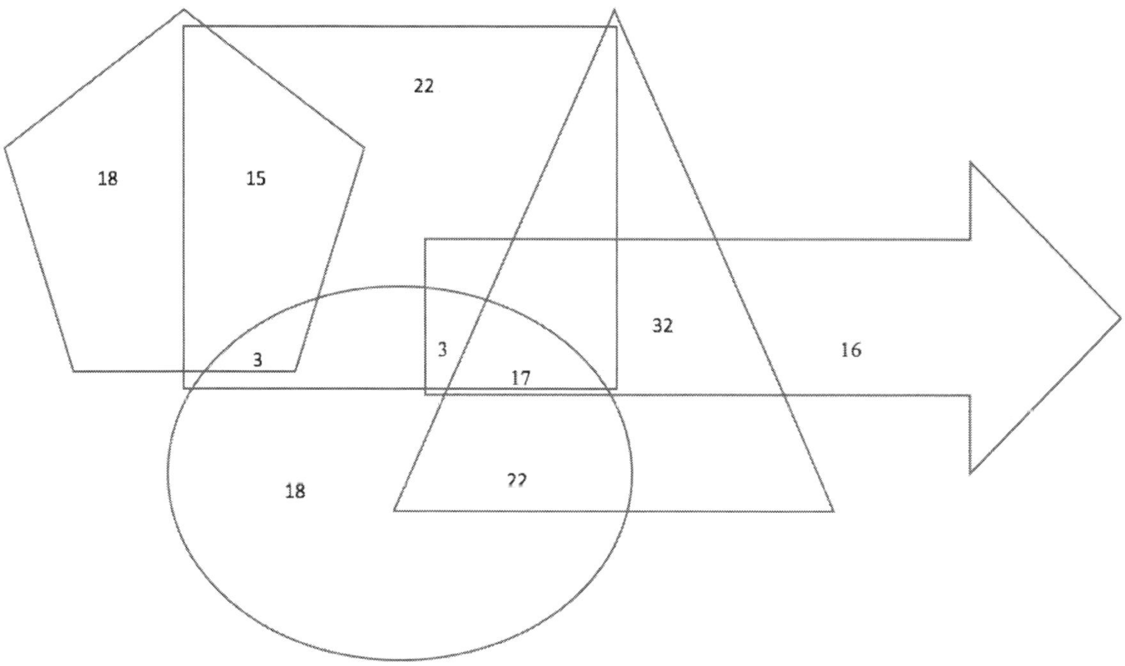

- The pentagon represents students studying Mathematics.
- The square represents students studying English.
- The triangle represents the students studying Sociology.
- The circle represents the students studying Biology.
- The arrow represents students studying Nursing.

Based on the above information, which of the following statements is true?

A. The number of students studying only Nursing, only Mathematics, and both Mathematics and English is 47.

B. There are more students studying a combination of English, Mathematics & Biology than those studying Biology, Nursing & Sociology.

C. The number of students studying only Nursing and only Biology is numerically equivalent to the number of students studying only Mathematics and only Nursing.

D. The number of students studying Sociology and Nursing represents the second highest combination of subjects chosen by students.

Question 7

To ensure the safety of younger children, should the speed limit in all school zones be reduced?

A. Yes, because a reduction in speed limit will ensure that fewer cars drive in speed zones.

B. Yes, because a reduction in the speed limit will ensure that drivers will become more careful while driving in such areas.

C. No, as accidents can be caused because of reasons other than speeding. Reducing the speed limit might reduce collisions but will not address the other causes of accidents.

D. No, because the speed limit in school zones is already low.

Question 8

The graph below shows the temperature across different cities in a country, taken on a particular day.

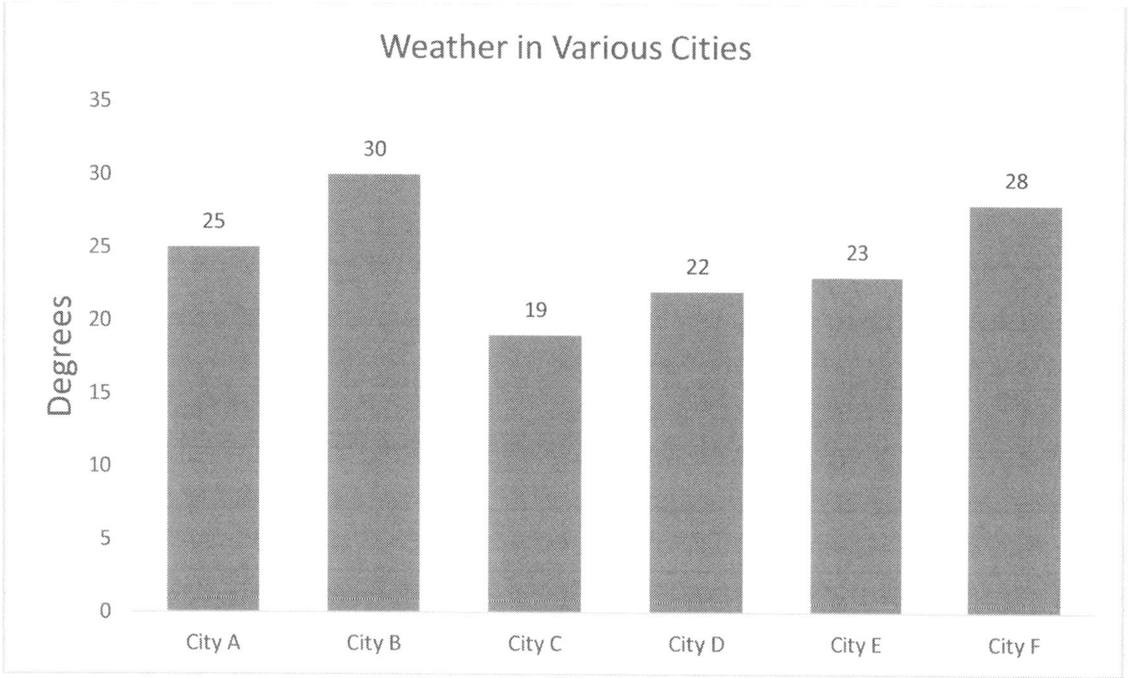

Place "Yes" if the conclusion follows. Place "No" if the conclusion does not follow.

A. The average temperature of City B, D and F is more than the average of City A, C and E. YES/NO
B. The average of the two cities with the highest temperatures differs from the average of the two cities with the lowest temperatures by 2 degrees. YES/NO
C. In this country, City B is the hottest city to live in. YES/NO
D. On this particular day, City C is the coldest city in this country. YES/NO
E. The temperatures of City B and City F usually differ by 2 degrees. YES/NO

Question 9

The diagram given below depicts the different combinations of A Level subjects chosen by students at this sixth form college.

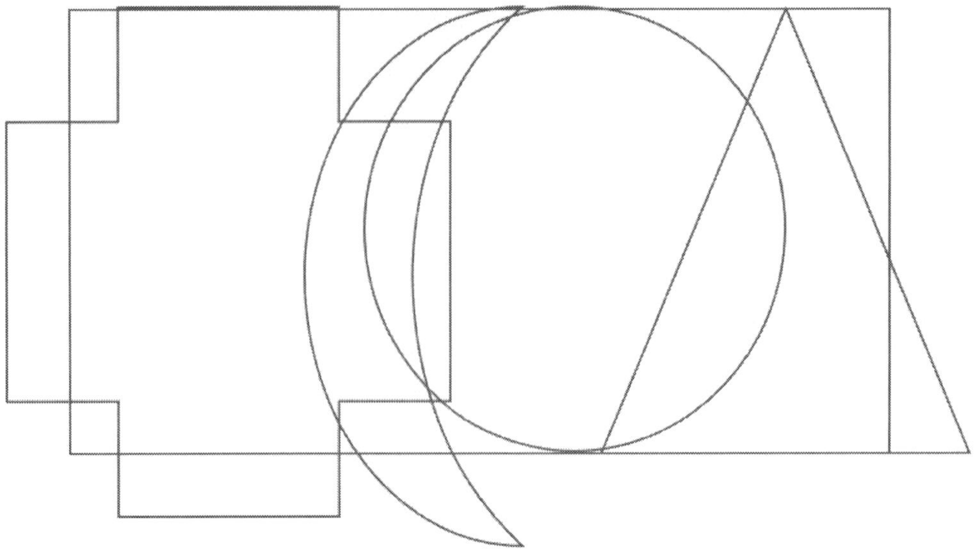

The following subjects are represented by these shapes:

The cross represents Mathematics.
The circle represents Biology.
The triangle represents Chemistry.
The crescent represents Psychology.
The rectangle represents English.

Which one of the following combinations of subjects is not represented by the above diagram?

A. Psychology, Mathematics and English.
B. Chemistry, English and Biology.
C. Mathematics, Chemistry and English.
D. Psychology, Biology and English.

Question 10

All tigers in the zoo are fast, and all sloths in this zoo are slow. This animal is not slow.

Place "Yes" if the conclusion follows. Place "No" if the conclusion does not follow.

A. This animal is a tiger. YES/NO
B. This animal is fast. YES/NO
C. Provided that this animal is not fast, it cannot belong to this zoo. YES/NO
D. If the animal is in this zoo and is a tiger, it must be fast. YES/NO
E. All sloths are slow. YES/NO

Question 11

The owner of a factory must determine which of two different wheat-processing machines he should buy to help him increase production.

Machine A requires maintenance twice in six days.
Machine B requires maintenance once in three days.
Machine A breaks down once in a month.
Machine B works at peak efficiency 95% of the time in a month.

Assume that one month consists of 30 days.

When the machines are working, they works at peak efficiency. Otherwise, they breaks down.

Considering the above-mentioned details, which machine should the owner choose for his factory?

A. Machine A, as it requires less maintenance.
B. Machine A, as it works at peak efficiency for a longer period.
C. Machine B, as it requires less maintenance.
D. Machine B, as it only breaks down 5% of the time per month.

Question 12

Rahul, Raheem, Richard and Rebecca went to four different countries during the summer holidays. These countries were either Japan, India, Brazil, or Germany. The prices were 640, 560, 650 and 970 in no particular order, and the price for a particular package to a country had to be paid in the currency of that country. Japan and India are in Asia, Brazil is in South America, while Germany is in Europe.

The currency conversion rates are as follows:

1 United States Dollar = 4.82 Brazilian Real

1 British Pound = 137.13 Japanese Yen
1 German Euro = 85.18 Indian Rupees
1 British Pound = 1.27 United States Dollar
1 Indian Rupee = 1.43 Japanese Yen

Rahul did not go to an Asian country, and spent the largest amount of money overall (in monetary value). Raheem went to Japan, and the amount of money spent by him in numerical value is 10 less than what was spent by Rebecca. Richard went to an Asian country.

Which of the combinations mentioned below is possible?

A. Rahul went to Brazil and spent 560 Reals.
B. Raheem went to Japan and spent 650 Yen.
C. Rebecca went to Brazil and spent 650 Reals.
D. Richard went to India and spent 970 Rupees.

Question 13

In view of the recent coronavirus pandemic, should all countries across the world enforce compulsory strict lockdowns?

A. Yes, because lockdowns can prevent the spread of the virus between people.
B. Yes, because that would lead to less people becoming sick, and more hospital beds available.
C. No, because restricting the movement of people is a violation to a fundamental human right.
D. No, as studies show that different countries have different infection rates, and while lockdowns may work in some countries, they might not necessarily work in another.

Question 14

In a particular country, there are 25 residents, and they read a combination of German, English and French newspapers.

4 residents read only German newspapers.
5 residents read German and English newspapers only.
3 residents read German, English and French newspapers.
2 residents read English and French newspapers.
4 residents read only French newspapers.
14 residents read English newspapers.
The rest read German and French newspapers only.

Based on the above information, how many residents read German and French newspapers only?

A. 3
B. 4
C. 5
D. 6

Question 15

All adults in this party are wearing a black hat. Rosie is wearing a black hat. Besides people, there are also pets in this congregation. The party serves beverages. Only those over the age of 18 are served an alcoholic beverage, and there are non-alcoholic beverages available for children.

Place "Yes" if the conclusion follows. Place "No" if the conclusion does not follow.

A. Stephanie is wearing a black hat, hence she must be an adult.	YES/NO
B. Rosie must be an adult.	YES/NO
C. Children cannot be above the age of 18.	YES/NO
D. There are dogs at the party.	YES/NO
E. Rajesh usually drinks alcoholic beverages, hence he must be above the age of 18.	YES/NO

Question 16

Arjun is playing a game with his friend, Becky. The rules of the game are as follows.

Arjun will have to pick a number from a box, which consists of the first 200 numbers.
If Arjun picks up a multiple of 6 or 8, Becky wins. Otherwise, Arjun wins.

Based on the above conditions, the probability of Arjun winning is thrice of that of Becky winning.

A. No, because the probability of Becky winning is 1/4.
B. No, because it cannot be said for certain that Arjun will not pick a multiple of 6 or 8.
C. Yes, because the probability of Arjun picking up a multiple of 6 or 8 is 1/4.
D. Yes, because since Arjun starts, he is more likely to win.

Question 17

To improve the quality of life of low-income workers, is it enough to just increase their wages?

A. Yes, because with an increased salary comes a better quality of life.
B. Yes, because increasing their wages would take care of all of the other aspects needed for a better quality of life.
C. No, because research shows that quality of life is decided by a plethora of factors.
D. No, because increasing their wages might not be economically feasible.

Question 18

Six students in a particular school are made to stand according to their height order, with the first in line being the shortest and the last in line being the tallest. These students are Becky, Rachel, Amy, Karen, Thomas and Holly. They study in years 4, 5, 6, 7, 8 and 9 in no particular order.

Karen stands between Amy and Thomas, and is not the eldest of them all.
Rachel stands between Becky and Amy, and is the youngest of all those standing.
The one standing between Karen and Holly is the oldest in the group.
The remaining students are standing in ascending order of their years of study.

Which of the following combinations is not possible?

A. Becky studies in year 5 and is placed first in the line.
B. Karen studies in year 7 and is placed fourth in the line.
C. Amy studies in year 5 and is placed third in the line.
D. Holly studies in year 8 and is placed last in the line.

Question 19

Richard and a few other members of his family are driving along the motorway in a car. A spectator claims that there are two fathers and two sons within the car. Another spectator claims that there are only three people in the car.

Is it possible for both the spectators to be saying the truth?

A. No, because two fathers two sons mean that there are a minimum of four people in the car.
B. No, because it is possible for spectators to make mistakes as the car could be going at high speeds.
C. Yes, it is possible for both the spectators to be telling the truth as there can be a family relation which satisfies the above-mentioned conditions.
D. Yes, because there is no reason for the spectators to lie about anything.

Question 20

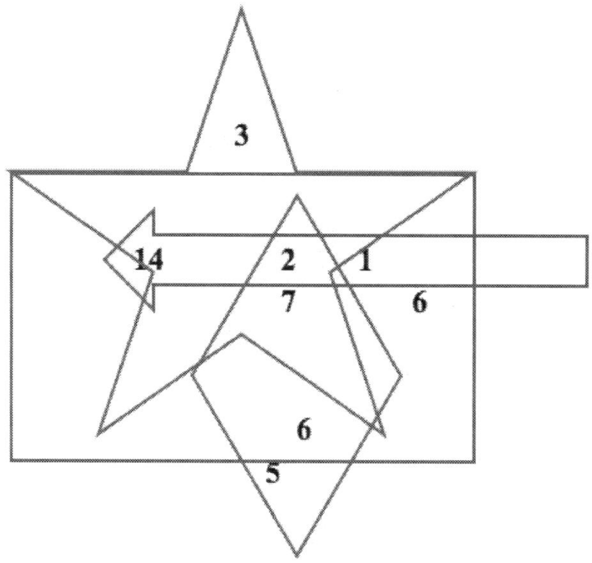

The diagram depicted above shows the number of people working in different sections of a hospital:

- The star represents those working in Cardiology.
- The diamond represents those working in Gynaecology.
- The rectangle represents those working in A&E.
- The arrow represents those working in Urology.

Based on the given information, which of the following observations is true?

A. The number of people working in all four sections of the hospital is 14 less than the number of people working in Urology and A&E, and A&E and Cardiology put together.

B. The number of people working in a minimum of 3 sections is less than the number of the number of people working in all four sections.

C. The number of people working in just one section is 14.

D. The number of people working in a maximum of two sections is 28.

Question 21

In order to reduce the number of plastic bags disposed daily worldwide, should the British population be forced to utilise biodegradable bags for shopping purposes?

A. No, because it might not be feasible for the entire UK population to switch over.

B. No, because the mandatory conversion in one country might not make much of a difference.

C. Yes, because it will cost less to produce a biodegradable bag compared to a plastic bag.

D. Yes, because it will reduce the number of plastic bags being used.

Question 22

In a company, the staff are required to undertake compulsory training as part of their employment contract. The training covers key areas such as effective communication, professionalism, work ethic, time management and safety training. According to the employment contract, all staff will be subjected to training during their tenure at the company. Only staff above the age of 55, and those who have worked for a minimum of 10 years at the company are exempt from some forms of training. However, if one of the training sessions fall on a Saturday, the employees who are married may be exempt with prior approval from the executive board.

Place "Yes" if the conclusion follows. Place "No" if the conclusion does not follow.

A. Dave is 56 years old, and hence is exempt from safety training. YES/NO
B. Ricky is 35 years old and has only joined the company this year; he is not exempt from any training sessions. YES/NO
C. The CEO of the company, who is a part of the executive board, has the authority to allow staff to be exempt from training sessions. YES/NO
D. All staff must be trained in order to work. YES/NO
E. There are 5 types of training sessions that staff have to participate in. YES/NO

Question 23

The diagram below shows the number of customers who purchased different products at a store.

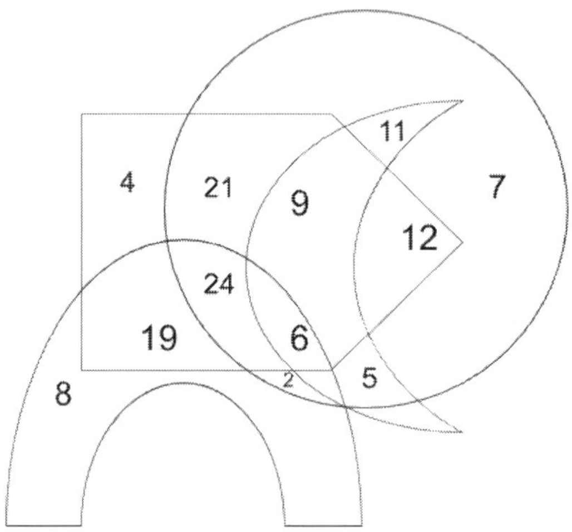

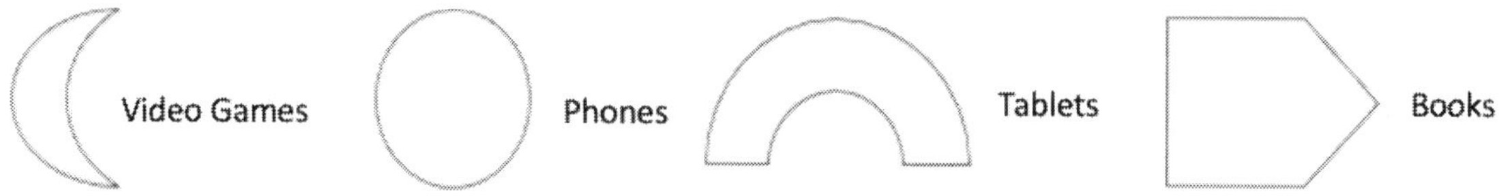

Based on the diagram, how many customers bought exactly 2 items?

A. 58
B. 70
C. 65
D. 68

Question 24

Asher flips 3 fair coins in a row.

The probability that 2 of the coins land on heads is 0.375.

A. No, because the coin is fair, so the probability is 0.5.
B. No, because if he flips it twice, you multiply the probability of each toss, so the probability is 0.25.
C. Yes, because he does not conduct any other event while flipping the coins.
D. Yes, because there are 8 possible outcomes, each with a 0.125 chance of occurring.

Question 25

Mr Simpson's class has an average score of 8.5 on their recent homework assignment. Of the twenty pupils in the class, ten got 8 on the assignment and five got 9.6 on the assignment.

Assuming the last five pupils all got the exact same score, what was their score?

A. 8.4
B. 8.2
C. 7.9
D. 7.6

Question 26

A social club has introduced 3 "event nights" to take place this week: movie night, book night and games night. The club has taken a poll of how many members will be attending each event. Of the 80 members, 29 will attend book night, 36 will attend games night, 52 will attend movie night, 8 will attend only movie night and book night, 10 will attend only book night and games night, 11 will attend only movie night and games night, 2 will attend only book night.

How many members will not attend any of the event nights?

A. 10
B. 8
C. 13
D. 15

Question 27

There are 53 video games in a store. All of the video games are either new or old. All of the video games are also either fun or boring. There are 11 more new games than there are old games. Of the 39 fun games, 12 are old.

How many games in the store are both boring and new?

A. 12
B. 9
C. 16
D. 5

Question 28

Adam, Bella, Clyde, Dan and Emil are all eating steaks. They eat their steaks either rare, medium or well-done. They also eat their steaks either with or without salt.

Only two steaks are with salt.
All steaks without salt are either rare or medium.
Bella and Dan don't eat their steaks without salt.
Of Adam, Clyde and Emil, Adam is the only one with his steak rare.
All steaks with salt are well-done.

Which of the following statements is correct?

A. Clyde is eating a medium steak with salt.
B. Three people have well-done steaks with salt.
C. Emil is eating a medium steak without salt.
D. Two people have rare steaks without salt.

Question 29

In a game, two fair dice are rolled once and the number on each die is multiplied by the number on the other die to get a final score.

Die X has numbers: 1, 2, 3, 4, 5, 6
Die Y has numbers: 5, 10, 15, 20, 25, 30

What is the probability of a player getting 30 as their final score?

A. 1/6
B. 1/12
C. 1/18
D. 1/9

Decision Making Answers

Question 1

After taking note of all the conditions placed, the numbers of each type of vehicle can be summarized using a table.

Car	Engine	Number
SUVs	2L	3
Sedans		5
Hatchbacks		4
Pickups	2L	3

A. No, the number of SUV's is less than the number of sedans, as shown above.
B. Yes, the difference in the number of sedans and pickups is 2, which is half the number of hatchbacks (4).
C. No, there were 4 hatchbacks put up for sale, but only 3 pickups.
D. No, it cannot be concluded as the data is insufficient. This question stem only talks about the number of vehicles put up on sale, not the number of vehicles in the showroom.
E. No, as only 4 types of vehicles are available in the showroom, and 4 are put up for sale, so there are no further types of vehicles that can be put up for sale.

Question 2

The correct answer is D.

This is because the *first* person to achieve the requirements will win the prize, and the players take one turn at a time. So whoever goes first is more likely to win, not because the numerical probability is altered, but simply because they are going first. As soon as they meet the requirement, the next person will not even have the chance to take their turn, resulting in the first person having one extra turn that the second did not.

Question 3

The correct answer is C.

A. Only discusses sustainability, does not mention the environment.
B. Only discusses the environment.

C. While the question talks about *all* countries, this option ensures to include all countries by mentioning the many countries that are not able to shift into this system. It provides a justification for why all countries cannot be *forced* to adapt this method, giving an evidence-based argument by discussing "studies".
D. Limits the argument to European countries.

Question 4

The correct answer is A.

If all frogs are amphibians, the circle for frogs should be contained within the circle for amphibians. All toads are also amphibians, so this should also be contained within the circle for amphibians. No frog is a toad, thus the two circles contained within the circle for amphibians should be distinct. Some cells are reptiles, frogs or toads, thus there should be another circle that overlaps all of these.

Question 5

The information can be summarised as follows:

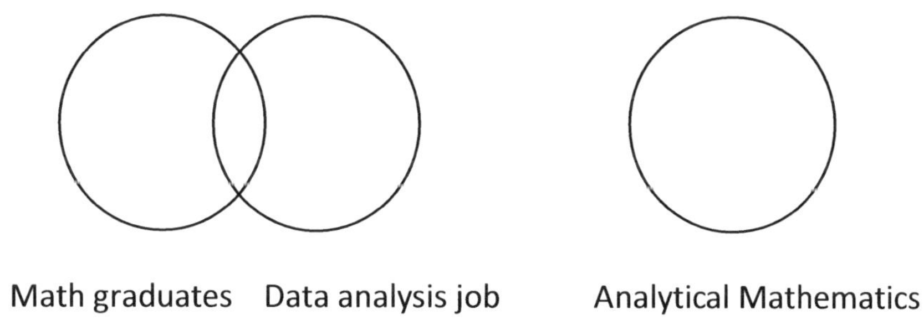

A. No, as it has not been mentioned that *only* mathematics graduates can work in that field.
B. No, while it has been mentioned that they do not work in this field, it does not say that they are not eligible.
C. Yes, as evidently some mathematics graduates are working in data analysis.
D. No, as those who studied *only* analytical mathematics do not work in data analysis, whereas David may have studied other forms of mathematics as well. This is not clear from the statement.
E. No, as no information about this has been mentioned.

Question 6

The correct answer is C.

Try to assess the options that can most easily be verified. You can easily calculate that the number of students studying only Nursing and only Biology is equal to those studying only Mathematics and only Nursing. If you try to analyse the options in sequential order, you would waste a significant amount of time trying to verify A and B and be disappointed not to get the correct answer.

Question 7

The correct answer is C.

The argument here backs up its premise very well. It mentions how accidents can be caused due to a plethora of reasons and not only speeding.

Question 8

A. No, the average of cities A, C and E is 26.6 (80/3), while that of B, D and F is 22.3 (67/3).
B. No, the average of the cities with the highest temperatures is 29 (58/2), whereas that of the lowest temperatures is 20.5 (41/2). They differ by more than 2 degrees.
C. No, as the data represents the temperature recorded only for a single day, so this generalisation cannot be made.
D. No, as there may be more cities in the country, which may be colder, but have not been shown on this graph.
E. No, such a generalisation cannot be made on the basis of data available from a single day.

Question 9

The correct answer is C.

This can be worked out from the diagram.

Question 10

A. No, as it could be any other animal that is not slow.
B. No, it could be medium paced.
C. No, as there could be medium paced animals in the zoo.
D. Yes, as all tigers in the zoo are fast.
E. No, a generalisation like that cannot be made based on the given data.

Question 11

The correct answer is B.

You can organise this information into a table:

Machine	Maintenance	Breakdown
A	2x/6days= every 3 days	Once a month= 96.7%
B	1x/3days= every 3 days	One and half times a month= 95%

Given that machine A only breaks down once a month, it must work at peak efficiency 96.7% of the time, which is more than machine B.

Given that the maintenance requirement is same, machine A is the better option.

Question 12

The correct answer is C.

The table, according to the conditions, can be summarised as follows.

Rahul	Brazil/Germany	
Raheem	Japan	640
Richard	India	
Rebecca	Brazil/Germany	650

If Raheem went to Japan, Richard went to the only other Asian country. We can fill in 640 and 650 in the table as we know that Raheem spent 10 less than Rebecca in numerical value.

Rahul and Rebecca went to either Brazil or Germany. We can first decide whether Rebecca went to Germany or Brazil. If Rebecca went to Brazil, and Rahul to Germany, using the values mentioned in the question, let us assume he spent 970 Euros. 970 Euros would be equal $1096.65.

If Rebecca went to Germany and Rahul went to Brazil, as the question mentions that Rahul spent the most amount of money, he would have spent 970 Reals. 970 Reals is equal to $192.65. Without even calculating this, you would know looking at the conversion rates that 970 Reals is worth far less than 970 Euros, therefore, Rahul would have gone to Germany and not to Brazil.

Question 13

The correct answer is D.

Option D gives a study-based answer and explains why lockdowns may not work in *all* countries. If they do not work in some countries, all countries should not have to enforce strict measures.

Question 14

The correct answer is A.

This can be visualised by using a Venn diagram as follows:

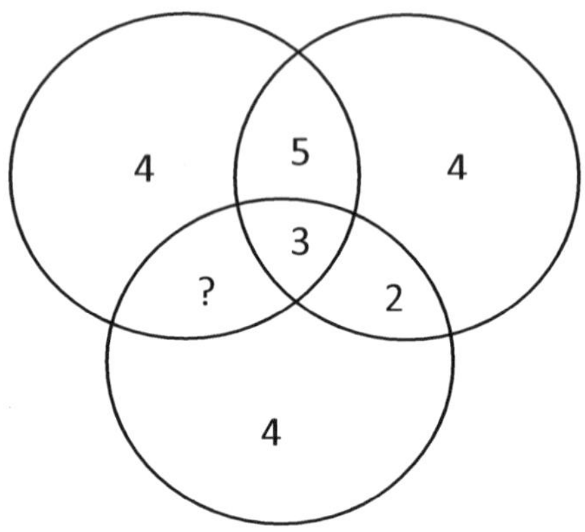

The total is 22 in the above diagram. We know from the question that there are 25 residents. 25 - 22 = 3.

Question 15

A. No, as the logic flows in one direction. If All A → B, this does not mean that All B → A.
B. No, same as above. Rosie could be a child who is also wearing a black hat or Rosie could even be the name of a pet with a black hat.
C. No, although it alters common logic, you must only base your answers according to the logic given in the question. It says that non-alcoholic beverages are given to children, and alcoholic beverages to those above 18. But it does not say that children are below 18, so there could be a 19-year-old child in the party!
D. No, we do not know for sure whether or not the pets include dogs.
E. No, Rajesh could be under 18 and still drink alcoholic beverage provided elsewhere. Just because this party does not serve alcoholic beverages to those under 18, this rule does not need to be applied everywhere.

Question 16

The correct answer is C.

The total number of multiples of 6 or 8 before 200 is 50. Hence the probability of Becky winning is 50/200, or 1/4, and hence that of Arjun winning is 3/4.

Question 17

The correct answer is C.

All the other statements are subjective and opinion based. Option C is objective and factual.

Question 18

The correct answer is C. The line order of the students can be finalised as below:

Becky: Year 5
Rachel: Year 4
Amy: Year 6
Karen: Year 7
Thomas: Year 9
Holly: Year 8

Question 19

The correct answer is C. If there is a Grandfather, Father and Son in one car, the claims of both spectators will be valid.

Question 20

The correct answer is C. This can be calculated from the diagram.

Question 21

The correct answer is B. Note the key word in the question – "worldwide". Making a change in Britain might not make such a great change unless efforts are seen in all nations across the globe.

Question 22

A. No, those above 55 are exempt from some forms of training, but whether safety training is a part of that is unknown.
B. No, if Ricky is married, he could be exempt from some training.
C. No, it has been mentioned that the executive board has the authority to make decisions, and the CEO might be a part of the board, but we do not know whether the CEO alone can make decisions.
D. Yes, this is explained in detail in the opening sentence of the passage.
E. No, it has not been mentioned anywhere that the five types of training given in the question are the only types of training that staff have to undertake.

Question 23

The correct answer is B. Since each shape represents an item that can be bought, areas where 2 shapes overlap represent how many people bought those 2 items. To find the total number of customers who bought 2 items, count the numbers in all of the areas where 2 shapes overlap. Careful not to count the people who bought more than 2 items (the areas where more than 2 shapes overlap)!

Question 24

The correct answer is D. The probability depends on how many ways we can possibly have 2 coins land on heads. Since there are 3 coins flipped, the possible outcomes of the three events are: HHH, HHT, HTH, THH, TTH, HTT, THT, TTT. You can draw a tree diagram to represent this. Since there are 8 possible outcomes, each one has a 0.125 chance of occurring (because 0.125 x 8 = 1.0). If we look at the 8 possible outcomes, 3 of them have 2 coins landed on heads; HHT, HTH, THH. Since each of these outcomes has a 0.125 chance of occurring, the total probability that 2 coins will land on heads is 0.125 x 3 = 0.375

Question 25

The correct answer is A. Since there are 20 pupils in the class and the average score is 8.5, 20 x 8.5 = 170 total points scored on the homework. Since 10 pupils got a score of 8, and 5 pupils got a score of 9.6, 10 x 8 = 80 points scored, and 5 x 9.6 = 48 points scored. So those 15 pupils collectively got 80 + 48 = 128 points. We already know that in total, the 20 pupils got 170 collective points. So 170 - 128 = 42 points scored by the last 5 pupils. 42 / 5 = 8.4 points on average for the last 5 pupils.

Question 26

The correct answer is A. It is easiest to draw a Venn diagram like the one below and to progressively fill it out with all the information that you are given.

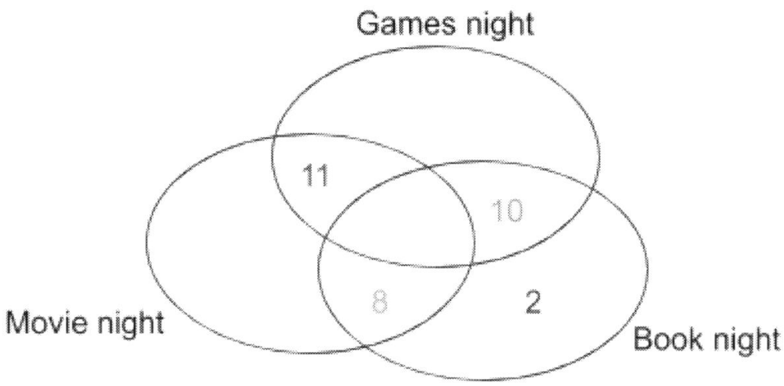

We can fill out the numbers above from the statements "8 will attend only movie night and book night", "10 will attend only book night and games night", "11 will attend only movie night and games night" and "2 will attend only book night". Once we have filled these numbers in, we can use the statement "Of the 80 members, 29 will attend book night (add 9), 36 will attend games night (add 6), 52 will attend movie night (add 24)" to fill the rest of the numbers in, as seen below.

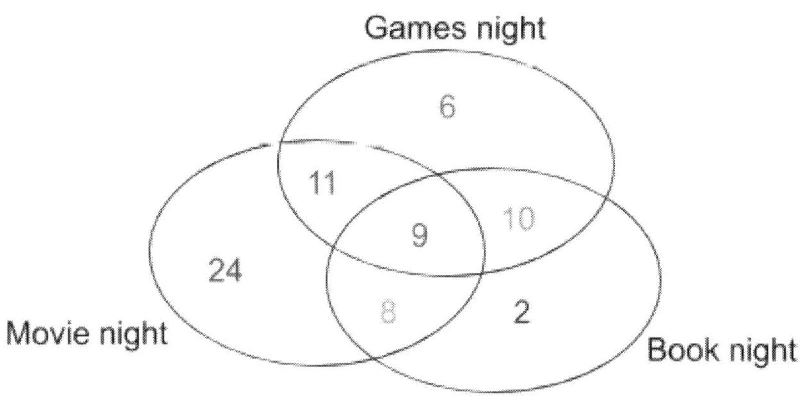

Once we have filled these in, we simply count-up all of the numbers and subtract them from 80, to find the number of people who did not attend any of the events.

Question 27

The correct answer is D. We know there are 53 games in total. Since there are 11 more new games than there are old games, we can say that "x" = old games and "x + 11" = new games. There are 53 games in total, so "x" + "x + 11" = 53. We can rearrange and solve this to find that x = 21. So there are 21 old games and 32 new games. We know that there are 39 fun games, of which 12 are old. So the other 27 fun games must be new. From the total of 32 new games, we know 27 were fun. So only 5 games remain which are both new and not fun (not fun = boring).

Question 28

The correct answer is C. Questions like this are best approached by making short logical deductions to make the large amount of information easier to comprehend. Since "Only two steaks are with salt" and "Bella and Dan don't eat their steaks without salt", we know that Bella and Dan are the two who eat their steaks with salt and everyone else has no salt. Also, "All steaks with salt are well-done", so Bella and Dan also eat their steaks well-done. Since "All steaks without salt are either rare or medium", Adam, Clyde and Emil must have either rare or medium steaks. "Of Adam, Clyde and Emil, Adam is the only one with his steak rare" means Clyde and Emil must eat their steaks medium.

Question 29

The correct answer is D. First, we must find all of the possible ways to get a score of 30. A score of 30 can be achieved with 1 x 30, 2 x 15, 3 x 10 or 6 x 5. Since the two dice have 6 sides and are fair, the odds of getting any particular number pair when rolling is (1/6) x (1/6) = (1/36). There are 4 possible combinations of number pairs needed to get a score of 30, so (1/36) x 4 = (1/9).

SECTION 3

Quantitative Reasoning

INTRODUCTION

Quantitative Reasoning is the third section of the UCAT. Although many students struggle with maths, this is generally one of the easier sections to score well in. Since 2016, this section has had the highest average every consecutive year. The average in this section score for the 2020 testing cycle was 664. This section is designed to test your numerical and problem-solving skills at GCSE standard.

You will have 24 minutes to answer 36 questions. This gives an average of 40 seconds per question. The questions will be of varying difficulty, randomly drawn from a database. Some may require simple calculations that can be completed within seconds, while others may be multi-step and more complex.

You will be given scenarios with 1-6 associated questions, although most scenarios will have around 3 follow-up questions. Scenarios may be associated with tables, diagrams, charts, graphs and other numerical presentations to use as reference when answering the questions. Normally, questions will have 5 answer choices, but in graphical analysis, you may be asked to identify if the given statement is "True", "False", or "Can't Tell" based on a graph.

In this section, you will learn how to tackle each question type in the timeliest manner. You will be given worked examples of common maths questions and formulae that you may have forgotten since GCSEs. You will also be introduced to additional topics such as tax and drug calculations, and learn key strategies that can be used to tackle them. There are various examples to help you understand the techniques taught, followed by a mock test of 36 Quantitative Reasoning questions at the end of the section.

Note: This section is intended to be applicable to everybody, regardless of maths ability. Some students may find the detailed explanations unnecessary and skip past them, while others will appreciate the step-by-step approach used to demonstrate each answer.

Types of Questions

The types of questions found in Quantitative Reasoning can roughly be classified into four main categories:

Ratios	Statistics	Day-to-Day Life	Geometry
Percentages Fractions Ratios	Averages Midpoints Interpreting graphs and charts	Converting units Speed, distance & time Midpoints Calculating taxes Time zone problems Drug calculations Probability	Area, volume and perimeter Pythagoras theorem

General Strategies

1. **Know what the question is asking for.** It is critical that you understand the question and identify the relevant information given. This may involve referring back to the scenario when answering the question.
    a. Often, long text and complicated graphs or charts can be distracting. With practice, your mind will be trained to notice the relevant information as quickly as possible.
2. **Eyeball (see page 158) if possible.** It might be possible to deduce the answer at times by simply doing mental maths or eyeballing the answers. This will help you save a lot of time!
3. Read quickly and with focus. Use the tips on speed reading and concentration from the Verbal Reasoning section of this eBook.
4. A couple of times in the exam, a stem may have a multi-step question prior to a different question that is simply one of the steps of the previous question. You can save time by answering the simpler question first – it will give you one of the values you need for the multi-step question. If you do the multi-step question first, you are likely to have rubbed out the steps or removed them from your calculator already, so you will have to redo this step to answer the following question. Therefore, it is worth skimming the questions before answering them to see if this is the case.
    - *Note*: This is not one of the biggest tips, as this may only happen a couple of times in your exam, so it should not be one of your biggest priorities.

5. Sometimes, a question will ask for an "approximate" answer. In this case, you can round the values given to be more easily manipulated using mental maths.
6. If you struggle with graph questions, you should practice these in your own time. Start with easier graphs, then move on to research papers that have more complex data and spend your time trying to interpret them. The better your interpretation and analysis skills get, the quicker you will be able to answer these types of questions.

Using the Calculator

The following diagram demonstrates the format of the UCAT calculator, annotated with functions and usage of each key.

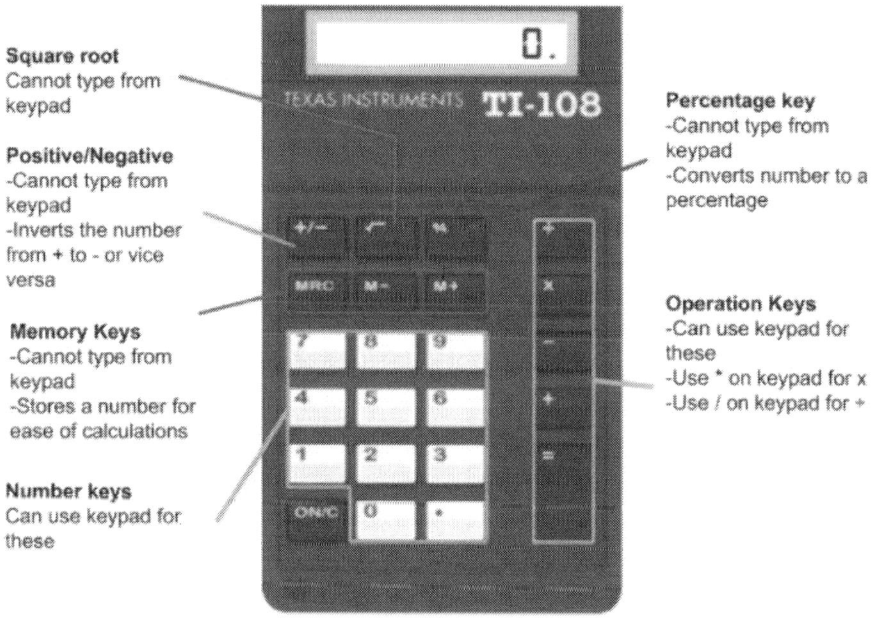

Adapted from: http://questions.ukcat.ac.uk/pages/calculator-ti108.aspx

Keys	Notes on operations
+ / -	**Function**: Toggles back and forth between the positive and negative of a value. The number must be on display for this function to work.
√	**Function**: Calculates the square root of the number. The number must be on display for this function to work.
M+	**Function**: adds the number to memory. The number must be on display for this function to work. You must first clear the memory if this function was used previously. *Note*: more on this key on page 158.
MRC	**Function**: Recalls the number from memory. The calculator will remember the same number until you manually clear the memory with the M- key.

	The number will be shown on screen. You can directly use it in your calculations. *Note*: more on this key on page 158.
M-	**Function:** Clears the number from memory. Must first use the MRC button to recall the number onto the display.
ON/C	**Function 1:** Turns the calculator on. **Function 2:** Clears the input. *Note:* If you press this button, or backspace on your keypad, you will lose your calculation!
=	**Function**: Equals key. Completes the calculation. Can be accessed by pressing "enter" on the keypad

You can practice using the UCAT calculator on https://questions.ucat.ac.uk/pages/calculator-ti108.aspx.

It is common to hear that the calculator should be avoided as much as possible. On the contrary, we would advise to use it with certain rules:

1. **Use it when you need to.** You will only be able to mentally calculate certain questions. Do not pressure yourself into doing everything in your head. Each individual has their own mental maths limits. Although it is beneficial to work on your mental maths, know your limits and adapt to them by practicing using the calculator as well.
2. **Avoid using your mouse!** Use the keypad for as many buttons as possible. This may seem obvious, but it will save you a **lot** of time.
3. **Practice keying in the numbers quickly and accurately.** If you can key in the numbers without looking down at the keypad, you will be able to watch the screen instead. This will allow you to ensure accuracy of your calculations and instantly correct your mistakes when necessary.
4. **Use the memory key if necessary.** It will remember the number you input and save you time from recalculating or writing it down. Alternatively, you can keep the numbers in the whiteboard or scratchpad.
5. **Only use the "equals" function at the end, if possible.** Try to make continuous calculations as much as possible. This is much faster than putting your answers onto the whiteboard/scratchpad. For example, you are asked to calculate the following:

   1080 - 679 - 28 - 9

   Instead of taking down the answer after 1080 - 679, then subtracting 28 from your answer, know that you don't have to stop! The calculator is able to carry out continuous calculations, so you can input the numbers and functions exactly as shown above, pressing the equals button, or "enter" on your keyboard, only at the end. Again, this simple tip will save you a lot of time! However, if there are multiple steps and functions in the calculation, be wary of this strategy. The calculator is not scientific and thus it does not follow the rules of BODMAS.

Limitations of the Calculator

This is not a scientific calculator. Therefore, it will carry out calculations in the exact order you key in the numbers and will not obey the mathematical laws of order, or "BODMAS". Thus, you must be careful of the order of operations.

There is no power button. Because there is no function to square or cube a number, you must repeatedly multiply by that number to achieve this. However, there is a square root button, so you can use this to double check you have done it correctly if you have any doubt.

Note 1: Learning some square and cube numbers will save you a lot of time in the exam. See the tables below.

Note 2: If you learn the square numbers but not the cube numbers, you can simply multiply the square number by the number being squared in order to reach the cube number.

- E.g. 5^3 = ?
  5^2 is 25, so 5^3 = 25 x 5
  = 125

First 20 Square Numbers

1^2	2^2	3^2	4^2	5^2	6^2	7^2	8^2	9^2	10^2
1	4	9	16	25	36	49	64	81	100
11^2	12^2	13^2	14^2	15^2	16^2	17^2	18^2	19^2	20^2
121	144	169	196	225	256	289	324	361	400

First 10 Cube Numbers

1^3	2^3	3^3	4^3	5^3	6^3	7^3	8^3	9^3	10^3
1	8	27	64	125	216	343	512	729	1000

There are no backspaces. If you make a mistake and/or press the delete button in the middle of your calculations, you will have to restart. Therefore, practice entering them correctly! If you make a mistake with a single function, you may not need to restart. Consider the example below.

- E.g. 3.95 + 1.25 – 0.75 + 6.25 =

If you get to the fourth step (+ 6.25) and accidentally hit (- 6.25), you would simply just need to hit (+ 6.25) twice to fix the problem, rather than restarting the entire calculator. You can apply the same rule to multiplying and dividing.

Saving Time

Avoid Clearing

> E.g. Publisher A in London has 6834 books that require printing. They printed 3802 of these last week, and the capacity of the printer this week is 4000. If Publisher B uses the remaining printer capacity after Publisher A finishes printing, how many books can Publisher B print this week?

Here, the steps would be:

1. Number of books Publisher A has left to print:
   6834 - 3802 = 3032

2. (Printer capacity) - (Number of books Publisher A needs to print) = (Number of books Publisher B can print)
   4000 - 3032 = 968

You might be tempted to clear the 3032 from the first step, or even write it on your whiteboard before starting the second step. Consider this method to speed up your calculations:

6834 - 3802 = 3032
3032 - 4000 = -968

This method saves a lot of time! You are solving for a magnitude, so you just need to ignore, or reverse, the " - " sign in front of 968. However, make sure you understand the question so you do not confuse yourself or make errors while using this tip.

Alternatively, you could use the " +/- " sign to change the sign on 3032 to -3032, then add 4000. This would give you the exact value, as (- 3032 + 4000) is the exact same as (4000 - 3032). However, this would take longer than the first suggestion as you would need to switch from your number pad to your mouse in order to use the +/- sign, and so, the first technique is a far more superior method of solving this question.

Memory Key

> E.g. Mickie recently bought a rare car for £125,925. The car increases in value by 9.5% each year as Mickie takes good care of it. What will the value of the car be after four years?

As the value increases by 9.5% annually, the *rate* at which the car would increase in value is 109.5%, or 1.095. This would be the multiplier of this question.

Note: If you simply multiply the car's value by 9.5%, you will get the value of the increase, but not the total value of the car after the increase! Thus, you must add 100% to the multiplier in order to obtain the value of the car.

To save yourself from entering the multiplier 4 times to obtain the value of the car in 4 years, you can simply add the multiplier to the calculator's memory. To answer this question using the memory key, you would make the following entries into your calculator:

1.	Start with the number you wish to save in your calculator's memory: 1.095
2.	Press M+ to store it in memory
3.	Multiply by the value of the car (125925) to obtain the value after 1 year: 1.095 x 125925
4.	Multiply by the memory (1.095) three more times to obtain the value in 4 years' time. x MRc x MRc x MRc
5.	= £181,037

Eyeballing Strategies

When you are short of time, you might need to calculate a question as quickly as possible. Sometimes, this is done without actually knowing the exact answer – what we call eyeballing.

This strategy usually only works if the numbers are different enough. If they are all very close together, you may not be able to eyeball.

Round the numbers to make them easily calculable

E.g. 18 x 21 (378) can be rounded to 20 x 20 (400)

This strategy will provide you with a close answer which may help you eliminate choices and make a more accurate guess.

Read the question to rule out impossible answers.

For example, if the question is asking for an answer in miles, and some answers are given in kilometres, you can easily rule these out. Further, if the question has a number and asks for a positive increase, whereas some answers have a lesser value than the original number, you can easily rule these out.

Order the numbers into ranges

E.g. Try to order the following numbers into 3 ranges based on their closeness in value.

A. 55
B. 98
C. 60
D. 100
E. 32

It is clear that there are three distinct ranges into which the numbers can be separated.

- **Range 1:** 32
- **Range 2:** 55, 60
- **Range 3:** 98, 100

This may appear to be slightly pointless, but once you are familiar with this technique, you will be able to apply it in seconds to improve your ability to eyeball the answer. Based on the numbers given in the question and the calculations needed, your options will be:

a) Guess any answer within the range that appears to be correct. For example, if you know which range the answer must in and there are only two numbers in the range, selecting one of them will give you a 50% chance of guessing the correct answer.
b) Work backwards. For example, if 60 seems to be too large, you can easily cancel out the other number within the same range. You would then choose an answer in a lower range. In this case, there is only one number in the lower range (32), so hopefully you

would have the correct answer! This would allow you to narrow down your guesses and is especially useful for long-winded, graph analysis questions.

c) Eyeball to double-check your answer. If you have completed a multi-step calculation and want to make sure you got the correct answer, rather than conducting the entire calculation again, you can estimate by looking at the question again and trying to eyeball the answer.

Mental Maths

Mental maths can be extremely daunting in a world where we are so focussed on using calculators for every simple problem we need to solve. Nonetheless, this is an extremely useful strategy to help increase your speed in Quantitative Reasoning, and it works best by slowly assimilating techniques into your practice.

Know your basics:

- Simple addition and subtraction
- Multiplication tables (from 1 to 10; optional from 11 onwards)

Multiplication:

Multiply by 10's, 100's, 1000's: just add the number of zeros behind "1" to the other number being multiplied.

E.g. 100 x 23

As there are 3 zeros in "100", so adding them to 23 = 2300

Division:

When dividing by 10's, 100's, 1000's, and so on, simply subtract the number of zeros in the numerator from the number of zeros in the denominator to find the number of zeros that will be present in your final answer.

Note: In division ($\frac{x}{y}$ or x / y), " x " is the numerator and " y " is the denominator

E.g. 23000 / 100:
There are 3 zeros in 23000 and 2 zeros in 10.
3 – 2 = 1, therefore the answer will have 1 zero
23000 / 100 = 230

These rules also apply to numbers that don't start with a 1 or end with a 0. However, you will have to conduct the non-zero calculations separately.

E.g. 1) 25 x 200

Information:

- 25 and 2 are non-zero digits.
- There are 2 zeros in 200.

Calculations:

- 25 x 2 = 50. Now we can add the 2 zeros that are in the original 200.
- 50 and 2 zeros = 5000

E.g. 2) $\frac{3300}{110}$

Information:

- 33 and 11 are non-zero digits.
- There are 2 zeros in 3300 and 1 zero in 110. If you subtract the number of zeros in the denominator from the number of zeros in the numerator, you find that the answer will have 1 zero.

Calculations:

- $\frac{33}{11} = 3$
- Add 1 zero = 30.

Place Values

Mental maths can be easier when separating numbers into "place values".

E.g. 37 + 56

Tens	Ones
3 (from 37)	7 (from 37)
5 (from 56)	6 (from 56)

- If you start by adding the "ones", 7 + 6 = 13.
- The number 3 (from 13) will be the value satisfying the "ones" in the answer, while the number 1 (from 13) will be added to the value of the tens.
- Now, adding the "tens", 3 + 5 (+ 1) = 9. This is now the first number, satisfying the tens in the answer, while 3 is the second number, satisfying the ones in the answer.

- Therefore, the answer is 93.

With multiplication, this strategy can be slightly more complex.

E.g. 12 x 9

- Separate 12 into 10 + 2
- Multiple 10 by 9, then 2 by 9
- = (10 x 9) + (2 x 9)
- = 90 + 18
- = 108

These strategies work well for mental maths. However, everyone has their own preferences. If you prefer just to multiply and carry the numbers across, and this has worked well for you for years, you can carry on doing what works for you.

Summary

The following diagram summarises the questions you should ask yourself before tackling any question:

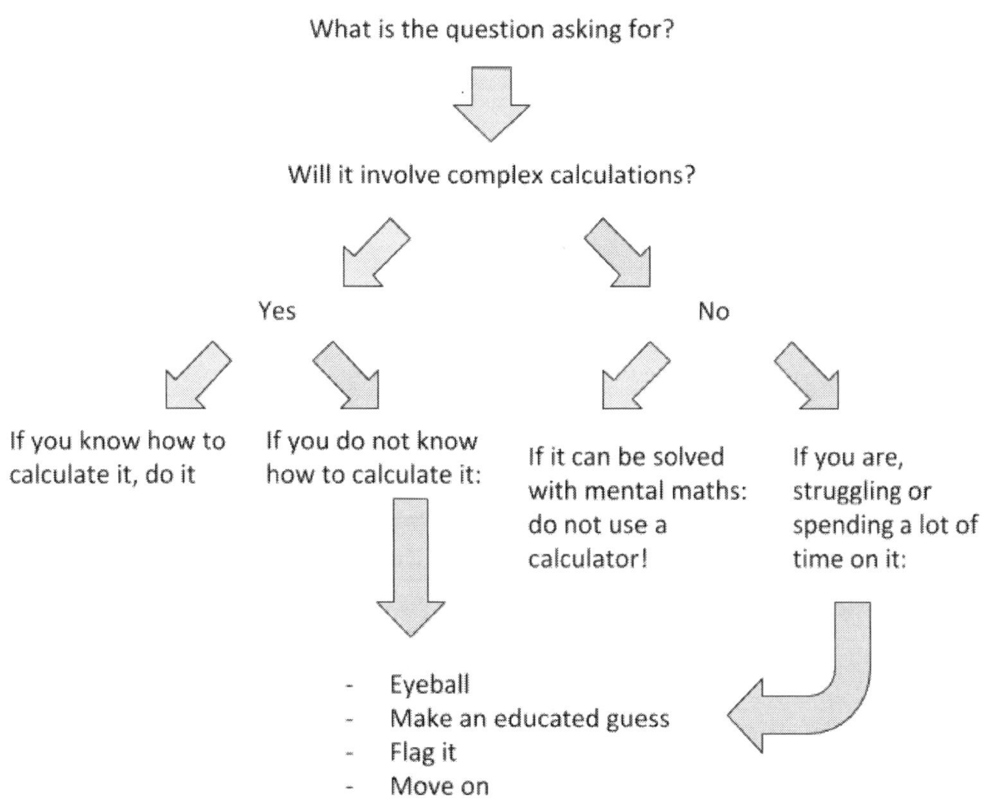

Percentages

"Cent" means hundred. "Percent" simply means "per cent" or "per hundred".

For example, 50% means 50 per 100. As such, 50% of a value is half of that value, just as 50 is half of 100. It is vital that you are comfortable with working out percentages, as many of the questions will involve percentage calculations.

Percentages on the Calculator

It is inevitable that you will need the calculator when working out percentages. However, there are a number of strategies that will save you time.

A fundamental concept of percentages is that they can be converted to decimals and fractions. Familiarity with this concept can help speed up your calculations, as precious time is wasted when multiplying by 100 or using the " % " button to obtain a whole number.

The following examples demonstrate different ways that a percentage can present:

$$33\% = \frac{33}{100} = 0.33$$

$$95\% = \frac{95}{100} = 0.95$$

Any percentage can be easily converted into a fraction by placing 100 in the denominator. You can also easily obtain a decimal from a percentage by moving the invisible decimal *after* the percentage 2 spaces to the left.

3 3 .0 % = 0.33

Shifted 2 places

Note: Each whole number has an invisible decimal with an infinite number of zeros after it. E.g. 33 is the same as 33.00000000. Each whole number also has an infinite number of zeros before it. E.g. 33 is the same is 00000000033. Therefore, shifting the decimal place will allow you to make visible the zeros in front of the number.

The following strategies will help you save time:

1. **Use decimals.** If you need to calculate a percentage of a number, the fastest way to do this is by multiplying the decimal form of the percentage. E.g. for 33% of a number, multiply the number by 0.33
2. **Omit the zero.** E.g. Instead of entering "0.33" on your calculator, you may enter ".33" and the same results will be produced. You will save time by omitting the 0 at the beginning.
3. **Practice converting words to decimals**. Percentages are often given in word form to confuse you. Becoming familiar with word forms and how to quickly interpret and convert them to numbers will save you time.

   E.g. 1) If something is tripled, the result is 300% of the original.

   E.g. 2) If something is reduced by a quarter, the result is 75% of the original.
4. **Divide to get a percentage.** Generally, we multiply to obtain a particular percentage. However, in some cases, you can divide. This will save you a lot of time, as dividing generally involves only a couple of clicks, whereas multiplying involves more. E.g. to type " x .25 " on your calculator would take 4 clicks. However, you can also find 25% of a number by simply dividing it by 4. " / 4 " only takes 2 clicks.
   a. Remember: To divide by x is the same as to multiply by $\frac{1}{x}$. For example, if you want to determine 12.5% of a number, rather than multiplying by 0.125, you can simply multiply by $\frac{1}{8}$ or divide by 8.

The following table summarises easy-to-learn fractions and decimals that will speed up your percentage calculations if committed to memory. That is not to say that these percentages will commonly or even definitely present, but if they do, you should not need your calculator to work out the decimal or fraction forms!

Decimals	Decimals Over 1	Fractions
1% = 0.01 10% = 0.1 20% = 0.2 25% = 0.25 50% = 0.5 75% = 0.75 100% = 1	100% = 1 110% = 1.1 125% = 1.25 150% = 1.5 175% = 1.75 200% = 2	12.5% = 0.125 = $\frac{1}{8}$ 25% = 0.25 = $\frac{1}{4}$ 33% = 0.33 = $\frac{1}{3}$ 50% = 0.5 = $\frac{1}{2}$ 100% = 1

To summarise, the following formulae describe the speediest methods of calculating percentages with a calculator:

1. **Number x percentage as decimal = x**

   E.g. 35% of 789 = 789 x .35 =

(Note: to save time, there is no zero before the decimal!)

2. **Number / the denominator of the percent's fraction form = x**
   E.g. 50% of 321 = 321 / 2 =

Using the strategies you have learnt, answer the questions below (Examples 1-5).

Example 1

Emmanuel earns a salary of £32,430.00 per annum.

At the beginning of the year, Emmanuel deposited £1,650 into the bank. He earns an interest of 7% on this amount per annum.

1. How much interest will he earn by the end of the year?
   A. £2,385.60
   B. £115.50
   C. £2,270.10
   D. £11.55
   E. £16.50

Answer 1

The correct answer is B.

Note: This question specifies that the interest is on "this amount", referring to the £1,650 that Emmanuel deposited in the bank. He did not deposit his entire salary.

Using the problem-solving method, we know that this question asks us to find the percentage of a given quantity. It is best to use the calculator here, as the calculation will involve a large value and a decimal. The method is as follows:

- Convert the percentage to its corresponding decimal.

$$7\% = \frac{7}{100} = 0.07$$

- Multiply the decimal with the original value.

  .07 x 1650 = £115.50

Example 2: Percent Decrease

2. Due to numerous mistakes in his work, Emmanuel now faces a 20% reduction from his annual salary. How much will he earn after this reduction?
   A. £25,944

B. £6,486
C. £38,916
D. £648.60
E. £2,594.40

Answer 2: Percent Decrease

The correct answer is A.

Here, the question asks for the amount remaining after a deduction. Again, it is easiest to use a calculator here due to the large values and decimals required in the equation. The method and calculations would thus be:

1.	Identify the percentage increase or decrease: He is now earning 20% less
2.	Find the new percentage equivalent with the original as 100%: 100% - 20% = 80%. His new salary is equivalent to 80% of his original salary.
3.	Convert the new percentage to a decimal: $80\% = \frac{80}{100} = 0.8$
4.	Multiply the decimal with the original value: 32430 x .8 = £25,944

Time-Saving Tips:

1. This question can easily be solved by eyeballing. If his salary of £32,430 is reduced by 20%, it is impossible for the answer to be **C. £38,916**, as this value is higher than the original. If we look at all of the other options, while roughly 50% of his salary would be £16,000, we can see that the rest of the options would mean a far greater than 20% reduction. Therefore, without even calculating, we can deduce that the answer should be **A. £25,944**.

2. Calculating 20% of Emmanuel's salary, then deducting this value from the original would also result in the same answer. However, this is a two-step approach, while simply calculating 80% of his salary saves a lot of time as it essentially skips the first step. When you become familiar with percentages and converting into decimals, you

should know in your head that subtracting 20% is the same as having 80% leftover, and 80% is equal to 0.8, thus, you can quickly type in " 32430 x .8 " to get your answer.

Example 3: Reversing Percent Increase

3. Due to inflation in 2020, Emmanuel's earnings per annum, i.e. £32,430.00 actually include a 10% bonus. What are his net earnings in 2020, without the bonus?
    A. £29,481.81
    B. £2,948.18
    C. £29,481.82
    D. £29,482.85
    E. £35,673

Answer 3: Reversing Percent Increase

The correct answer is C.

The calculations are as follows:

1.	Deduce the percentage increase: +10%
2.	Deduce the percentage value of the increased salary, where the original salary is 100% of his earnings: Increased salary = original salary + bonus = 100% + 10% = 110% The increased salary is 110% of his earnings.
3.	Divide the increased salary (£32430) buy its percentage value (110%): £32,430.00 = 110% of the original salary 110% = $\frac{110}{100}$ = 1.1 (you should be familiar with converting percentages into decimals by now! 32430 / 1.1 = 29481.818
4.	29,481.818 ≈ £29,481.82 The answer is thus **C**, not A!

Example 4: Reversing Percent Decrease

This example is separate to the above example. Do not include any information about the 10% bonus

4. Emmanuel signed up for a work scheme that would donate 15% of his earnings to COVID-19 relief funds. Therefore, Emmanuel's earnings per annum, i.e. £32,430.00 are reduced by 15%. What is his net annual income before the reduction?
   A. £29,150
   B. £2,915
   C. £3,815
   D. £38,150
   E. £38,153

Answer 4: Reversing Percent Decrease

The correct answer is E.

The calculations are as follows:

1.	Deduce the percentage decrease: -15%
2.	Deduce the percentage value of the decreased salary, where the original salary is 100% of his earnings: Decreased salary=original salary - reduction = 100% - 15% = 85% The decreased salary is 85% of his earnings.
3.	Divide the decreased salary (£32430) buy its percentage value (85%): £32,430.00 = 85% of the original salary 85% = $\frac{85}{100}$ = 0.85 (you should be familiar with converting percentages into decimals by now! $\frac{32430}{.85}$ = 38,152.94
4.	38,152.94 ≈ £38,153

Example 5: Total from a Percentage

5. Emmanuel earns £32,430.00, which is 46% of his entire household's income. What is the entire household income in pounds?
    A. £149,178
    B. £14,917.80
    C. £64,860
    D. £38,070
    E. £70,500

Answer 5: Total from a Percentage

The correct answer is E.

The calculations are as follows:

1.	Identify the percentage of the total amount: The total household income is 100%. Emmanuel's income is 46%.
2.	Identify the numerical value equivalent to this percentage: Emmanuel's earnings (46% of the total) = £32,430.00
3.	Divide this numerical value by its corresponding percentage in order to find the original value. 32430 / 0.46 = 70500

Time-Saving Tips:

This question can also be easily answered by eyeballing.

- If you look at the answers, there are some that you can clearly cross out. 46% is close to 50%, so you can look for values that are almost double that of Emmanuel's salary (as the *total* household income will be *double* the value of *50%* of the household income).
- 64,860 and 70,500 seem to be around double Emmanuel's salary.
- To decide the better value between these two, realise that ~32,000 (Emmanuel's salary) is **exactly** half of ~64,000. However, it is **less than** half of ~70,000. It is not a **lot** less than half (which is why A is incorrect – it is too far off) so it would make sense that ~32,000 is about 46% of ~70,000.

Note: If you actually calculate these rounded numbers, 32,000 is 45.7% of 70,000. You would not need calculate if you are eyeballing like this, but this is to demonstrate that this method of is effective.

Tax Calculations

It is common to ask about taxes in Quantitative Reasoning – generally about how much tax someone owes, given their income. However, you can be expected to work out the reverse of this – someone's income, given how much tax they pay. For either scenario, it is important to understand how tax bands work.

Tax is always given as a percentage of someone's income, where the percentage changes depending on how much is earned. This "change of percentage" is known as "bands". The tax bands for 2019/2020 in the U.K. (but not necessarily in the UCAT) were as follows:

Tax Rate	Taxable Income
0%	£0 - £12,500
20%	£12,501 - £50,000
40%	£50,001 - £150,000
45%	£150,001 and over

A common misconception is that income can only fall into a single band or category. E.g. Someone with an income of £60,000 will pay 40% tax, or £24,000. **This is completely incorrect!** Taxes add up. Individuals fall into a certain tax band, but also fall into every tax band before this. Therefore, an individual earning £60,000, would pay 0% tax on their first £12,500 of income, 20% tax on the next £37,499, and 40% tax on the final £9,999 of income. The total would then come to £11,499.40 – significantly less than the miscalculated £24,000.

Example 6: Tax Paid

Income	Tax Paid
£0 - £ 10,000	0%
£10,001 - £25,000	10%
£25,001 - £35,000	15%
£35,001 - £70,000	20%
≥ £75,001	30%

Based on the above table, how much tax should a person with £39,000 income pay, rounded to the nearest pound?

A. £3,800
B. £780
C. £1499.90
D. £7,550
E. £75.50

Answer 6: Tax Paid

The correct answer is A.

It might be useful to use your scratchpad or whiteboard here to make a short list with the help of your calculator.

Income	Tax Paid	Calculations
£0 - £ 10,000	0%	£0
£10,001 - £25,000	10%	25,000 – 10,001 = 14,999 14,999 x 10% = **£1,499.90 tax**
£25,001 - £35,000	15%	35,000 – 25,001 = 9,999 15% x 9,999 = **£1,499.85 tax**
£35,001 - £70,000	20%	39,000 - 35,001 = 3,999 20% x 3,999 = **£799.80**
≥ £75,001	30%	£0

Note: To calculate the tax taken within the final band (£35,001 - £70,000), you must first calculate how much of the income applies to this band. Do this by subtracting the total income from the minimum value of that band (39,000 - 35,001).

Therefore, the total amount of tax someone with an income of £39,000 will pay is:

£0 + £1,499.90 + £1,499.85 + £799.80 = £3,799.55

The question asks for the answer to be rounded to the nearest pound:

£3,799.55≈ £3,800

Example 7: Tax Reversal

Income	Tax Paid
£0 - £ 10,000	0%
£10,000 - £20,000	10%
£20,000 - £30,000	15%
£30,000 - £40,000	20%
£40,000 - £100,000	25%
≥ £100,000	50%

Based on the table above, If Yusuf pays £900 income tax per month, how much does he earn annually?

A. £102,400
B. £65,200
C. £41,000
D. £98,400
E. £66,000

Answer 7: Tax Reversal

The correct answer is B.

1.	Calculate how much tax he pays per year: £900 (per months) x 12 months = £10,800 in taxes per year
2.	Determine which tax band he falls into by calculating the amount of tax paid in each band (you should know how to do this by now! If not, see the previous question's working out.) Band 1 (0-10,000): £0 tax Band 2 (10,000-20,000): £1000 tax Band 3 (20,000-30,000): £1500 tax Band 4 (30,000-40,000): £2000 tax Band 5 (40,000-100,000): £15,000 tax Band 6 (100,000+): Unknown, as no maximum
3.	Add up the taxes in each band to determine where Yusuf's salary (£10,800) lies:

	Band 2 (1000) + Band 3 (1500) = 2500: His salary is more than this! So, it cannot lie in Band 3. 2500 + Band 4 (2000) = 4500: Still more than this! So it cannot lie in Band 4. 4500 + Band 5 (15000) = 19,500: This, the maximum paid for someone in Band 5, is now more than Yusuf's salary. Therefore, Yusuf's salary must lie within Band 5 (£40,000 - £100,000)
4.	Now, calculate how much of the £10,800 he pays lies within this tax band: 10,800 – 4500 (total tax from the previous bands) = 6300 This means that he will be paying £6300 worth of tax in the £40,000-£100,000 bracket.
5.	How can we use this information to calculate how much he earns: Information: • Tax within Band 5 = £6300 • Tax percentage of Band 5 = 25% Therefore, 25% of x = 6300, where x is his salary in this band.
6.	Rearrange the equation to solve for x: x = 6300 / 25% = 6300 / 0.25 x = 25200
7.	If his salary in Band 5 is £25,200, add the minimum salary of the band to find his total salary. 40,000 + 25,200 = £65,200

As you can see, this type of question is very taxing and has a multitude of steps. If you do not have time, do not waste precious minutes! Flag, guess and go with these questions whilst using your eyeballing skills. For example, you could have quickly determined what band he falls into, and crossed out any answers that are outside of that band to give you a better chance of getting the correct answer. Do not get caught up in long calculations when you could be answering many easier questions with fewer steps in the same amount of time.

Ratios

A ratio is a method of demonstrating proportions, or how many times one "thing" exists in comparison to another.

Ratios can be written in many different ways. For example, the ratio of 7 girls to 14 boys in a classroom can be expressed:

- In words: 7 to 14
- In odds notation: 7:14 or 1:2
- In fractions: $\frac{7}{14}$ or $\frac{1}{2}$

It is evident from the above example that ratios can be simplified, as the proportion may be demonstrated without mentioning the whole number of boys or girls present. The following statements describe the same ratio:

- For every 1 girl in a classroom, there are 2 boys.
- For every 7 girls in a classroom, there are 14 boys.

It is essential to respect the order in which the numbers appear. For example, the ratio of girls to boys is 7 to 14. It cannot be 14 to 7, as there are not double the number of girls as there are boys. The numbers in the ratio must correspond directly to the wording of the statement they relate to.

Ratios can present in the UCAT in various ways. For example, you may be given a ratio and be asked to calculate the total number of items in the ratio. In the example above, if there are 7 girls to 14 boys in the classroom, the total number of students in the classroom is 21. Although the number 21 is not mentioned anywhere in the ratio, you should be familiar with the concept of adding both parts of a ratio to obtain the total.

Example 8

Bertha's year group recently had an English test. They achieved a pass:fail ratio of 5:1.

1. If there are 60 people in her year group, how many people passed the test?
   A. 12
   B. 10
   C. 6
   D. 48

E. 50

2. It was found that 15 people failed the test. How many people are there in her year group?
    A. 75
    B. 60
    C. 20
    D. 90
    E. 55

Answer 8

1. The correct answer is E. Remember that the ratio accounts for the entirety of the year group. Thus, a ratio of 5:1 divides the year group into 6 equal portions, where 5 portions passed the test and 1 portion failed. With this knowledge, it would be useful to know how many students belong to each portion, then simply multiply that number by 5 to determine how many belong to the 5 portions that passed the test. The calculations are as follows:

- 5 portions passed + 1 portion failed = 6 portions total
- $\frac{60 \text{ students}}{6 \text{ portions}}$ = 10 students per portion
- 10 students per portion x 5 portions who passed = 50 students passed the test

2. The correct answer is D. We are told that out of the 6 equal portions, 1 portion of students failed the test. This is equivalent to 15 students. As each portion is equal to the others in a ratio, we simply need to multiply the value of 1 portion by 6 in order to determine the value of 6 portions. The calculations can be demonstrated as follows:

- 15 students = 1 portion
- Each portion has the same number of students. There are 6 portions total.
- 15 students x 6 portions = 90 students total.

Example 9

A pet shop is selling cats, guinea pigs, bunnies and fish. The pie chart below demonstrates the percentages of each of the animals.

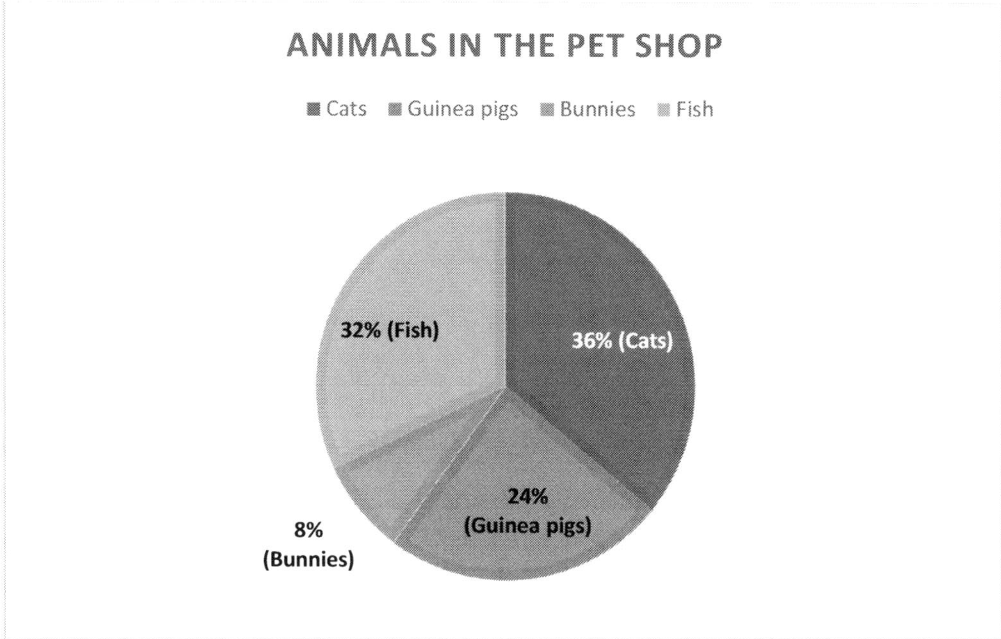

1. There were 200 animals in total, but someone bought 17 of the fish. What is the remaining percentage of cats to the nearest whole number?
   A. 34
   B. 39
   C. 30
   D. 40
   E. 55

2. If the pet shop has 30 guinea pigs, how many bunnies does it have?
   A. 18
   B. 8
   C. 24
   D. 10
   E. 9

Answer 9

1. The correct answer is B. This is a two-step problem. Given that there are 200 animals in the original pie chart, the number of cats is 36% of 200. 200 x 0.36 = 72. The number of cats does not change. However, 17 of the animals have been sold, so the total number of pets is reduced from 200 to 183. The new percentage of cats will be 72/183 = 0.393, or 39%

2. The correct answer is D. This can be solved by cross multiplication. If you are unfamiliar with this strategy, you can learn about it on page 181.

$$\frac{\text{30 guinea pigs}}{24\%} = \frac{x \text{ bunnies}}{8\%}$$

Therefore, x = (30x8)/24 = 10

Converting Units

The majority of questions will involve some sort of unit conversion. It is important to be comfortable with this skill, be able to perform conversions quickly and accurately, and memorise some of the basic formulae, as follows:

Length	1 km = 1000 m 1 m = 100 cm
Mass	1 kg = 1000 g 1 tonne = 1000 kg
Volume	1 litre = 1000 ml 1 m^3 = 1,000,000 cm^3 1 cm^3 = 1 ml

Some main points to note are:

- To convert a *larger* unit to a *smaller* unit, multiply. E.g. 10m → cm = 10 x 100 = 1000cm
- To convert a *smaller* unit to a *larger* unit, divide. E.g. 1000 cm → m = 1000 / 100 = 10m

The following diagram may help you to visualise the basic calculations needed for converting between the most common metric units.

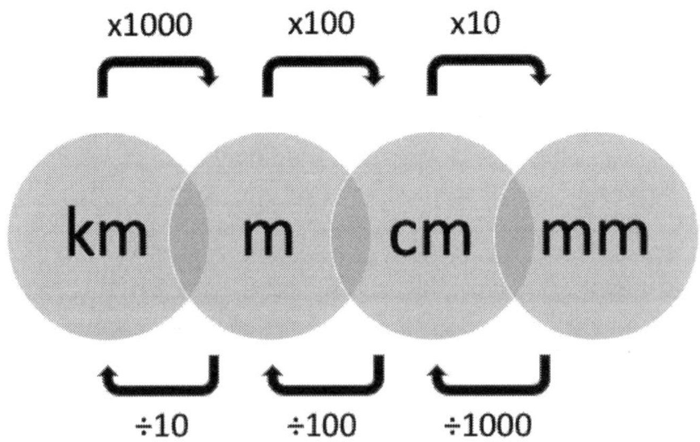

You should also memorise how to convert units of time. To go from hours (larger unit) to minutes or seconds (smaller units), multiply. To go from seconds (smaller unit) to minutes or hours (larger units), divide.

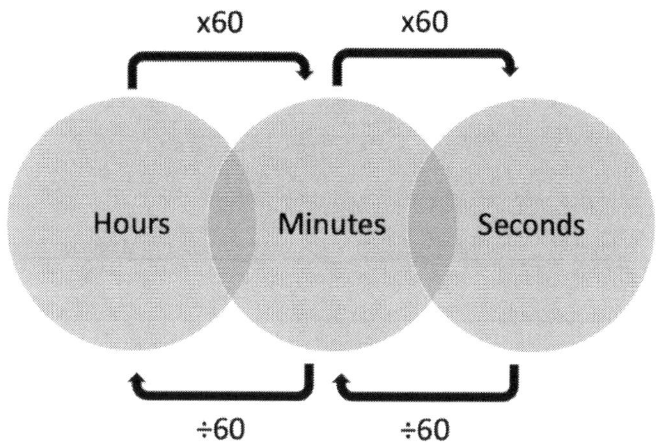

Averages

Average refers to the mean of a set of data, i.e. the sum of the values, divided by the number of values.

$$\text{Average} = \frac{\text{the sum of all values}}{\text{number of values}}$$

Some important points to note about averages are:

- When each of the numbers in a data increases by a certain value, the average of that data will increase by the same value.
- If only one number increases in a set of data, the average of that data will not increase by that same value. Rather, only the numerator (sum of values) will increase by that value. Thus, the average will still increase, but to a lesser degree.
- You should be comfortable with rearranging formulae, as you may need to solve for other than the average, such as one of the values in the dataset, given the average.

To implement these points in practice, try the questions below.

Example 10

The average of three numbers is 140.

1. If all three numbers increase by 5, what is the average now?
    A. 140
    B. 145

C. 141.67

2. One of the three numbers increases by 6. What is the average now?
   A. 146
   B. 142
   C. 140

3. If two of the numbers are 122 and 157, what is the third number?
   A. 140
   B. 141
   C. 138

Answer 10

1. The correct answer is B.

The diagrams below may be helpful. The three bars represent the numbers in the dataset, while the dotted line represents the average of the three numbers.

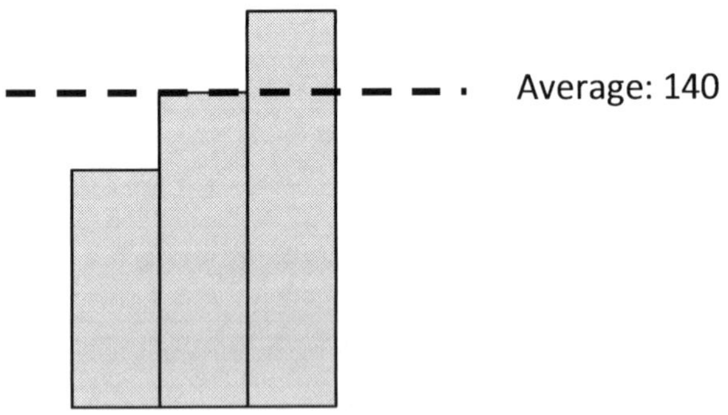

This visual diagram can be modified to represent an even increase in all of the values. The pink bars show the increase, whereas the dotted line towards the top shows the new average.

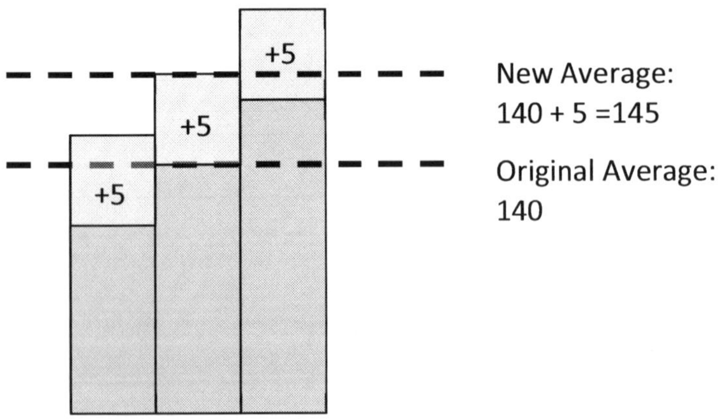

When all of the numbers increase, the average value will increase by the same amount. The reason for this is as follows:

- If each number in a set of 3 numbers increases by 5, the total increase is 15.
- The average increase is (sum of the increase) / (number of values) = 5 (average)

Therefore, the new average is 140 + 5 = 145.

2. The correct answer is B.

In this question, there is not enough information given to calculate an answer using the formula provided for averages. However, the answer can be obtained simply by distributing the increase across all of the values. The diagrams below should help explain this concept.

The blue bars represent the original values, while the pink bar represents the increase in a single value. The shift in average has not been demonstrated here.

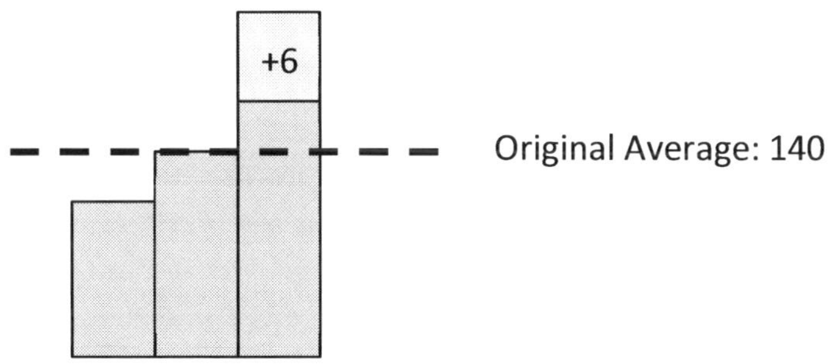

The increase of 6 in a single value will not increase the average by 6, as the other two values have not increased by 6. The first example demonstrated that an increase in each value by the same number will increase the average by that number. This example shows that an increase in a single value will increase the average by a lesser value.

This is due to the formula: average = (sum of values / number of values). In this case, the sum of the values has increased by 6, and the number of values remains the same. The average increase would then be 6 / 3 values = an average increase of 2 for each value. This method demonstrates how this increase in 6 can be distributed across each of the values. Then, as you already know, if each value increases by 2, the average will also increase by 2 → 140 + 2 = 142.

The diagram below shows how the increase in a single value can be distributed across each of the values in order to obtain a new average.

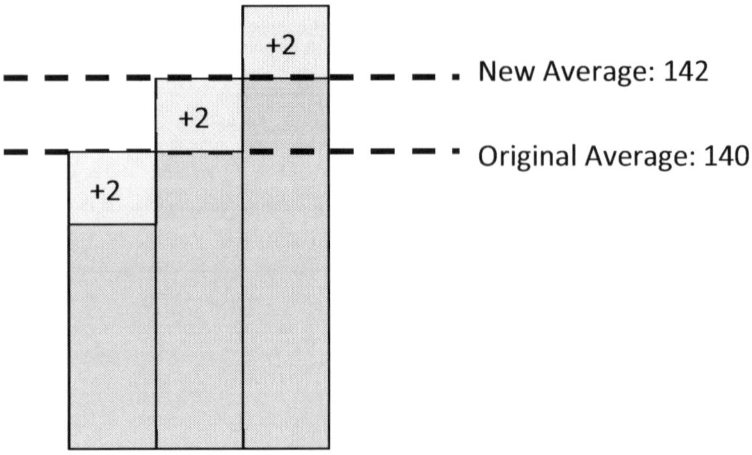

Remember: The principle of averages is to obtain an "evened out" number to represent all of the values. Therefore, distributing the single increase across all of the values is an effective method of determining the average increase if there is not enough information provided to calculate this using the formula.

3. The correct answer is B.

This a "reverse" question, as it requires you to rearrange the formula to solve for one of the values in the dataset, rather than solving for the average. The calculations are as follows:

1.	$\text{Average} = \dfrac{\text{the sum of all values}}{\text{number of values}}$
2.	$140 = \dfrac{122 + 157 + x}{3}$
3.	$140 \text{ x } 3 = 122 + 157 + x$
4.	$420 = 279 + x$
5.	Subtract 279 from both sides: $141 = x$

Cross-Multiplication

Cross multiplication is a brilliant strategy that can be used to answer many different types of equations that involve a variable. If you have not come across this strategy before, it may take some time to get your head around. However, it is highly recommended that you learn and understand how to implement this strategy, as it will prove very useful in Quantitative Reasoning and in real-life scenarios.

Cross multiplication is a way of rearranging fractions to solve for a missing value, or variable.

- E.g. $\frac{2}{x} = \frac{8}{6}$
- To solve for x, you need to rearrange the fraction by cross multiplying. The numerator (top number) of each fraction is multiplied by the denominator (bottom number) of the other fraction. This equation would become:
- $\frac{2}{x} = \frac{8}{6} \rightarrow 2 \times 6 = 8x$
- You can see from this example that cross multiplication is named as such due to the numbers crossing over to the other side.
- Note: This only works when two fractions equal each other, and, as with any algebra, there can only be one variable to achieve a numerical solution.

Let us practice this with some simple problems.

> E.g. If 1 litre of milk is needed to make 10 cups of tea, how many litres are needed to make 37 cups of tea?

You need to lay out the ratios correctly for this to work. The ratio of litres of milk to cup of tea is 1:10, as demonstrated by the scenario. Therefore:

$$\frac{\text{1 litre}}{\text{10 cups of tea}}$$

On the other side of the equation, you should use the same units in the numerator and denominator, and add your variable/missing value where needed.

$$\frac{\text{1 litre}}{\text{10 cups of tea}} = \frac{x \text{ litres}}{\text{37 cups of tea}}$$

If you do not like this method, you can try the other method below.

$$\frac{\text{1 litre}}{x \text{ litres}} = \frac{\text{10 cups of tea}}{\text{37 cups of tea}}$$

This layout will work in the exact same way. You are still using the same ratios: 1 litre makes 10 cups of tea, and *x* litres make 37 cups of tea. Let us now cross-multiply. Whichever layout you choose to utilise will result in the following calculations:

1.	1 litre x 37 cups of tea = x 10 cups of tea
2.	Remove the units for ease of calculation: 1 x 37 = 10 x
3.	Divide both sides by 10: $\frac{1 \times 37}{10} = x$
4.	$x = 3.7$ litres

If this is your first time learning cross multiplication, you may feel that it is too complex to utilise on such a simple equation. However, learning this strategy will prove useful for a variety of problems. Take unit conversions, for example.

Example 11

Kelly and her partner decided to go on a road trip across the United States and Canada. Their car is able to take them from Florida to New Mexico in 3 days – a distance of 1770 miles. There are another 3701 kilometres to go until they reach British Columbia.

Travelling at the same rate, at least how many more days will it take to reach British Columbia? (1 mile = 1.61km)

A. 3 days
B. 4 days
C. 2 days
D. 5 days

Answer 11

The correct answer is B.

Let us firstly convert the kilometres (that they intend to travel further) into miles by cross multiplying. The number of miles will be our variable.

1 mile = 1.61km
x miles = 3701km

1.	Our format will be: $\frac{1 \text{ mile}}{1.61\text{km}} = \frac{x \text{ miles}}{3701 \text{ km}}$

2.	Cross-multiply: 3701 km x 1 mile = x *miles* x 1.61 km
3.	Isolate the x by dividing both sides by 1.61 km: $\frac{3701 \text{ km x 1 mile}}{1.61 \text{ km}} = x \text{ miles}$
4.	Cross out the repeating units in the numerator and denominator: $\frac{3701 \text{ x 1 mile}}{1.61} = x \text{ miles}$
5.	Therefore, x miles = 3701 / 1.61 = 2298.76 miles

So, we now know that 3701 km is equal to 2298.76 miles. Therefore, they have 2298.76 miles left to go.

Let us remind ourselves of the information given in the question, replacing it with the converted units:

- If Kelly and her partner can travel 1770 miles in 3 days, it will take them x days to travel a further 2298.76 miles.

We can solve for x by cross-multiplying again.

1.	Our format will be: $\frac{1770 \text{ miles}}{3 \text{ days}} = \frac{2298.76 \text{ miles}}{x \text{ days}}$
2.	Cross multiply: x 1770 miles = 2298.76 miles x 3 days
3.	Isolate the x by dividing both sides by 1770 miles: $x = \frac{2298.76 \text{ miles x 3 days}}{1770 \text{ miles}}$
4.	Cross out the repeating units in the numerator and denominator: $x = \frac{2298.76 \text{ x 3 days}}{1770}$
5.	Therefore, x = 3.9 days

It will take 3.9 days to reach British Columbia. The question asks *at least* how many more days it will take, therefore, the answer is 4 days.

Speed, Distance and Time

The relationship between speed, distance and time can be summarised with the following triangle:

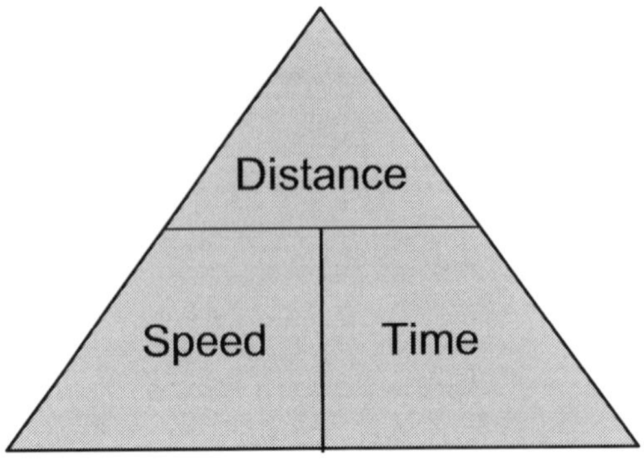

The three formulae that can be devised from this triangle are:

- Distance = Speed x Time
- Speed = Distance / Time
- Time = Distance / Speed

Using these formulae, you can solve a number of questions. Your exam questions will not solely fall into a category such as "speed, distance, time calculation", "unit conversion", or "percent calculation." The questions in Quantitative Reasoning will require you to apply knowledge of the various different topics, formulae, and calculations you are required to know.

Try the question below to see this in practice.

Example 12

Every morning, Amy walks at a speed of 15 km/h for 45 minutes from her house to school without passing by the pond. The diagram below details the relationship between Amy's house and her surroundings.

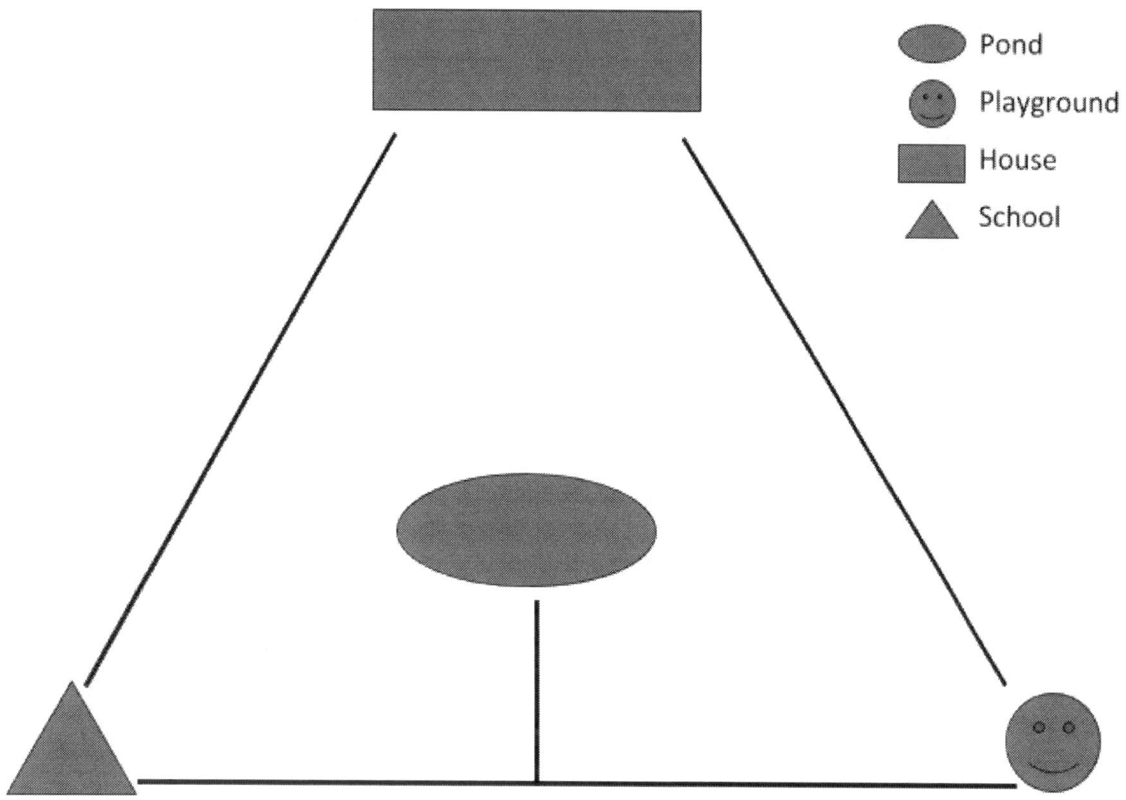

What is the distance between her house and the school? (1 mile = 1.61 kilometres)

A. 0.75 miles
B. 11.25 miles
C. 6.99 miles
D. 7.14 miles
E. 15 miles

Answer 12

The correct answer is C.

The question is asking for the distance in miles between Amy's house and the school - that is, between the rectangle and the triangle.

Some traps to watch out for:

- **Legend and representation of shapes:** The legend is often presented in a random order in comparison to the image given. This makes interpreting the image much more difficult. Practicing questions with legends and watching out for this trick can help save you from making mistakes in the time-pressured environment of your exam.

- **Unit of time:** Speed is given per hour while time is given in minutes. The units need to match before you can do any calculations!
- **Unit of distance:** You are given both kilometres and miles – again, the units need to match! You should convert your units early on to save yourself from performing calculations with mixed units. In your exam, you will not have much time to write out the units associated with every number, therefore, maintain a single unit for each part of the formula to prevent any errors.

The calculations are as follows:

1.	The question asks for distance. The information we have so far is: Distance = Speed x Time Speed = 15 km/hour Time = 45 minutes
2.	It is clear that the time needs conversion. It would be wise to convert the time as it has a single unit, rather than the speed which has two units (km/hr). Thus, we will convert minutes into hours as shown below: 1 hour = 60 minutes $\frac{45\text{ minutes}}{60\text{ minutes}} = 0.75\text{ hours}$ It takes her 0.75 hours to travel to her school.
3.	Therefore: Distance = 15 km/hour x 0.75 hours Distance = 11.25 km

There is more! All of the answer options are in miles, so we will have to convert the answer we have. If you forget to do this, you may incorrectly answer option B, which has the same numerical value as our answer in kilometres.

If you are comfortable with cross-multiplication, you can use this strategy to convert the units. We are told in the question that 1 mile = 1.61 kilometres, and we know how many kilometres we have, so we just need to solve for miles.

1.	1 mile = 1.61 km x miles = 11.25 km

2.	Cross-multiply: $11.25 \times 1 = 1.61\,x$
3.	Now, isolate the x by dividing both sides by 1.61: $\frac{11.25}{1.61} = x$
4.	$x = 6.987$ miles ≈ 6.99 miles

Alternatively, if you wish to memorise the formulae for interconverting kilometres and miles, they are as follows:

Miles = Number of kilometres / 1.61
Kilometres = Number of miles x 1.61

Although using these formulae can be quicker, it is still recommended that you become comfortable with cross-multiplication. If you happen to forget a formula under the time pressure of the exam, cross-multiplication will prove extremely beneficial. When you gain practice with cross-multiplication, you will be able to skip steps by answering them in your head, further increasing your speed.

Using the concepts you have learnt thus far, answer the following question.

Example 13

Vanessa starts her bike ride at 9:00 am. She bikes 8.5 miles before getting weary and taking a break. She stops for 9 minutes and resumes her bike journey at 9:52 am. Over the next 35 minutes, she is able to bike a further 5 miles.

From the start of her journey to the end, what is her average speed in kilometres per hour, rounded to the nearest kilometre?

A. 15 km/hour
B. 18 km/hour
C. 9 km/hour
D. 21 km/hour
E. 35 km/hour

Answer 13

The correct answer is A.

The calculations are as follows:

1.	Vanessa's average speed must take into account the break that she had. You may be tempted to spend time working out what time it was when she started her break, given that it was 9:52 when she restarted her journey. However, the final information informs you that her journey ended 35 minutes after 9:52. 52 + 35 minutes = 87 87 - 60 minutes in an hour = 27 Therefore, her journey ended at 10:27.
2.	If her journey started at 9am, we can conclude that her journey was 1 hour and 27 minutes long. Because the speed will be in km/hour, we must convert this to a decimal value. • 27 minutes/60 minutes in an hour = 0.45 • So, 27 minutes is 45% or 0.45 of an hour. • Therefore, 1 hour and 27 minutes = 1.45 hours
3.	The next part is determining the total distance: 8.5 miles + 5 miles = 13.5 miles. This can be converted into kilometres as follows: 13.5 miles x 1.61 = 21.74 km Therefore, the distance is 21.74 km and the time taken is 1.45 hours
4.	$\text{Average speed} = \frac{\text{total distance}}{\text{total time taken}} = \frac{21.74}{1.45} = 14.99 \approx 15 \text{ km/hour}$

Another way to answer this question is to leave the time conversion until the very end. The calculations are as follows:

1.	Information we have: Speed = Distance/Time Time= 87 minutes Distance= 21.74km Speed= ?
2.	Therefore, speed = 21.74km / 87 minutes = 0.249885 km/minute ≈ 0.25 km/minutes
3.	To convert from km/minute to km/hour, you can simply multiply by 60: 0.25 km/minute x 60 minutes/hour = 15 km/hour

Calculating Midpoints

A midpoint refers to the midway coordinates between two points, either on a graph, or simply in terms of distance.

The midpoint formula is:

$$\left(\frac{x_1 + x_2}{2}, \frac{y_1 + y_2}{2}\right)$$

This type of question is not usually complex, as you simply need to fill the values into the formula to solve the question.

Example 14

Amina and Jasmine realise that they are at the same campsite with their families. They decide to meet at the halfway point between their tents. Amina's tent is at (1, -4) and Jasmine's tent is at (-5, 8). The graph below shows their campsite.

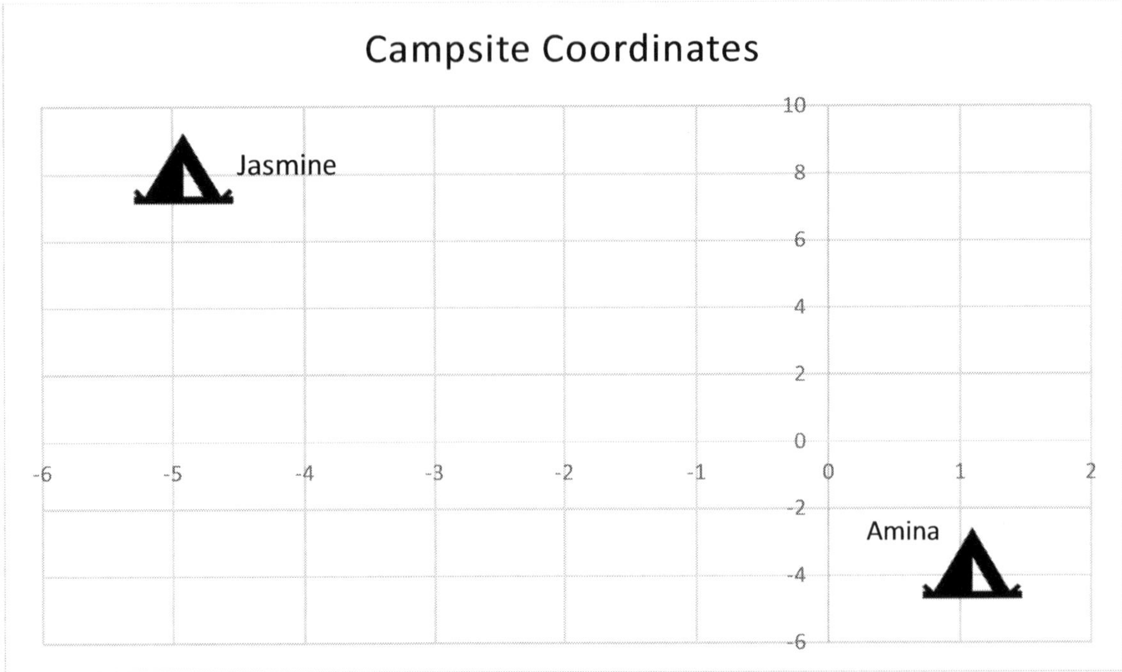

What are the coordinates of their meetup point?

A. (3, 4)
B. (-3, 2)
C. (-2, 2)
D. (2, -2)
E. (-6, -12)

Answer 14

The correct answer is C.

Coordinates are always formatted as (x, y). Whether Amina's coordinates are x_1 and y_1 or whether Jasmine's are, the answer will remain the same. In this case, the answer will be demonstrated using Amina's coordinates as x_1 and y_1.

$x_1 = 1$

$x_2 = -5$

$y_1 = -4$

$y_2 = 8$

You will simply have to substitute the numbers into the formula to obtain the answer.

1.	The formula is: $(\frac{x_1 + x_2}{2}, \frac{y_1 + y_2}{2})$

2.	Let us firstly solve for the x coordinate: $x: \frac{(1 \pm 5)}{2} = \frac{-4}{2} = -2$
3.	Let us now solve for the y coordinate. $y: \frac{(-4 + 8)}{2} = \frac{4}{2} = 2$
4.	Therefore, the midpoint = (-2, 2).

Example 15

Sharon took a road trip with her friends a few days ago. From Sharon's house, they travelled at 56 km/hour for a total of 2.5 hours, before reaching town A. They then left for town B, travelling at 90 km/hour for 1 hour. They then stopped to fill up the petrol and left for their final destination at noon, spending a further 3 hours on the road, travelling 120 km. Where during the journey is the midpoint located?

A. Town A
B. On the way to town A
C. On the way to town B
D. On the way to their final destination
F. Town B

Answer 15

As the question mentions no returns on the journey, we can conclude that it is a straight, one-way trip.

From the question, we are able to create the diagram below:

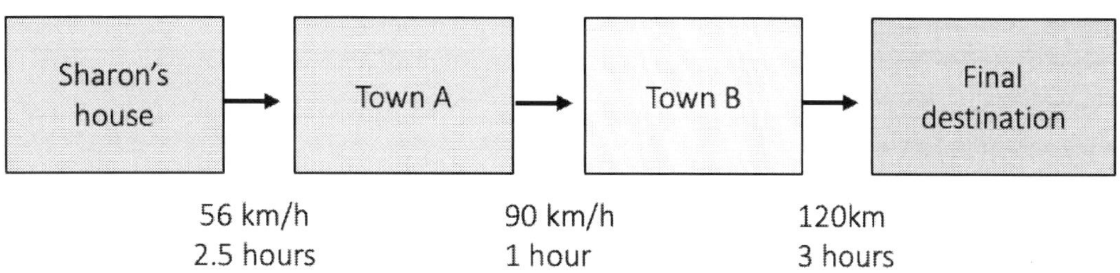

The calculations are as follows:

1.	The question asks for the midpoint during this journey, for which we will need the total distance travelled, as the midpoint will be half of that. We will thus need to calculate for the distance travelled first from Sharon's house to town A, then from Town A to Town B. The distance from town B to the final destination is already given, so we do not need to calculate that.
2.	Distance = Speed x Time From Sharon's house to Town A: 56 km/hour x 2.5 hours = 140 km From Town A to Town B: 90 km/hour x 1 hour = 90 km
3.	The total distance travelled = 140 km + 90 km + 120 km (Town B → final destination) = 350 km
4.	The midpoint would be half of the distance travelled: 350 km / 2 = 175 km
5.	To find which part of the journey the midpoint is on, let us take a look again at the diagram, this time labelled with distances:

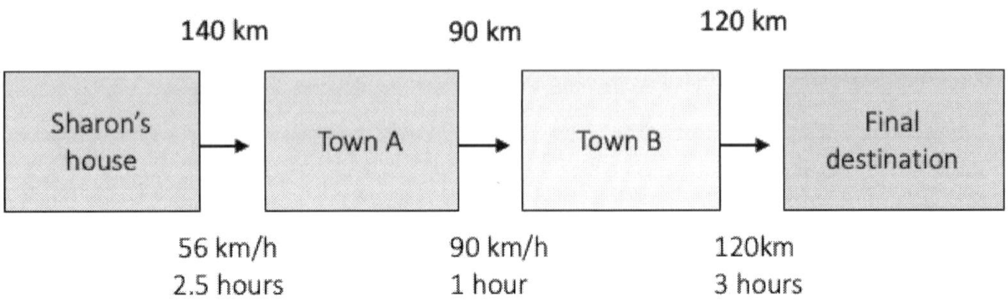

6.	The midpoint = 175 km 175 km is more than the 140 km from Sharon's house to town A, but is less than the distance of 230 km (a further 90km to town B) Thus, the midpoint is during the journey from town A to town B.

Time Zone Problems

Occasionally, you may be given questions that require you to convert time from one time zone to another in order to solve problems. Besides casual use of this skill, you may need to convert time zones as a doctor. Healthcare professionals are often responsible for making phone calls to family members of patients. If a family member is abroad, it is important to note the time zone difference and determine an appropriate time to make a call.

The following strategies will aid you in answering the upcoming questions:

1. If the question involves multiple different cities or time zones, it can get very complex. The best thing to do is select either the *earliest* or the *latest* time zone and convert every other time zone to match up with the one you have chosen.
2. Use a 24-hour format for time, rather than 12-hour.
    a. In a time-pressured exam, you may accidentally interchange afternoon and morning times of the same value using a 12-hour format, therefore, it is best to remain safe. For example, if it is 6am for one person in the scenario, and 8pm (the day before) for another person, you do not want to get confused and think one person is at 6pm, or the other is at 8am, or think that they are both within the same day!
    b. The 24-hour format allows you to easily add and subtract values in your calculations.
3. Do not use outside knowledge. The time zones in the exam will not necessarily represent real-life time zones.
4. If you are given a visual representation, such as a world map with time zones, you may be able to simply count the number of time zones between two locations.
5. Practice, as with everything else. Most smartphones allow you to download various time zones within the "Clock" application. There is no use memorising these time zones, but you can practice time conversions in your head using the following strategy:
    a. Download a few different time zones, remembering what the difference in hours is between your time and the time in the locations you have added to your "Clock". Select locations that are ahead of you in time as well as behind you (i.e. cities in the east as well as in the west).
    b. Throughout the day, try to calculate in your head what time it is in various locations.
    c. Check the application on your phone to confirm.
    d. This kind of practice will help you to convert time zones in your head, thus easing the difficulty of these questions in your exam.

Example 16

The diagram below shows various time zones across the world.

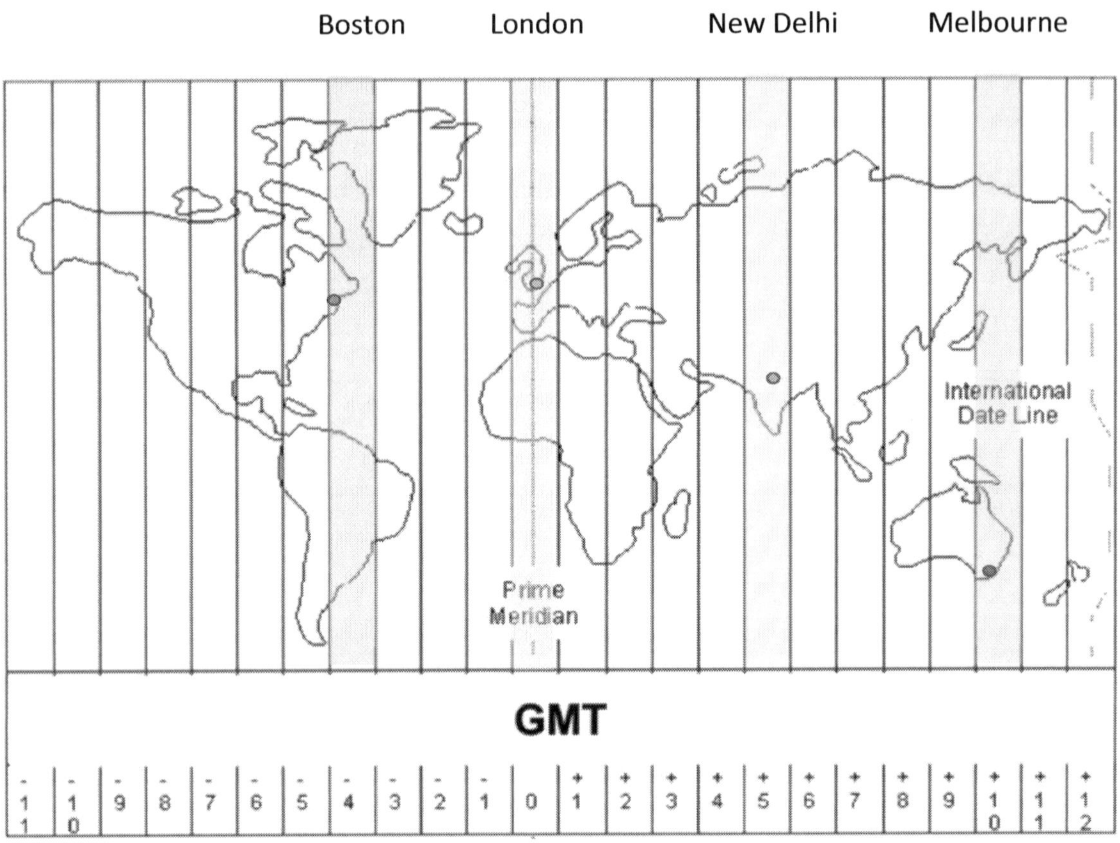

Altered from: https://www.chegg.com/homework-help/questions-and-answers/vuljiiuitj-use-time-zone-map-answer-following-questions-international-date-line-prime-meri-q45747149

Genevieve will be flying from Melbourne to London and transiting in New Delhi, India. Emily, Genevieve's friend, calls Genevieve during her layover. Emily resides in Boston, USA, and makes the call at 8pm her time.

What time it for Genevieve when Emily calls?

A. 3am
B. 5am
C. 12am
D. 11am
E. 5pm

Answer 16

The correct answer is B.

Genevieve's layover is in New Delhi. The question is therefore asking you to convert from 8pm Boston time to New Delhi time.

Two methods can be used to tackle this problem.

1. **Count the number of bars from one zone to another.**

The diagram shows a world map. It should be widely known that time goes forward as you move towards the east, or right side of a map, and goes backwards as you move towards the west, or left side of the back.

There is a difference of one hour between each time zone, as demonstrated by the diagram. If you simply count the time zones, or the bars, between Boston and New Delhi, you will find that New Delhi is 9 time zones ahead of Boston. This means that the time in New Delhi is 9 hours ahead of Boston.

You can add this up in your head to work out what 8pm + 9 hours is.

Alternatively, see the calculations below. Hopefully, with practice, you should be able to skip some of these and work out the answer using mental maths.

1.	8pm can be written as 20:00
2.	20:00 + 9 hours = 29:00
3.	There are only 24 hours in a day, so it is clear that at the time of the phone call, New Delhi was a day ahead of Boston. Therefore, the time in New Delhi was: 29:00 - 24:00 = 5:00 or 5am

2. **Use an analogy to understand**

Referring to GMT, which is the number 0 in the chart, we can see that:

- New Delhi is 5 hours ahead of GMT.
- Boston is 4 hours behind GMT.

This means that New Delhi is 9 hours ahead of Boston. This is the sum of their differences compared to GMT. We will have to add 9 hours to Boston time in order to get New Delhi time.

You can use the analogy of a high building with many underground floors.

- The Ground floor in this analogy would be GMT, 0, as labelled above on the map.
- The underground floors are every zone that is behind, i.e. to the left of the map

- The overground floors of the building are the zones ahead of GMT, i.e. to the right of the map.

We have been given Boston time, a time that is behind GMT by 4 hours (floor -4 of the building). We need to obtain New Delhi time which is 5 hours ahead of GMT (floor 5 of the building).

Consider the diagram below. If you are in a lift starting on the floor -4, how many floors would the lift need to elevate to reach the 5th floor?

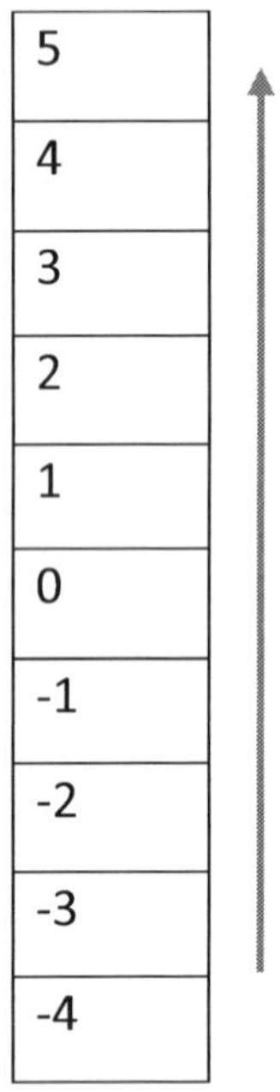

You can see that an elevation of 9 floors is required to reach the 5th floor. As such, to travel from the time zone in Boston, which is at -4, to the time zone in New Delhi, which is at +5, you need to "elevate" by 9 hours. Therefore, when it is 8pm in Boston, the time in New Delhi is 5am on the following day.

Example 17

Genevieve took off when it was 7am in Melbourne. Her flight to New Delhi was 3 hours long, had an hour-long layover, and landed in London at 8am GMT. Genevieve's mother who was in Melbourne called Genevieve as soon as she landed.

What time was it for Genevieve's mother when she made the phone call?

A. 6am
B. 5am
C. 12pm
D. 4pm

E. 6pm

Answer 17

The correct answer is E.

This question uses **durations** to try to confuse you. It may appear that you need to calculate the duration of the flight, as many details are given that would point towards working this out. However, if you read closely, you will find that Genevieve's landing time is given in GMT and the question is only asking you to convert it to Melbourne time.

From the graph, Melbourne is 10 hours ahead of GMT. As GMT is the reference point, we can now directly proceed to calculations.

1.	Melbourne time = GMT + 10 hours
2.	8:00 + 10 hours = 18:00
3.	18:00 = 6pm Remember: to convert from 24-hour format to 12-hour format, you must subtract 12 hours from any number greater than 12. E.g. 18:00 - 12 hours = 6:00pm

Drug Calculations

Drug calculations are not very common in Quantitative Reasoning, but do appear from time to time. It is beneficial to gain practice doing such calculations, as they can appear in your interviews, as well.

These questions can broadly be divided into two categories:

1. Volume
2. Concentration

Often, drugs are administered in liquid form, where part of the liquid is the drug and the other part is made up of non-active elements. In such questions, you may be required to interconvert between mass and volume units.

Mass Units	Interconversion	Volume Units
1 kg = 1000 g 1 g = 1000 mg 1 mg = 1000 μg 1 μg = 1000 ng	1 kg = 1 litre 1 g = 1 millilitre	1 l = 1000 ml

Try the questions below, using the table above for reference.

Example 18: Volume

You are asked to prescribe insulin to a patient weighing 75kg. 7mg of insulin is needed per 5 kg of body weight and you have a syringe measuring in millilitres.

What is the amount of insulin needed in millilitres?

A. 105 ml
B. 525 mg
C. 0.105 ml
D. 1.05 ml
E. 0.525 ml

Answer 18: Volume

The correct answer is C.

Cross multiplication is a very handy tool for drug calculations. Below is a step-by-step method for solving for the mass of the drug needed. Hopefully, you will become comfortable enough with cross-multiplication to be able to perform most of these steps in your head.

1.	The information we have is as follows: 7 **mg** needed for every 5kg x **ml** needed for 75 kg.
2.	We can alter the question to firstly solve for how many milligrams of insulin are needed for a 75kg patient. We can later convert this to millilitres. 7 **mg** needed for every 5kg x **mg** needed for 75 kg.
3.	We can lay this out in the following format:

	$\frac{7\text{mg}}{5\text{kg}} = \frac{x}{75\text{kg}}$
4.	Now, cross multiply: 7 x 75 = 5 x
5.	Divide by 5 on both sides to solve for x. (7 x 75) / 5 = 105
6.	Therefore, x = 105mg

We now know how many mg of insulin this 75kg patient would require. We must convert this into ml to answer the question. You can cross multiply again to convert the units. See the calculations below.

1.	The information we have is as follows: 1000mg = 1g 1g = 1ml Therefore, 1000mg = 1ml
2.	If 1000mg = 1ml, 105mg = x ml We must solve for x to determine how many ml of the drug the patient will need.
3.	Format: $\frac{1000\text{mg}}{1\text{ml}} = \frac{105\text{mg}}{x\text{ ml}}$
4.	Cross multiply: 1000 x = 105 x 1
5.	Divide by 1000 on both sides to solve for x. x = 105 / 1000
6.	Therefore, x = 0.105 ml

Example 19: Concentration

An aqueous drug comes in 75ml syringes but only 3% of its contents are the active ingredient of the drug. A patient requires 9 ml of the active ingredient.

How many syringes do you need to give?

A. 3 syringes
B. 3.5 syringes

C. 0.12 of a syringe
D. 4 syringes
E. 1.2 syringes

Answer 19: Concentration

The correct answer is D.

This question demonstrates how the Quantitative Reasoning section combines various skills in each question you are asked. This question requires you to have a good understanding of percentages, as well as drugs.

1.	The information we have is as follows: The active ingredient in each 75ml syringe is 3% of the total volume.
2.	3% of 75ml = 75ml x 0.03 = 2.25 ml Therefore, each 75ml syringe has 2.25ml of the active ingredient.
3.	How many lots of 2.25ml do we need to deliver 9ml total of the active ingredient? This is a simple division calculation. 9ml/2.25ml = 4 lots of 2.25 ml
4.	Therefore, if each syringe contains 2.25ml of active ingredients, and we need 4 lots of 2.25ml, we need 4 syringes.

Probability

Probability can be defined as the likelihood of an event occurring, with a maximum value of 1 which represents an event that will definitely occur.

Probability can be a complex topic which students often struggle with. This section will attempt to explain and simplify probability concepts using a mathematical approach. Once you understand the maths behind probability, we would recommend using tree diagrams to solve questions, as a visual representation is easier to process for most people. However, tree diagrams are not useful if you do not understand the concepts that they represent. Tree diagrams are covered in detail in the Decision Making section of this book.
A basic concept that needs to be understood is the measurement of probability.

- If an event will definitely occur, the probability is said to be 1.
- Probability can never be higher than 1.
- If an event is less likely to occur, the probability value will decrease. E.g. a probability of 0.4 means that the event is less likely to occur than if the probability was 0.6.
- If the probability of an event occurring is x, the probability of it not occurring is 1 - x. E.g. if the probability of it raining today is 0.4, the probability of it not raining today is 0.6.
- Probability is comparable to ratios as it is given in either a percent, a decimal, or a fraction format.

It is also important to note that probability questions must be based on the assumption that the events in question are not biased. For example, if you are picking different coloured sweets out of a bag, in order for each sweet to have equal probability:

- You must not look at which sweet is being picked.
- Each sweet must be the same size and texture.
- The sweets cannot be distinguishable from each other in any way during the selection process.

If there is some sort of bias, then probability equations automatically cannot be applicable.

Example 20

There are 5 red marbles in a bag, and you randomly pick out a marble. What is the probability that it will be red?

A. 1/5
B. 4/5
C. 1
D. 1/6
E. 5/6

Answer 20

The correct answer is C.

There are only red marbles, so if you pick out a marble, it will definitely be red.

Single events

The probability of an event occurring can be defined by the equation:

$$P = \frac{\text{Number of ways the event can occur}}{\text{Total number of events/outcomes}}$$

E.g. What is the probability of getting a 4 when rolling an unbiased 6-sided die once?

The event in question: Rolling a 4
Number of ways the event can occur: 1
Total number of outcomes/events: 6, as there are 6 numbers on a die.

Therefore, if we fill in the formula above, the probability of rolling a 4 on a 6-sided die is $\frac{1}{6}$.

Multiple Events: Independent

An independent event is not affected by the occurrence of another event.

This means that two events independent of each other will always have the same probability, regardless of whether or not the other event occurs. To find the combined probability of two independent events occurring, the following formula can be used:

Probability of event A and event B = Probability of A x Probability of B.

This can be simplified as follows:

P(A and B) = P(A) x P(B)

Try the following example using the formula provided.

Example 21

If you flip a coin, then roll a die, what is the probability of getting heads and rolling a 6?

A. 1/12
B. 3/4
C. 7/8
D. 1/16
E. 1/8

Answer 21

Let us first define each event.

Event A = Heads

Event B = 6

The individual probability of getting heads is $\frac{1}{2}$.

The individual probability of rolling a 6 is $\frac{1}{6}$.

You should be familiar enough with flipping a coin and rolling a die to be able to quickly deduce the probability of a single event occurring when either of these actions is conducted.

The probability of *both* events occurring can be calculated as follows:

1.	The information we have is as follows: $P(A) = \frac{1}{2}$ and $P(B) = \frac{1}{6}$
2.	Substitute the information into the equation provided: $P(A \text{ and } B) = \frac{1}{2} \times \frac{1}{6}$
3.	Therefore, $P(A \text{ and } B) = \frac{1}{12}$

Thus, the probability of getting heads and rolling a 6 is $\frac{1}{12}$.

To better understand this, think about all of the 12 possible combinations of events that could have occurred when flipping a coin and rolling a die. These are demonstrated in the table below.

- Event number is displayed first (1-12)
- H representing heads on a coin.
- T representing tails on a coin.
- Numbers 1-6 represent the number on a die.

Event	1	2	3	4	5	6	7	8	9	10	11	12

Coin	T	T	T	T	T	T	H	H	H	H	H	H
Die	1	2	3	4	5	6	1	2	3	4	5	6

Take event 1 for example: You could have gotten tails and rolled a 1. Event 2 shows that you could have gotten tails and rolled a 2, and so on.

Out of the 12 possibilities, one of them shows that you could get heads and roll a 6. This means that the possibility of this combination of events occurring is 1/12.

To summarise this example, please understand that the number rolled on the die and the side flipped on the coin are completely independent of each other, and thus, what you roll on the die will not impact what you flip on the coin.

Multiple Events: Dependent

A dependent event is affected by the occurrence of another event.

This leads to "conditional" probability, where the probability of an event is conditional or dependent on another event happening. If the first event happens, the probability of the dependent event will change.

When you have an event whose probability is dependent on an event occurring prior to it, you need to use a different formula to calculate the joint probabilities. This is due to the fact that the probability of the second event will change depending on whether or not the first event occurs. Therefore, if a question asks for the probability of a dependent event occurring alongside the event that it depends on, the following equation can be used:

Probability of A and B = Probability of A x Probability of B, given that A has occurred.

This can be simplified as follows:

P(A and B) = P(A) x P(B|A)
Note: The symbol "|" is used to represent "given".

To better understand dependent events and conditional probabilities, attempt the following question using the formula provided.

Example 22

A box contains 4 red and 2 yellow balls. Two balls are randomly selected from the box without being replaced.

What is the probability that the first ball is red and the second is yellow?

A. 8/12
B. 2/3
C. 11/15
D. 4/15

E. 1/12

Answer 22

The correct answer is D.

*Note: When the answers are in fraction format, **do not** use your calculator! It will not give you a fraction answer. Thus, it is essential to be comfortable with solving with fractions by hand.*

In this case, you must understand that there is no replacement – i.e. the balls are not being put back into the box. Therefore, the total number of balls in the box will decrease after each ball is taken out.

Let us define the events:

Event A: red ball
Event B: yellow ball
Condition: The yellow ball is picked after already picking a red ball

The calculations are as follows:

1.	The formula for dependent events is: P(A and B) = P(A) x P(B|A)
2.	Define the probability of event A $P(A) = \frac{\text{number of red balls}}{\text{total number of balls}} = \frac{4}{6}$
3.	Define the probability of B, given that A has already occurred. Note: If A has already occurred, there is 1 less ball in the box now. Therefore, the total number of balls has decreased and the denominator needs to be changed. $P(B\|A) = \frac{\text{number of yellow balls}}{\text{total number of balls - 1}} = \frac{2}{5}$
4.	Substitute both into the equation: $P(A \text{ and } B) = \frac{4}{6} \times \frac{2}{5} = \frac{4}{15}$

Therefore, the probability of first picking a red ball, not replacing it, then picking a yellow ball is 4/15.

To further understand why event B is dependent on event A, consider event B prior to event A occurring. The probability of selecting a yellow ball would normally be $\frac{2}{6}$ or $\frac{1}{3}$ if it was to be selected first. Given that a ball is taken out prior to selecting the yellow ball, the total number of outcomes is reduced by 1.

Using the basic calculation for probability of an event occurring, we know that:

- P(B) = (number of ways B can occur / total number of outcomes)

The probability changes to $\frac{2}{5}$ following the occurrence of event A, thus demonstrating event B's dependence on event A.

The calculations can further be demonstrated using a tree diagram.

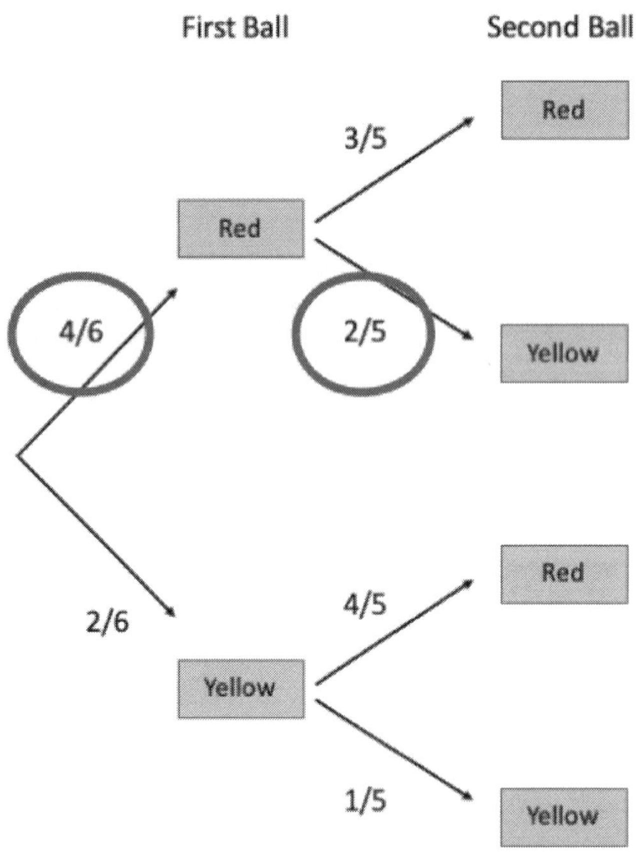

Given the probability of the first ball being red is 4/6, and the next ball being yellow is 2/5, the probability of both is (4/6) x (2/5) = 8/30, or 4/15.

Note: The Decision Making section of this book covers tree diagrams in further detail.

Example 23

Jannah has a bag with 18 marbles. 13 of them are green, 3 are blue and 2 are orange. She decides to randomly select a marble to give to her sister and one to give to her brother.

Rounded to two decimal places, what is the probability that she will pick out a blue marble for her brother after already picking out a blue marble for her sister?

A. 0.21
B. 0.09
C. 0.01
D. 0.14
E. 0.02

Answer 23

The correct answer is E.

As explained earlier, probability can be defined in various formats. This question is asking for an answer in decimals. Thus, you are able to use your calculator for this question.

This is a conditional probability question, i.e. one event is dependent on another.

Let us first define the events A and B.
Event A: Jannah picks out a blue marble
Event B: Jannah picks out a blue marble.
Condition: The first blue marble is not replaced in the bag.

1.	The formula for dependent events is: P(A and B) = P(A) x P(B|A)
2.	Define the probability of event A $P(A) = \frac{\text{number of blue marbles}}{\text{total number of marbles}} = \frac{3}{18}$
3.	Define the probability of B, given that A has already occurred.

	Note: If A has already occurred, there is 1 less blue marble in the bag now. Therefore, the numerator (blue marbles) and the denominator (total number of marbles) have both changed. $$P(B\|A) = \frac{\text{number of blue marbles - 1}}{\text{total number of marbles - 1}} = \frac{2}{17}$$
4.	Substitute both A and B into the equation: $$P(A \text{ and } B) = \frac{3}{18} \times \frac{2}{17}$$
5.	Therefore, P(A and B) = 0.0196

Notice how in this question, the same option (blue marble) was selected twice. Always remember to subtract from both the numerator and the denominator if this is the case.

Statistics

Essential Terms

For the UCAT, you are expected to know and implement the following terms and their respective formulae:

Term	Definition
Mean	The average of the data set. Mean = $\frac{\text{sum of the values}}{\text{number of values}}$
Median	The middle number of a list that is ordered from highest to lowest or vice versa. The median number separates the upper half from the lower half. *Note*: If the dataset has an even number of items, and thus there is no middle number, then the median will be the average of the two middle numbers.
Mode	The value in the data set that appears most often. E.g. The mode of "5, 5, 7, 5" would be 5 as it is the most repeated in this data set.

Range	The difference between the maximum and the minimum values in a data set. E.g. "5, 12, 2, 8." The range of this data set = 12 - 2 = 10.

Example 24

The following table demonstrates the number of students in each of 5 schools that speak the given languages.

	Spanish	Mandarin	English	French	Arabic
Students in School 1	72	44	107	29	63
Students in School 2	37	88	61	19	8
Students in School 3	44	13	49	77	21
Students in School 4	114	88	47	61	52
Students in School 5	18	30	51	49	103

1. Which school has the median number of English speakers?
    A. School 1
    B. School 2
    C. School 3
    D. School 4
    E. School 5

2. Which school has the mode number of Mandarin speakers?
    A. School 1
    B. School 2
    C. School 3
    D. School 5
    E. None of the schools

3. What is the mean number of students studying Arabic across the 5 schools?
    A. 103
    B. 52
    C. 49.4
    D. 247

E. 95

Answer 25

1. The correct answer is E. Arrange the numbers in order to determine the median number: 47, 49, 51, 61, 107. The median, or the middle number of this data set, is 51. School 5 has 51 students who speak English, hence the correct answer is E.

2. The correct answer is B. The mode is the number that is most frequently repeated. The only number repeated in the data set for "Mandarin" is 88. There are 88 students who speak Mandarin in School 2 and School 4. Because School 4 was not an option, School 2 is the correct answer.

3. The correct answer is C. The mean can be calculated as follows:

$$\frac{\text{sum of the values}}{\text{number of values}} = \frac{63 + 8 + 21 + 52 + 103}{5} = 49.4$$

Data Interpretation

Often, you will be required to interpret a data set, such as a chart or a graph, without necessarily performing any calculations. The data is followed by a series of statements, and your role is to decipher which of them are true or untrue based on the data given.

Usually, two types of questions regarding data interpretation will be present during the exam.

1. You will be asked to identify the correct (or incorrect) statement.
2. You will be asked to identify whether the statement given is True, False, or Can't tell.

Both of these question types may possess statements that are "Can't tell". The question-writers have various tricks they can implement in these types of questions. There are various tricks that the question-writers can use. These are comparable to tricks used in Verbal Reasoning, and would often point towards the answer being "Can't tell".

1. **Qualifiers of necessity and generalisations**: E.g. "The graph shows that men above the age of 65 **must** be bald." It is important to watch out for such examples, as data in graphs often only include *sample sets*, and so, even if this applies to every individual in the data set, it is not appropriate to generalise and apply it to **all** men.
2. **Unclear adverbs**: E.g. "The number of bald men over the age of 65 is very high." This is a very subjective statement, as there is no quantification of "very". Who is to determine what "very high" refers to? Your interpretation of this term could be entirely different to someone else's, and thus, a statement like this cannot be true. It needs to be objectively correct.

3. **Incomplete data**: E.g. If the graph only has data for men in London, yet the statement refers to "men in the U.K." you will not be able to accept this statement as the data has not accounted for all men in the U.K.
4. **Assumptions and outside information:** E.g. A statement might refer to these men over 65 being retired, and you may assume this based on outside knowledge. However, if the information does not say that they are retired, there is no evidence for this. Be careful not to make any assumptions, and use only the information that has been provided.

Statements are only false if they are *directly contradicted* by the data given. Consider the example of a diagram that shows that all men above the age of 65 in London are bald. Statements from this diagram may be categorised as follows:

Can't tell:

- "All men above the age of 65 are bald." The statement generalises a conclusion based on limited data.
- "Men above the age of 65 in London are very bald." The statement has subjectivity.
- "All women above the age of 65 in London are bald." Or "All men above the age of 65 are retired." These statement does not match the data from the supposed diagram, and may require outside knowledge. However, they are not contradicted by the data.

False:

- "All men above the age of 65 in London are not bald". This is directly contradicted by the data.
- Check the statement! Sometimes there are differences in words or spellings. E.g. In a time-pressured environment, you may mistakenly read "Iran" as "Iraq" – a mistake the question-writer may have wanted you to make.

Example 26

Miners are at risk of developing a lung disease called pneumoconiosis (CWP) because of their regular exposure to airborne respirable dust. Miners with 5 or more years of mining experience, who are exposed to exhaust from diesel engines, have an increased risk of dying from lung cancer.

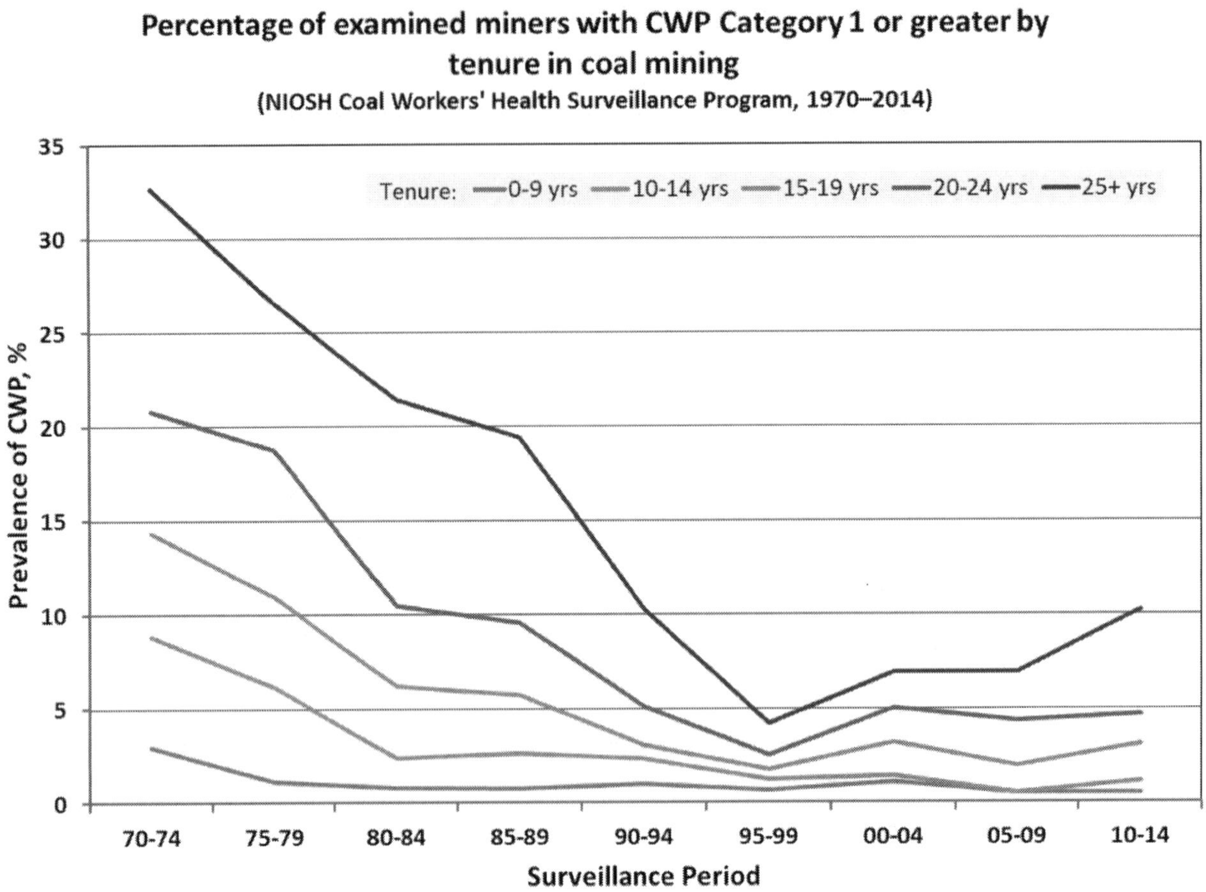

Source:
https://www.cdc.gov/niosh/mining/topics/RespiratoryDiseases.html#:~:text=Miners%20are%20at%20risk%20of,of%20dying%20from%20lung%20cancer

1. Based on the information given above and in the chart, which of the following statements is correct?
    A. Miners with 25+ years of experience are at an increased risk of dying from CWP compared to miners with 10 years of experience.
    B. In the surveillance period of 95-99, prevalence of CWP in miners is at its all-time low.
    C. CWP is not very prevalent in miners with 0-9 years of experience.
    D. The prevalence of CWP in miners has an overall decrease during the period of this survey.
    E. Among all of the miners in the study, prevalence of CWP in miners with 0-9 years of experience was the highest.

2. Miners with 20-24 years of tenure have always had less CWP prevalence compared to those with 25+ years of tenure
    A. True
    B. False
    C. Can't tell

Answer 26

1. The correct answer is D. Although the lines start to rise again after a certain point, this is not a large rise, so there is an overall decrease throughout the time period on the graph.

   All of the other options are incorrect because they are either "can't tell" or false.

   Statement A is "can't tell". The information given prior to the graph mentioned an increased risk of dying when years of mining experience are also associated with exposure to exhaust from diesel engines. There is no information in the graph to suggest that the miners have had such exposure. Further, the y-axis shows an increased risk of CWP, with no further information to indicate an increased risk of dying from CWP. We would need extra information to validate or contradict this answer, so it is "can't tell".

   Statement B is "can't tell". It mentions an "all-time" low, but this data only includes 1970-2014. The statement is not contradicted. More information is required to be certain, so it is "can't tell".

   Statement C is "can't tell". The adverb "very" cannot be quantified, as it is subjective. Furthermore, there is no specification of a time period given in the statement. The data includes only 1970-2014, thus it would be difficult to make a statement as such, unless specifying the time period being referred to. E.g. "Between 1970 and 2000, miners with 0-9 years had the lowest prevalence of CWP." Notice how "not very prevalent" is changed to a more specific statement – the lowest prevalence. This statement can be proven, as the time period being referred to is also specified.

   Statement E is false. The prevalence of CWP is the lowest in miners with 0-9 years of experience, and the statement is limited to the miners investigated in this study only. As such, the statement directly contradicts the data represented by the graph.

2. The correct answer is C. This question tests your ability to notice minute details, such as incomplete data and qualifiers of necessity. The data given is only from 1970 – 2014, thus, we have no way to ascertain that these miners "always" had less prevalence.

Geometry

Geometry questions involve area, perimeter and volume of common shapes. It is important to memorise the formulae and be comfortable recalling them to apply to any questions. The formulae you need to know are summarised below:

2D Shapes

Shape	Perimeter	Area
Square	4 x length of any side	$(\text{length of any side})^2$
Rectangle	2 (length + width)	length x width
Triangle	sum of the 3 sides	$\frac{1}{2}$ (base x height)
Circle	$2\pi r$	πr^2

This is rarely asked, though might be helpful to review:

Parallelogram	sum of the 4 sides	base x height

The questions are not always as straight-forward as entering numbers into an equation. You may also be asked to answer questions that require you to rearrange equations.

It would also be a good idea to remind yourself of simple conversions and the easiest ways to convert between units (page 177).

Example 27

A rectangle has a perimeter of 30 metres and a width of 6 metres.

What is the length of the rectangle, in metres?

A. 9
B. 72
C. 5
D. 32,400
E. 90

Answer 27

The correct answer is A.

Hopefully, this should be a straight-forward question. The detailed calculations are as follows:

1.	The formula is: Perimeter of rectangle = 2 (length + width)
2.	Substitute the numbers in: 30m = 2 (length + 6m)
3.	Divide by 2 on both sides: 15m = (length + 6m)
4.	The brackets can now be removed. Isolate the variable (length) by subtracting 6 on both sides. 15m - 6m = length
5.	Therefore, the length of the rectangle = 9m

3D Shapes

For 3D shapes, you need to understand how to calculate:

1. **Surface area:** the combined area, in units^2, of each surface.
2. **Volume**: the amount of space, in units^3, that an object occupies, or that can be enclosed within an object.

Surface Area

The surface area of any shape can be calculated by adding up the individual areas of each surface. The area formulae are given in the previous table.

Try the following question.

Example 28

Jonathon is wrapping a gift for his wife and needs to determine how much wrapping paper he needs. The gift is placed in a box as demonstrated by the diagram below.

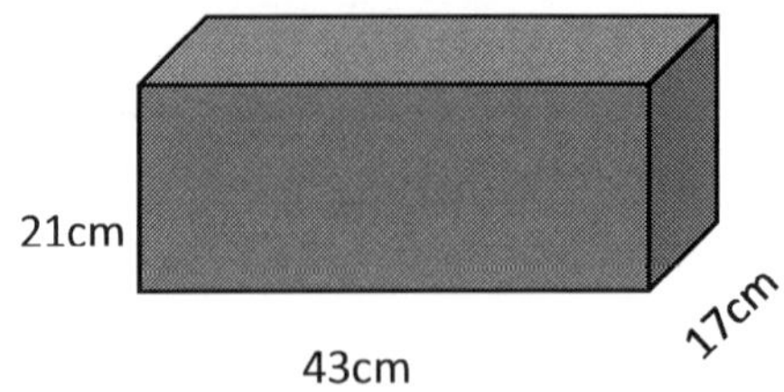

Based on the measurements given, how much wrapping paper does Jonathon need to fully cover each surface of the box?

A. $982cm^2$
B. $15,351cm^2$
C. $8902cm^2$
D. $3982cm^2$
E. $382cm^2$

Answer 28

The correct answer is D.

This is a surface area question. Hopefully, this should be straight-forward as well! The detailed calculations are as follows:

1.	The information we have is: Length = 43cm Width = 17cm Height = 21cm
2.	A rectangle has 6 sides. Because each of the 3 measurements are distinct, the rectangle will 3 different area calculations applicable to the sides. Side 1: length x height Side 2: length x width Side 3: width x height Remember that each side has an identical counterpart.
3.	Fill in the numbers to calculate the area of each surface: Side 1: 43 x 21 = 903cm Side 2: 43 x 17 = 731cm Side 3: 17 x 21 = 357cm

4.	To calculate the surface area, you must add up the areas of each side. There are 6 sides total (2 sides with each of the areas calculated above) Surface area = (903 x 2) + (731 x 2) + (357 x 2)
5.	Therefore, the surface area of this rectangle = 3982cm^2

Jonathon will need 3982cm^2 of wrapping paper.

Volume

The volume formulae you need to know are summarised below. Other shapes are rarely used, and equations may be provided for irregular ones.

Shape	Volume
Cube 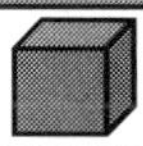	length^3 (length x length x length)
Cuboid 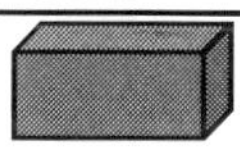	length x width x height
Cylinder 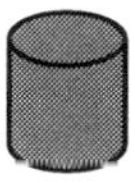	$\pi r^2 h$ (i.e. the area of the circular base x height)
Sphere 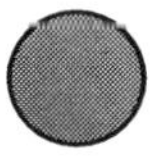	$\frac{4}{3}\pi r^3$ Note: for a hemisphere (half of a sphere), multiply the above by $\frac{1}{2}$, or divide by 2

Density

Some of the more difficult questions can also involve density.

Density = mass / volume

This describes how heavy an object is for its size, allowing a comparison to be made between objects of a similar size. For example, the density of a 30cm^3 brick is much higher than the density of a 30cm^3 container of candy floss.

It is important to note that there are various units for mass (mg, g, kg, tonnes) and various units for volume (cm^3, m^3, ml, l).

E.g. The density of a $500cm^3$ tub of flour is $0.6g/cm^3$. What is its mass?

You can solve for this by rearranging the formula.
Mass = density x volume.
Therefore, mass = 0.6 x 500 = 300g.

Example 29

Gabriel is installing a small cylinder-shaped baby bath in his side room. The measurements of the bath are as follows:

Radius = 12cm
Height = 30cm

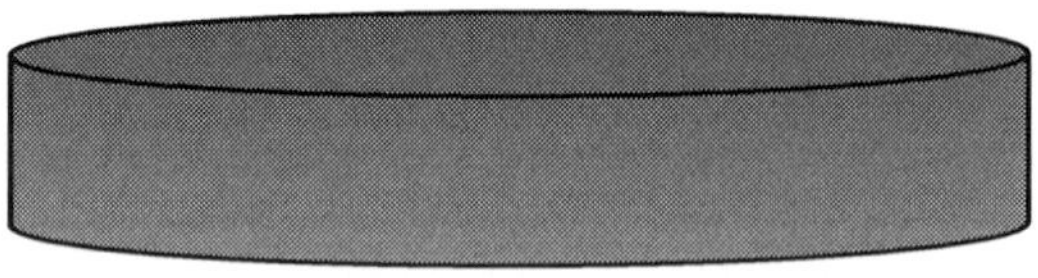

1. To fill the bath to the brim, what volume of water should he add? 1 litre = $1000cm^3$
   A. 13.6 litres
   B. 1.4 litres
   C. 32 litres
   D. 16.6 litres
   E. 19.1 litres

2. The bath is very light, weighing only 720 grams. When he adds 2 litres of water, he notices that the weight of the bath increases to 2714 grams. What is the density of the water?
   A. 1.34 g/cm^2
   B. 0.997 g/cm^2
   C. 39.1 g/cm^2
   D. 4.32 g/cm^2
   E. 0.32 g/cm^2

Answer 29

1. The correct answer is A.

The calculations are as follows:

1.	The formula for volume of a cylinder is:

	$\pi r^2 h$
2.	Substitute the numbers in: $3.14 \times 12^2 \times 30 = 13{,}564.8\ cm^3$
3.	Convert to litres, as the answers are all in litres. 1 litre = 1000 cm^3 You can cross multiply to solve this. Otherwise, simply divide 13,563.8 by 1000. 13,563.8 / 1000 = 13.56 litres

2. The correct answer is B.

The calculations are as follows:

1.	The information we have is: Mass of water = the difference between the mass of the tub with the water and the mass of the tub without the water. Therefore, mass of water = 2714 - 720 = 1994 g. Volume of water: 2 litres Mass of water: 1994 g Density of water: ?
2.	The formula for density is: Density = mass / volume
3.	The answers are all in g/cm^3 so we should convert our volume to cm^3. 1 litre = 1000 cm^3 Therefore, 2 litres = 2000 cm^3
4.	Substitute in the numbers:

Density = 1994 g / 2000 cm^3= 0.997 g/cm^3

The Pythagoras Theorem

This theorem, applicable only to right angle triangles, allows us to calculate the length of an unknown side given information about the other two sides. Given a triangle such as below, the theorem states that:

$$a^2 + b^2 = c^2$$

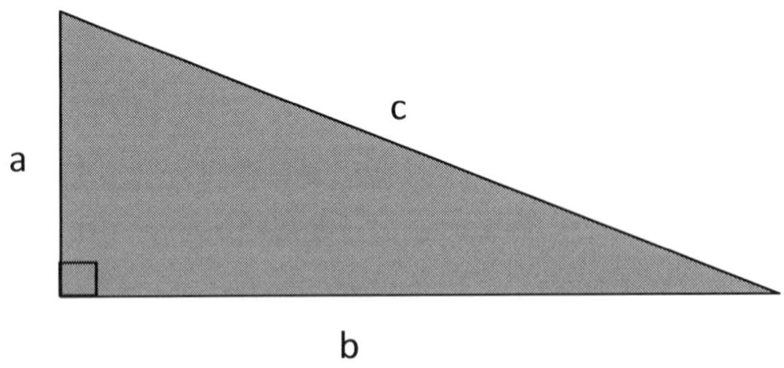

This can be written out as: *"The squared length of the hypotenuse of a right angle triangle is equal to the sum of the squares of the other two sides."*

This equation will not be given to you in the exam. You must memorise it and learn how to apply to it scenarios.

It is also very crucial that you know how to identify each side, as this will allow you to apply the theorem correctly:

- The **hypotenuse** is the longest side in the triangle, ***c***. It is directly opposite the right angle.
- The two sides making the right angle are interchangeably ***a*** and ***b***, although once you begin your calculations, the letters cannot be exchanged.

Example 30

James has a farm in the shape of a triangle. It has two straight edges and one diagonal edge. The straight edges are fenced, as shown in bold on the diagram below. The diagonal edge is not fenced, although someone is moving in on the other side of the diagonal edge so James wishes to fence this side as well.

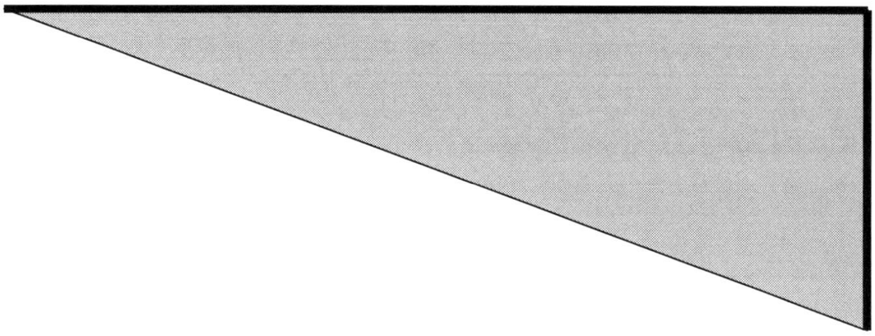

Given that one fenced side is 15m long and the other is 7m long, how many metres of fencing should James buy for the diagonal side?

A. 16 metres
B. 17 metres
C. 22 metres
D. 15 metres
E. 8 metres

Answer 30

The correct answer is B. From the diagram above, we can see that the remaining, fenceless side is the longest side and opposite the right angle. As each fence corresponds to the length of its respective side, it is the length of the hypotenuse the question is asking for.

The calculations are as follows:

<table>
<tr><td>1.</td><td colspan="2">The information we have is:

$a = 15$ m
$b = 7$ m
$c = ?$ where c is the hypotenuse

The formula is: $a^2 + b^2 = c^2$</td></tr>
<tr><td>2.</td><td>Method 1
Substitute the numbers into the equation:

$15^2 + 7^2 = c^2$
$225 + 49 = c^2$
$274 = c^2$</td><td>Method 2
You can alter the equation and start to solve for c if you square root both sides:

$\sqrt{a^2 + b^2} = \sqrt{c^2}$, therefore:
$\sqrt{a^2 + b^2} = c$

Substitute the numbers into the equation:</td></tr>
</table>

		$\sqrt{15^2 + 7^2} = c$ $\sqrt{274} = c$
3.	To obtain the length of the hypotenuse, c, we would need to square root both sides. $\sqrt{274} = \sqrt{c^2}$ Therefore, c = 16.55 m	Therefore, c = 16.55 m

Using method 2, students may mistakenly make the assumption that the squares on the numbers 15 and 17 are cancelled out by the square root sign, thus resulting in an answer of C. 22m. This is incorrect, as the square root applies to the whole of the equation. If there was a single number under the square root sign, then the square and square root symbols would cancel out. Because there is a full equation under the square root sign (i.e. numbers being added) and each square applies to its respective number, this rule cannot apply.

- *Note*: If the equation was within brackets, and the square applied to the whole equation, then the square root sign would cancel it out. E.g. $\sqrt{(15 + 7)^2}$
  Please note that this is completely different to $\sqrt{15^2 + 7^2}$. The value here is $\sqrt{247}$ whereas the value of $\sqrt{(15 + 7)^2}$ is $\sqrt{484}$.

The solution to our equation is 16.55m. This is not found within any of the answer options, so we need to select the best option. If you select A. 16m, James will be left with 0.55m unfenced. The question is asking how many metres James should **buy**. Thus, it is logical to buy slightly more than necessary in order to fully fence the area.

Therefore, James should buy 17 metres of fencing.

Example 31

Salma usually travels to the supermarket using the most direct route from her home, which is 5km in distance, as marked on the diagram below. Today, she plans to go to Rita's house first so they can travel to the supermarket together.

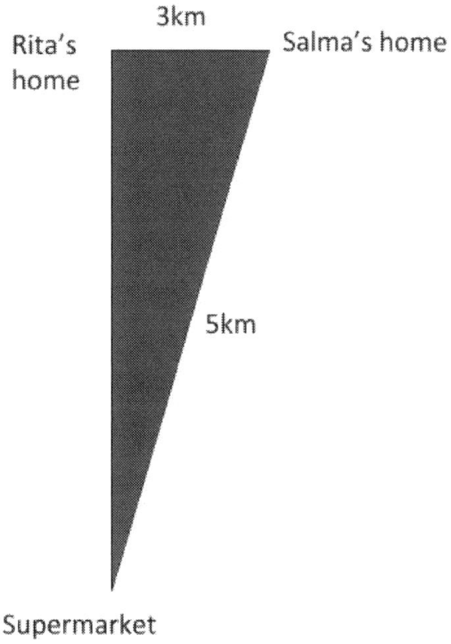

What distance will Salma and Rita will have to travel together to get to the supermarket?

A. 3 km
B. 3.5 km
C. 2 km
D. 4 km
E. 8 km

Answer 31

The correct answer is D. Based on the diagram, it is evident that Salma normally travels the length of the hypotenuse when she goes to the supermarket, i.e. the 5km path. Today, she will be travelling the other two lengths of the triangle.

However, it is important to note the wording of the question. It asks for the distance that the two will travel **together**, i.e. the length of the missing side. Ensure that you do not add the 3 km side to this. We must rearrange the equation, as we are *not* solving for the length of the hypotenuse, c.

We can either name the unknown side *a* or *b*. In this case, we will go with *a*, and rearrange the equation to solve for the length of *a*.

The calculations are as follows:

1.	The information we have is:

	$c = 5$ km $b = 3$ km $a = ?$
2.	The equation is: $a^2 + b^2 = c^2$
3.	Rearrange to solve for a: $a^2 = c^2 - b^2$ $a = \sqrt{c^2 - b^2}$
4.	Substitute in the numbers: $a = \sqrt{(5)^2 - (3)^2}$ $a = \sqrt{25 - 9}$ $a = \sqrt{16}$ $a = 4$

Therefore, the distance they will travel together is 4 kilometres.

Important Things to Remember

To sum up, here are some important things to remember when practicing for Quantitative Reasoning:

1. **Practice mental maths every day.** Start practicing simple mental calculations within 100. This will improve your timing significantly as you will not have to waste time using the calculator for calculations that you can complete accurately in your head within 2-3 seconds.
2. Beside the calculator and yourself, the **whiteboard** may be the most useful tool you can use during the exam. Here are a few tips on how to make the most of it.

   You should receive multiple laminated paper sheets as whiteboards, as well as markers and erasers. **Before you start, check that you have everything and they are all working**: take care to ensure that your markers have ink and that you have enough sheets to work with. Have the whiteboard handy and practice with it.
   - You may use it to illustrate multi-step calculations to better understand them.
   - Sometimes, a diagram given may not illustrate all of the necessary details. You can redraw diagrams to better understand them.
   - It may also be useful to write down numbers which you may need for future references, as the calculator is only able to remember one number at a time. However, make sure to write down a small "note" beside it, explaining what the number represents so you are not confused. This note does not have to be long, so you're not wasting a lot of time on it.

   Try not to rub anything out during your timed test. Clear the board during the 1-minute break in between tests instead.

3. **Practice with the required electronic hardware and software.** This may seem counterintuitive to the first tip, but it is important that you know how to use them when you need to.
   - **If you can, obtain a keyboard with a number pad**. The numbers are closer together on the number pad compared to the row of numbers above the alphabet, so using the number pad is far more time efficient. The keyboards in Pearson test centres are also equipped with number pads so you will have the opportunity to use one on the day.
   - **On the scratchpad:** If you do not have a whiteboard at home, you can use the scratchpad. It can be launched by clicking the icon at the top of the screen or using the shortcut alt+D.
     - It launches as a pop-up window which can be repositioned and resized
     - You can take notes and plan answers by typing into it.

- You can cut, copy and paste within the pad but not from the question to the pad.
- It will close when you move to the next questions but the text will still be there if you reopen it. The contents of the scratch pad are wiped at the end of each subtest.

If you plan to use it on the day, use it will you prepare as well. It may be especially useful for questions with difficult numbers, and may help you sort out your thoughts.

4. **Know your equations.** This section thoroughly explores nearly all of the concepts tested within the UCAT exam, and provides you with the necessary equations needed to solve the problems. Remember them! The exam will not provide you with any formulae other than the mile → kilometres conversion.
5. **Know your shortcuts.** It might only take a few milliseconds for you to use a mouse to click on the calculator, but when the milliseconds from all of the questions add up, you might be losing more time than you think. Therefore, try to memorise these shortcuts and incorporate them into your practice!

Alt + N	Next Question
Alt + P	Previous Question
Alt + F	Flag current question
Alt + C	Calculator
Alt + D	Scratchpad

6. **Eyeball whenever possible**!

Quantitative Reasoning Mock Test

Scenario 1

The following table shows the distribution of birthdays in a class of 30 students:

Month	Frequency
January	3
February	5
March	3
April	3
May	2
June	2
July	4
August	0
September	2
October	1
November	3
December	2

1. What percentage of students are born in the second half of the year?
    A. 50%
    B. 33.3%
    C. 40%
    D. 23%
    E. 38%

2. What is the ratio of students born in July to December to students born in January to June?
    A. 2:3
    B. 5:2
    C. 4.2:1
    D. 3:2

E. 5:3

3. What is the probability of the birthdays of two randomly selected students being in May?
    A. 0.00230
    B. 0.00444
    C. 0.00228
    D. 0.00460
    E. 0.00273

4. Which combination of months accounts for 40% of all birthdays in the class?
    A. January, February, March, May
    B. January, February, July
    C. February, July, September
    D. February, October, November, December
    E. February, July, October, November

Scenario 2

A car hire company offers a number of different types of vehicles. Insurance and hire cost are always charged at an hourly rate, while the deposit is refundable given there is no damage to the car when returned.

Type of Vehicle	Deposit	Insurance (per hour)	Hire Cost (per hour)
Standard	£50	£5	£8.50
Small SUV	£72.50	£8.20	£13.50
4x4	£80	£11.15	£16.35
Luxury	£125	£17.50	£22.65
Sport	£115	£17.50	£20.65

5. Tom hires a vehicle for 5 hours and returns it with no damage. His total bill is £67.50. Which type of vehicle did he rent?
    A. Standard
    B. Small SUV
    C. 4x4
    D. Luxury
    E. Sport

6. Assuming there is no damage, how much more expensive would it be to rent a luxury vehicle for 4 hours than a 4x4, given as a percentage?
   A. 42.5%
   B. 146%
   C. 142.5%
   D. 46%
   E. 4.6%

7. Tom comes back to hire another vehicle the next day. He hires it for 4 hours, and his final bill is £104. Which type of vehicle did he rent?
   A. Standard
   B. Small SUV
   C. 4x4
   D. Luxury
   E. Sport

8. There is a 15% markup on all hourly rates for each car. The insurance and deposit stay the same. How much does it now cost to rent a 4x4 for 6 hours (assuming no damage to the car)?
   A. £244.62
   B. £189.75
   C. £150.00
   D. £192.56
   E. £192.74

Scenario 3

The shape of a water container is a perfect cylinder, with height 1m and diameter 50cm.

The formula for the volume of the cylinder (V) is $V = \pi r^2 h$, where r is the radius and h is the total height of the cylinder.

The formula for the surface area of the cylinder (A) is $A = 2\pi rh + 2\pi r^2$

1 litre = 1 cubic decimetre (dm^3) = $1000cm^3$

9. What is the volume of the cylinder to 3 significant figures?
   A. 196 cm^3
   B. $1.96 \times 10^5\ cm^3$
   C. $7.85 \times 10^5\ cm^3$
   D. 785 cm^3

E. $1960cm^3$

10. What is the surface area:volume ratio?
    A. 2:1
    B. 1:1
    C. 1.55:1
    D. 1.62:1.32
    E. 1.83:1.94

11. If the diameter of the cylinder changed to 25cm, how would the height need to change to keep the volume the same?
    A. The height would be doubled
    B. The height would be squared
    C. The height would be multiplied by 4
    D. The height would be halved
    E. The height would be tripled

12. Water pours into the cylinder at a rate of 2 litres per second. How long would it take to fill the container?
    A. 19.6 seconds
    B. 22.2 seconds
    C. 98.0 seconds
    D. 12.2 seconds
    E. 9.8 seconds

Scenario 4

The following table shows the tax rates on annual income:

Band	Taxable Income	Tax Rate
Personal Allowance	Up to £12,500	0%
Basic Rate	£12,501 to £50,000	20%
Higher Rate	£50,001 to £150,000	40%
Additional Rate	Over £150,000	45%

13. How much income tax would someone earning £75,000 a year pay?
    A. £17,500
    B. £25,000
    C. £30,000
    D. £15,500
    E. £19,850

14. Lucy pays £12,500 income tax per year. How much is her annual salary before tax?
    A. £50,000
    B. £62,500
    C. £72,250
    D. £56,250
    E. £64,270

15. Alex pays £12,000 income tax per year. As a percentage of his monthly salary, how much does he need to save per month in order to have enough to pay his income tax?
    A. 1.63%
    B. 9.6%
    C. 20.0%
    D. 19.6%
    E. 18.3%

16. A change to the tax system means that any income between £100,000 - £150,000 will now be taxed at 45%, with the Additional rate moving up to 55%. Under the new system, how much would somebody earning £200,000 a year have to pay in income tax?
    A. £75,000
    B. £77,500
    C. £80,000
    D. £110,000
    E. £128,000

Scenario 5

A lorry driver needs to drive from London to Edinburgh, a distance of 402 miles. His average fuel economy is 6.8 miles per gallon (mpg).
1 gallon = 4.54 litres
1 litre of fuel = £1.14

17. If the lorry driver drives at an average speed of 55mph, how long does it take to reach Edinburgh?

A. 6.82 hours
B. 7.31 hours
C. 4.02 hours
D. 8.01 hours
E. 9.02 hours

18. How much would this journey cost in terms of fuel?
    A. £300
    B. £312
    C. £292
    D. £306
    E. £442

19. What would be the latest time that the driver could leave London at to still arrive in Edinburgh by 5pm?
    A. 08:30
    B. 09:20
    C. 09:40
    D. 10:15
    E. 10:45

20. The lorry has to make a diversion en route, causing the length of the journey to increase by another 10 miles. How much more fuel would the driver need in pounds?
    A. £7.00
    B. £7.61
    C. £5.57
    D. £6.46
    E. £7.74

Scenario 6

The following table shows the distances between 4 major cities in Italy:

	Rome	Florence	Milan	Naples
Rome	/	125 miles	200 miles	210 miles
Florence	125 miles	/	120 miles	85 miles
Milan	200 miles	120 miles	/	45 miles
Naples	210 miles	85 miles	45 miles	/

1 mile = 1.6 kilometres

21. It takes Adam exactly 4 hours to drive from Florence to Milan. What is his average speed in miles per hour?
    A. 30 miles/hour
    B. 40 miles/hour
    C. 45 miles/hour
    D. 60 miles/hour
    E. 70 miles/hour

22. The drive between Rome and Milan usually takes 4 hours. However, increased traffic means that the journey will take 5 hours on a given day. What is the difference in average speed between the two journeys?
    A. 5 miles/hour
    B. 10 miles/hour
    C. 15 miles/hour
    D. 20 miles/hour
    E. 25 miles/hour

23. Zakariya sets off on a drive between two cities, averaging a speed of 50mph. He breaks down 1.5 hours into the drive, meaning that he is 60% of the way to his destination. Which two cities is he travelling between?
    A. Milan and Rome
    B. Florence and Milan
    C. Rome and Milan
    D. Florence and Rome
    E. Florence and Naples

24. Gracie decides to travel from Rome to Milan via Florence. Assuming on the way back she travels directly from Milan to Rome, how long would the round trip take if she traveled at an average of 50mph?
    A. 8.6 hours
    B. 8.7 hours
    C. 8.8 hours
    D. 8.9 hours
    E. 9.0 hours

Scenario 7

A bank offers two different long-term investment accounts with two different types of interest: fixed-rate simple interest and compound interest. They also offer Lifetime ISA accounts, which have their interest calculated and altered yearly. Below are the standard interest rates for two of their accounts.

Fixed-Rate Simple Interest Account	5%
Compound Interest Account	3.5%

25. Sam invests £1000 into both accounts. After 5 years, what is the difference in value between the two accounts to the nearest pound?
    A. £55
    B. £62
    C. £78
    D. £65
    E. £66

26. How many years would it take for the Compound Interest Account to grow larger than the Fixed-Rate Account?
    A. 18 years
    B. 21 years
    C. 25 years
    D. 30 years
    E. 7 years

27. Sophie wants to invest £20,000 in one of these accounts, but is not sure which one to go with. Which would give her the greatest return after 10 years, and by how much (to the nearest thousand)?
    A. The Fixed-Rate account, by £2000
    B. The Fixed-Rate account, by £5000
    C. The Compound Interest account, by £2000
    D. The Compound Interest account by £5000
    E. They would be worth the same

28. Sophie decides to go with the Compound Interest account. How long would it take for her to make a 25% return on her investment?
    A. 6 years
    B. 5 years
    C. 7 years
    D. 8 years
    E. 9 years

Scenario 8

A sphere has a diameter of 1m.

29. What is the volume of the sphere in cm^3?
    A. 5.24×10^5 cm^3
    B. $1.48x10^6$ cm^3
    C. $148cm^3$
    D. $5240cm^3$
    E. $524cm^3$

30. What is the surface area of the sphere, to the nearest thousand cm^3?
    A. 30,000 cm^3
    B. 31,000 cm^3
    C. 32,000 cm^3
    D. 33,000 cm^3
    E. 34,000cm^3

31. A different sphere has volume 25,000cm^3. What is the diameter of the sphere to 3 significant figures?
    A. $36.1cm^3$
    B. $64.2cm^3$
    C. $18.2cm^3$
    D. $36.3cm^3$
    E. $37.4cm^3$

32. What is the surface area to volume ratio of the second sphere to 3 significant figures?
    A. 0.151
    B. 0.165
    C. 0.142
    D. 0.231
    E. 0.823

Scenario 9

The following pie chart shows the distribution of degrees held by 140 employees at a particular financial institution

Degree Subject

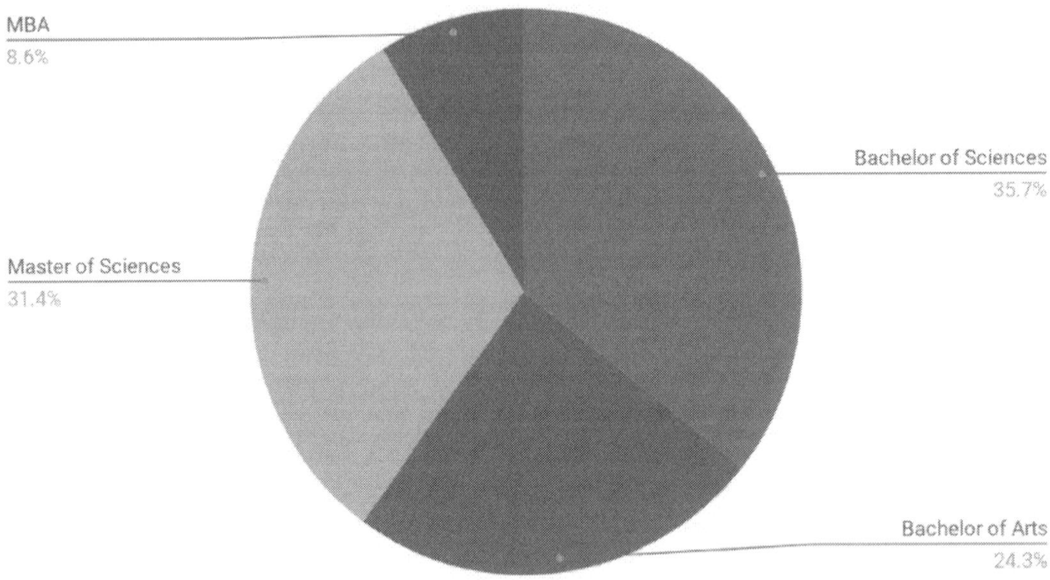

33. How many employees do not hold a degree in a scientific field?
    A. 42
    B. 44
    C. 46
    D. 48
    E. 50

34. What is the probability of randomly selecting two employees with MBA degrees out of the pool of 140 employees?
    A. 0.00678
    B. 0.678
    C. 0.00735
    D. 0.735
    E. 0.768

35. The firm hired 5 new employees. Two held MBAs and three held Bachelor of Arts degrees. What is the new percentage of employees holding MBAs to the nearest whole percentile?
    A. 10%
    B. 9%
    C. 12%
    D. 8%
    E. 6.5%

36. Including the 5 new employees, what would be the probability of randomly selecting three employees with Bachelor of Sciences degrees out of the new pool of employees?
    A. 0.0339
    B. 0.0394
    C. 0.0401
    D. 0.0422
    E. 0.3394

Quantitative Reasoning Answers

Scenario 1

1. The correct answer is C. Adding up all of the values from July to December will give you 12. 12 / 30 = 0.4 → 40%
2. The correct answer is A. Make sure you read the question carefully – it is asking for the ratio of July-December : January-June, not the other way round. 12:18 can be simplified into 2:3 by the division of 6 on both sides.
3. The correct answer is A. This question can easily catch you out. In order to find the probability of one person in the class having a birthday in May, you would use 2/30 as the probability. However, once this person is selected, the number of remaining students is 29, and the number of remaining students born in May is 1. Therefore, the second value you need is 1/29. (2/30) x (1/29) will give you the correct answer.
4. The correct answer is B. From the first question, we already know that 12 students make up 40% of the class. Therefore, we need to try the given combinations until one adds up to 12, in this case B.

Scenario 2

5. The correct answer is A. For this question, the most important thing to do is to read the question carefully. By doing that, you will know that the insurance needs to be added up hourly like the hourly rate, but the deposit is returned when the car is returned without any damage. You can add the insurance and the hourly rate together to get a "total" hourly rate of £13.50, and 13.5 x 5 = £67.50
6. The correct answer is D. By working out the total cost of hiring the two vehicles, you would then divide the value of the luxury car by the value of the 4x4. This would give you the number 1.46 → 46% increase.
7. The correct answer is A. By looking at the numbers of the other cars, you would be able to see that multiplying the hourly rates by 4 would not give a whole number because of their decimal places. Note how the question does not mention any damage on the car – all of the other questions specified that there was no damage and so the deposit was returned. In this case, the deposit was not returned and the answer is A – £54 hourly fee + insurance and £50 deposit.
8. The correct answer is B. All you need to do in this question is make the same calculation as you would when working out the cost of hiring any of the cars, but multiply the "hourly rate" number by 1.15 to reflect the 15% markup.

Scenario 3

9. The correct answer is B. Here, you want to use the formula $V = \pi r^2 h$. Be careful to convert 1 m when plugging in the numbers into the formula as the answers are in cm^3. Also, make sure that you use 25 cm as the radius instead of 50cm, as this is the diameter.
10. The correct answer is B. To work out the surface area, use the formula $A = 2\pi rh+2\pi r^2$. You will see that the surface area equals the volume, and so the ratio is 1:1.
11. The correct answer is C. If you cannot tell this by looking at the formula, the best strategy would be to see what happens when you halve the radius. Try out the different options given until one of them works. Alternatively, as you are dividing a square number by 2, you will need to multiply the other number by 2^2 (4) to get to your original value.

    $3.142(12.5^2) \times h = 3.142 \times (25^2) \times h$

    $156.25 \times h = 625 \times 100$

    $h = 400$ which is 4x more.
12. The correct answer is C. Use the information given to convert the volume into litres so you have smaller numbers to work with. 196 litres / 2 litres per second = 98 seconds.

Scenario 4

13. The correct answer is A. The maximum tax that can be charged from £12,500 to £50,000 is £7500 (37,500 x 0.2). The person in question earns £25,000 over the band of £50,000, so that £25,000 is taxed at 40%. 25,000 x 0.4 = 10,000, and 10,000 + 7,500 = £17,500.
14. The correct answer is B. This question is asking for the same thinking as the previous question, but in reverse. We have established that the maximum tax that can be charged from £12,500 to £50,000 is £7500 (37,500 x 0.2), and so we can take that number away from her total tax (£12,500) to get £5000. We know that the £5000 is 40% of her earnings above £50k, and so we can do £5000 / 0.4 to get £12,500. £50k + £12,500 is £62,500 → the answer is B.
15. The correct answer is D. We can use the same working as the previous question to work out how much he earns a year (£61,250). Dividing this by 12 will give his monthly salary of ~£5104. He needs to save £12k a year to pay his tax, which works out at £1k a month. £1k a month as a percentage of his total monthly salary is 19.6%, hence the answer is D.
16. The correct answer is B. Using the same style of working as the first question in this branch will give you the answer. Make sure to read the question carefully and use the correct tax bands, instead of the ones initially given in the table

Scenario 5

17. The correct answer is B. Rearranging the formula speed = distance / time to get time = distance / speed will give you the answer here.
18. The correct answer is D. You need to use the information given to you in the question to answer this one. The first step would be converting the miles per gallon value into miles per litre, which is 1.497 miles per litre. Then, divide the total miles driven by this number to work out the volume of fuel required, and convert to pence using the value given. Then, divide by 100 to get the value in pounds.
19. The correct answer is C. You can use the answer that you worked out in the first question to help you here. Be careful – 7.3 hours does not mean 7 and a half hours. Multiply the value in the first question by 60 to get the minutes, then take away the closest multiple of 60 to find the time in hours:minutes.
20. The correct answer is B. It is the same working as the second question, but without the initial step of working out miles per litre.

Scenario 6

21. The correct answer is A. Use the formula speed = distance / time to find your answer.
22. The correct answer is B. Calculate the two average speeds and subtract the larger from the smaller.
23. The correct answer is D. Calculate the miles he would have travelled in 1.5 hours, which is 75 miles. Then you are left with an inverse percentage calculation – 60% is 75 miles, so 100% of the distance is 125 miles.
24. The correct answer is D. Calculate the total miles she will do and divide by her average speed to get the time.

Scenario 7

25. The correct answer is B. The key thing here is to understand the meaning of simple interest vs compound interest. Simple interest gives you a fixed rate of interest on your initial deposit. For example, in this case the account holder would receive £50 per year. However, compound interest gives you interest on your entire account value, including interest you have previously earned. This means that the amount of interest you generate each year will increase the longer you keep the money in the account. To calculate the value of the simple interest account, add £50 to the account for every year it is held. For the compound interest account, you would want to multiply the £1000 by 1.035 for every year it is held in the account. Here, that would be £1000 x 1.035^5.

26. The correct answer is B. Using the above information, you just need to calculate a point where the compound interest account will be worth more than £1000 + (50 x the number of years). In this case, it would be 21 years.
27. The correct answer is A. Using the same logic as the previous two questions, work out how much each account will be worth after 10 years and compare the values.
28. The correct answer is C. Her initial investment is £20,000, so a 25% return would mean an increase of £5000. This happens after 7 years, and so the answer is C.

Scenario 8

29. The correct answer is A. Here, you want to use the formula $V=4/3(\pi r^3)$ to work out the formula. Be careful to convert 1 m to 100 cm and then divide by 2 when plugging in the numbers into the formula as the answers are in cm^3.
30. The correct answer is B. The formula $A = 4\pi r^2$ will give you the answer.
31. The correct answer is D. Use the formula for the volume of the sphere and rearrange it to make the radius the subject. Then, multiply the radius by 2 to find the diameter.
32. The correct answer is B. Previously, we have seen ratios given in A:B form. The numbers given are just another way of showing a ratio – A / B. In this context, they are the surface areas of the spheres divided by the volumes.

Scenario 9

33. The correct answer is C. Adding the percentages of the employees with an MBA and with a BA would give you 32.9%. 140 x 32.9 is equal to ~46 employees.
34. The correct answer is A. Similar to the question in the first block of questions, it is easy to be caught out here. Make sure that when you consider the two separate employees, you recognise that the first one is taken out of the pool of employees. In this case, you would want to use 12/140 x 11/139 for your answer - 12 being the number of employees with an MBA.
35. The correct answer is A. Adding 2 to the number of employees with an MBA and adding 5 to the overall number of employees would give you 14/145 as the required fraction, which equates to roughly 9.8%. Rounded, this would give you 10% → option A.
36. The correct answer is B. You can use the same logic as in question 42 - just make sure you use the updated figure of total employees.

SECTION 4

Abstract Reasoning

INTRODUCTION

Abstract Reasoning is the fourth section of the UCAT. It consists of 55 questions that are to be completed in 13 minutes. This gives roughly 14 seconds per question. Although students find this section to be particularly difficult at first, the questions tend to get easier with practice. Abstract Reasoning has the second highest average in most years, with the average being 653 in 2020.

This subtest assesses your ability to scrutinise patterns, deduce relationships from abstract figures, derive hypotheses, and to predict the next sequence in a pattern. The data within the questions presents in the form of abstract shapes, patterns and designs. The majority of questions are in sets of 5, while some are standalone questions. Each question is independent of other questions, and is associated with the pattern provided.

This section of the book focusses on identifying the key strategies that can be used to answer each type of question in Abstract Reasoning, with the main focus being on the various characteristics of patterns. Once you familiarise yourself with characteristics of patterns and how to spot them, pattern identification will become much easier for you. To help you out, there are many written examples, tables, diagrams, and a mock test towards the end.

Types of Questions

An overview of the types of Abstract Reasoning Questions:

Question Type	Time Needed	Description
Type 1	~70 seconds	There are 2 sets of shapes given (Set A and Set B), each with 6 boxes representing the same pattern. 5 associated questions each show 1 box. You must decide whether the box demonstrates the same pattern as Set A or Set B.
Type 2	~10-15 seconds	There is a specific change that is applied to a series of boxes that contain shapes. You must identify the change in order to select the next box in the series.
Type 3	~20 seconds	A specific change is made to one box. You must identify the change and apply it to another box.
Type 4	~70 seconds	Similar to Type 1 questions. Rather than 5 questions with 1 box each, you are given 5 questions with 4 boxes each, and you must identify which box in each of the questions belongs to either Set A or Set B.

Type 1 Questions: Sets

Type 1 Questions

Type 1 questions require you to analyse two sets (A and B) which each contain 6 boxes of shapes. The pattern in one set will apply to each of the boxes in the set and will be unlike the pattern in the other set. Once you identify the pattern, you can answer each of the 5 associated questions – simply determining whether each test shape given holds the same pattern as set A or set B.

Note: For the correct answer to be Set A, the test shape in question *cannot* also apply to Set B, and vice versa. If it happens to apply to both, you are either missing one of the patterns, or you must say that it applies to neither.

Example 1

Set A

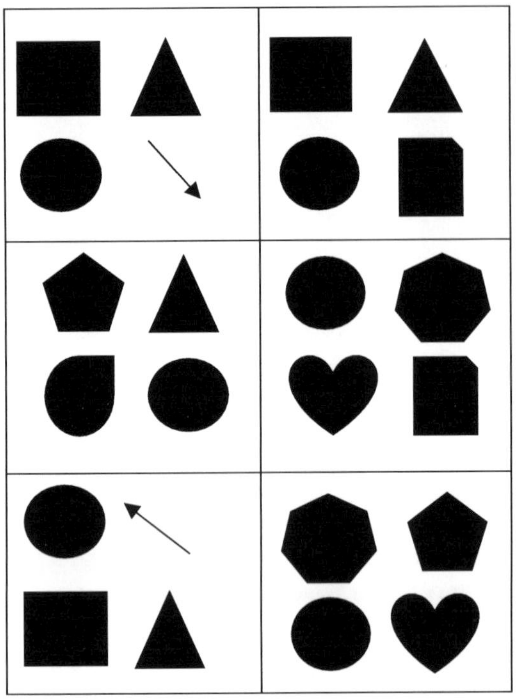

Set B

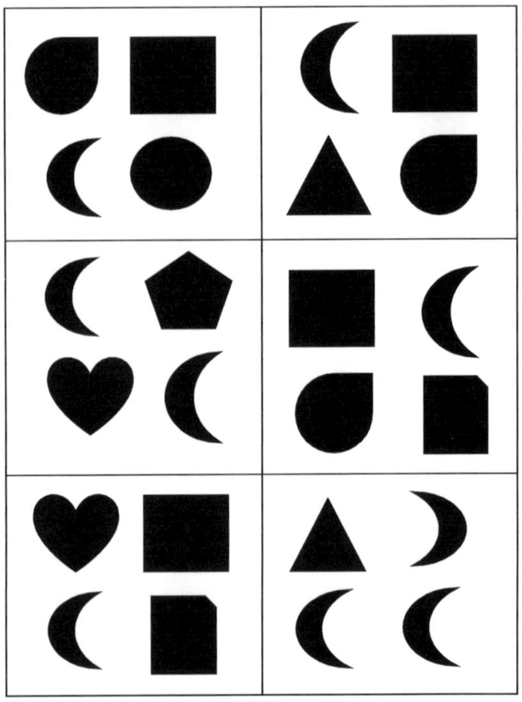

Determine whether the test shapes (1-5) belong to Set A, Set B or neither.

Test Shape 1 | Test Shape 2 | Test Shape 3 | Test Shape 4 | Test Shape 5

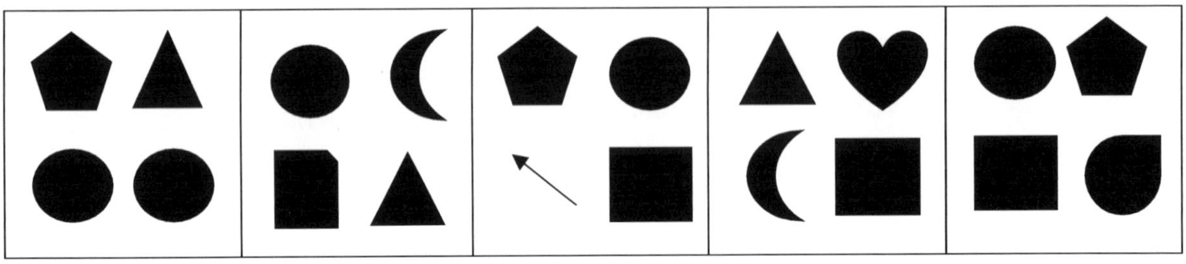

Test Shape 1	Test Shape 2	Test Shape 3	Test Shape 4	Test Shape 5
A. Set A	A. Set A	A. Set A	A. Set A	A. Set A
B. Set B	B. Set B	B. Set B	B. Set B	B. Set B
C. Neither	C. Neither	C. Neither	C. Neither	C. Neither

Answer 1

If this is your first time looking at Abstract Reasoning, you will find it very difficult to find the pattern here. Throughout this book, you will learn various strategies that will help you in pattern recognition. For now, understand the pattern is as follows:

Set A: There are 3 shapes in each box which have an odd numbers of sides (triangle has 3, circle has 1, arrow has 1, pentagon has 5, etc.) and 1 shape which has an even number of sides (square has 4, heart has 2, leaf has 2, etc.).

Set B: There are 3 shapes in each box which have an even number of sides and 1 shape which has an odd number of sides.

Notice how the pattern in Set B is the "inverse" of Set A. You will commonly see this type of relationship between Sets A and B throughout Abstract Reasoning. So, once you decipher the pattern in one set, it becomes much easier to find the pattern in the other. Furthermore, once you have found the patterns, it becomes easy to answer the 5 associated questions. If you keep in your mind, or potentially on your whiteboard, "**A= 3 odd, 1 even; B= 3 even, 1 odd**" you can answer the questions as follows:

1. The correct answer is C. Each of the 4 shapes has an odd number of sides, therefore, it does not fit into either Set A or Set B.
2. The correct answer is A. 3 shapes have an odd number of sides, while the crescent moon has an even number of sides.
3. The correct answer is A. The square has an even number of sides, while the other 3 shapes have an odd number of sides.
4. The correct answer is B. There are 3 shapes with an even number of sides, and the triangle has an odd number of sides.
5. The correct answer is C. You can see that the circle and the pentagon have an odd number of sides, while the square and the leaf have an even number of sides. This does not fit in with any of the patterns.

If this does not make sense to you, do not worry! You will understand it much more as you progress through this section of the book.

Type 1 Questions: General Strategy

When you first look at a pattern, you should always do so from a slight distance. Move your head back and take a quick overall glance at both sets to see whether anything obvious stands out. This makes much more sense when your brain is trained to recognise patterns, so you are unlikely to be able to apply this "quick glance" method when you are just starting your revision. If you see nothing at a quick glance, move on to the *simplest box rule*.

1. Locate the simplest box. This can be something that has the least number of shapes, the least number of lines, the least number of colours, the least variety, or whatever looks simplest to you.

2. The simplest box can be in either Set A or Set B, or both may have an equally simple box. It does not matter which set you look at first, as you will have to determine the pattern in the other set regardless.
3. If you feel like you may recognise a pattern within the simplest box you have chosen, look at the next simplest box to test your theory. The pattern must apply to every single box in the set in order to be valid, therefore, if it does not apply, you must try again.
4. If you cannot see any pattern in the simplest box, compare the two simplest boxes and see whether there is a similarity between the two.
5. *Note:* If you are short on time, see if the pattern applies to at least 3 of the boxes, rather than going through all of them. If it does apply to at least 3, there is a good chance that you have discovered the pattern.

Type 1 Questions: Finding the Pattern With SCANOS

SCANOS: Shape, Colour, Arrangement, Number, Orientation, Symmetry

To the untrained eye, finding patterns is extremely daunting. SCANOS covers the characteristics that many patterns consist of, giving you insight into what you should look for. It is important to note that you will not be given enough time in the UCAT to go through an exhaustive list of characteristics based on the SCANOS technique. However, with practice, you should adapt to identifying patterns based on the features of this acronym, and possibly develop your own preferred methods.

Shape

While trying to identify patterns, first try to locate whether there are certain subtle differences noticeable between the shapes present.

1. **Is there a specific shape present in each box?**

E.g. 1) Every box in Set A has 1 circle in it, whereas box in Set B has 1 square in it.

If you happen to notice this pattern, you can simply look through the 5 test shapes given and select "Set A" for the boxes that contain a circle, "Set B" for the boxes that contain a square, and "Neither" for the boxes that have none or both.

Note: There are usually 2 patterns in each set, so it will not be as simple as this. However, this is a good starting point!

2. **Are two shapes always present together?**

E.g. Every box in Set A has a circle and a diamond. There are no boxes without these two shapes, and no boxes with just one of these shapes. They are always present in a pair.

If you are able to recognise this, you can decide that any of the test shapes in the questions that have a diamond or a circle *alone,* without its respective partner shape, cannot belong to Set A.

3. **Is there a particular stand-out rule that applies to *each* of the shapes present in each of the boxes in a particular set?**

E.g. 1) Every shape in Set A has only straight lines, whereas every shape in set B has only curved lines.

For example, squares, triangles, pentagons, and octagons all have *only* straight lines. Circles, crescents, clouds, hearts, etc. have curved lines only. If a shape in the questions contains a semi-circle, you will know that this can belong to neither of the sets, as it contains both a curved *and* a straight line.

E.g. 2) Every shape in Set A has only concave shapes, whereas every shape in set B has only convex shapes.

This can be slightly difficult to define. When you learn about concave and convex shapes, you often think of a curve either going outwards (convex) or caving inwards (concave). Understand that these terms can also apply to polygons (shapes with straight edges, such as a square, cross, arrow or star). See the examples below:

Convex Shapes	Concave Shapes
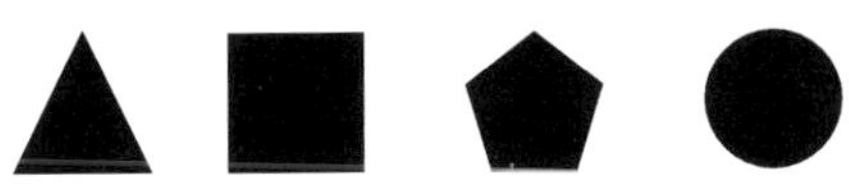	

Convex shapes cannot have any angles cutting into the bulk of the shape. You will notice that each concave shape has a "chunk", or multiple chunks, taken out of it. The cross shape is essentially a square with 4 angles cutting into each corner of it. The heart would be convex were it not for the inwards point at the top. The arrow has two inwards chunks, one on either side of it. These missing "chunks" are demonstrated in red in the table below.

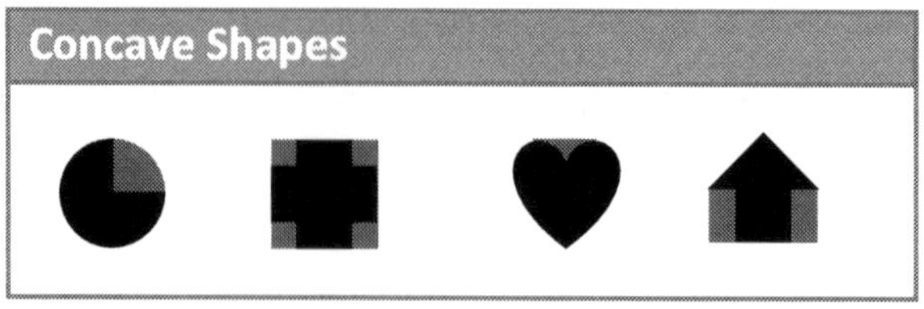

You will notice that the convex shapes are whole – they have no inwards caving or points, and no chunks missing out of them.

Note: If a shape appears to have both a convex and a concave side, it will be classified as ***concave***, as convex shapes cannot contain anything that is concave.

4. **What type of triangle is present?**

E.g. Set A only has right-angle triangles present, whereas Set B only has isosceles triangles present.

This is a common pattern to be aware of. Triangles can all look the same when you are not specifically looking for differences in them. It is important to determine whether there is a right angle (90°) or no right angle, as this could be the basis of the pattern.

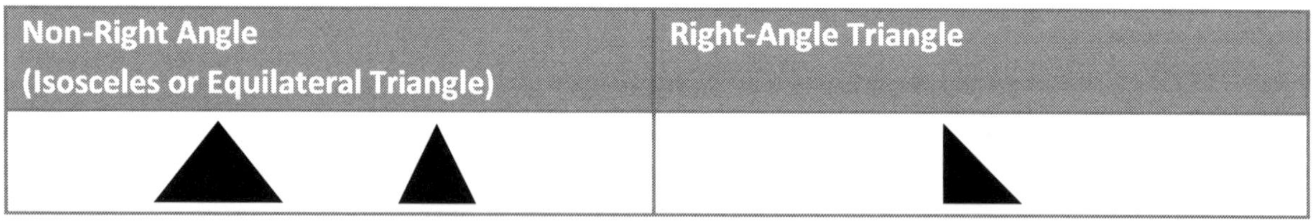

5. **Is there any irregularity in the shapes?**

E.g. Set A only has regular shapes, whereas Set B only has irregular shapes.

Regular shapes have a common internal angle in each of their sides and corners, whereas irregular shapes have varying internal angles. For example, a right-angle triangle is irregular, because it has one 90° angle and two 45°angles. However, an equilateral triangle is regular because each angle is 60°. A square is regular because each angle is 90°.

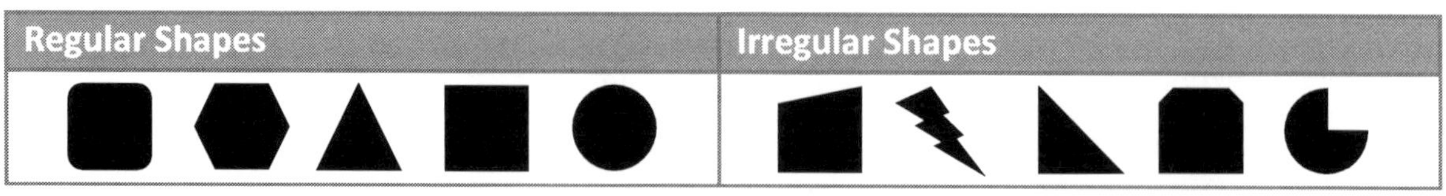

6. **Are there different sizes of shapes?**

E.g. Set A has 1 large shape in each box, whereas Set B has no large shapes at all.

Often, size differences between shapes are not very noticeable. However, if there is a pattern based on size, there will be at least 1 shape that has a clearly larger size than the shapes around it. If you see such a case, you will recognise that there are differences in size throughout the boxes, and these differences may lead you to finding the pattern.

Example 2

There is no question associated with this example. Simply determine the pattern in each of the following sets:

Set A

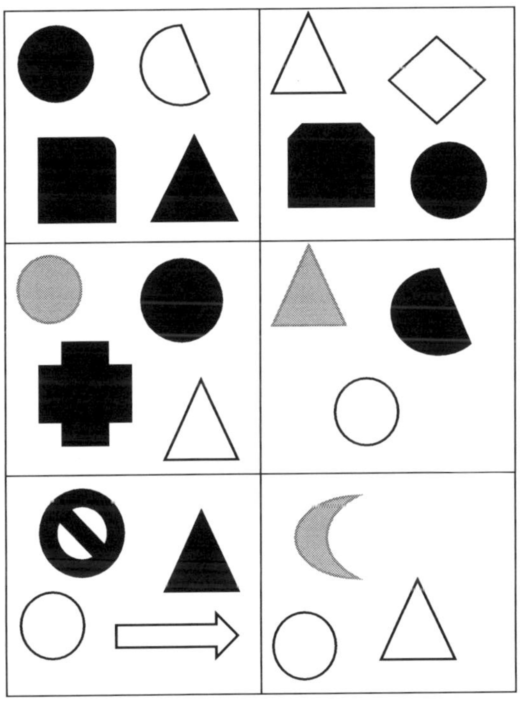

Set B

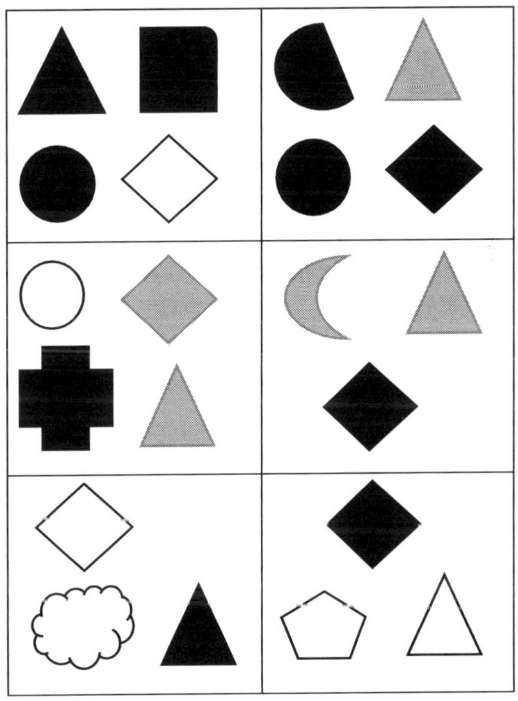

Answer 2

Following the rule of the simplest box, you will notice that most boxes have 4 shapes, while a couple in each set only have 3 shapes. In Set A, the 2 boxes with 3 shapes (middle right and bottom right) contain the following shapes:

- Box 1: Triangle, semi-circle, circle
- Box 2: Crescent moon, triangle, circle

You will notice that both boxes contain a triangle *and* a circle. If you look at the remaining boxes in Set A, you will notice that each of them contains a triangle and a circle. This rule applies across the whole set, so we have identified the pattern!

Now, let us look at Set B. As you know, the patterns in each set are usually related to the other set. So, in Set B, it would be wise to also look for shapes that are present in each of the boxes. Starting with the two boxes at the bottom which both contain only 3 shapes, you will find:

- Box 1: Diamond, cloud, triangle
- Box 2: Diamond, pentagon, triangle

Notice that both boxes contain a diamond *and* a triangle. If you check the remainder of the boxes in the set, you will notice that the rule holds true!

The colours of the shapes are not relevant in this section – they are simply there to distract you. You will learn more about distractors on page 276. However, sometimes colour can be relevant. The next section will explain this in more detail.

Colour

Identifying differences between colours of objects can certainly help in pattern recognition. In Abstract Reasoning, colour is generally limited to black, white and grey. Shapes can also contain patterns, such as stripes, which represent the colour of that shape. To identify patterns based on colour, you can ask yourself the following questions:

1. **Is there a specific colour allocated to a shape?**

E.g. 1) In Set A, the squares are always white, whereas in Set B, the squares are always black.

Remember, for a pattern to apply to the set, it needs to be present in every single box. So if there is a box without a square in it, this cannot be the pattern!

E.g. 2) In Set A, the squares are always white, whereas in Set B, the circles are always black.

This is another example of a pattern that is not directly inverse, but has a common theme across the sets. Again, every box in Set A would have to have at least one square, and every box in Set B would have to have at least one circle.

2. **Does the colour of a shape influence its size?**

E.g. In Set A, black shapes are always bigger than white shapes, whereas in Set B, white shapes are always bigger than black shapes.

Size can often be difficult to spot, as the difference between "big" and "small" may be minute. However, there is usually at least one box with a very clear difference in size. When you notice such a box, you should assess the pattern in that box.

3. **Does a specific colour correlate to the number of sides in a shape?**

E.g. In Set A, every shape with an even number of sides (square, hexagon, etc.) is white and every shape with an odd number of sides (circle, triangle, arrow, etc.) is black.

You can find more on the number of sides of a shape on page 256.

4. **Are there a certain number or ratio of coloured shapes to uncoloured shapes?**

E.g. 1) In Set A, there are 5 black shapes and 3 white shapes in each box. In Set B, there are 3 white shapes and 5 black shapes in each box.

This example demonstrates a simple inverse pattern between the sets. When deciphering the pattern in the next set, you should always check for the inverse. It will not always hold true, but the pattern will still be of similar nature to the pattern in the other set.

E.g. 2) In Set A, there are always double the number of white shapes as there are black shapes. In set B, there are always triple the number of white shapes as there are black shapes.

This example demonstrates how the pattern may not always be the inverse, but will still be of similar nature.

5. **Is there a relationship between the shape of an object, and where an arrow or a triangle in the box is pointing?**

E.g. In Set A, every time there is a black circle, the arrow points upwards, whereas every time there is a white circle, the arrow points downwards.

This is an example of a dependent relationship. The direction of the arrow is dependent on the colour of a specific shape. You can find more on dependent relationships on page 274 and more on orientation/direction of shapes on page 262.

This is not an exhaustive list of questions, but it should give you a good starting point. The more you progress through this book, the greater your understanding of key characteristics of patterns will become, and the better you will get at pattern identification.

Example 3

There is no question associated with this example. Simply determine the pattern in each of the following sets:

Set A

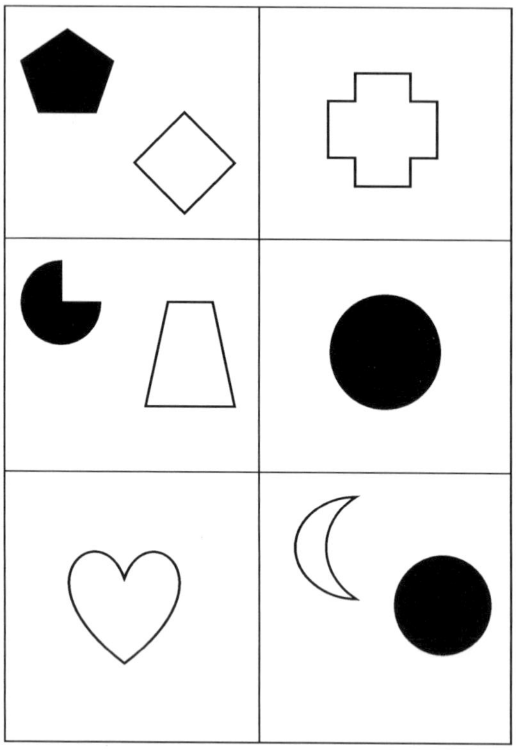

Set B

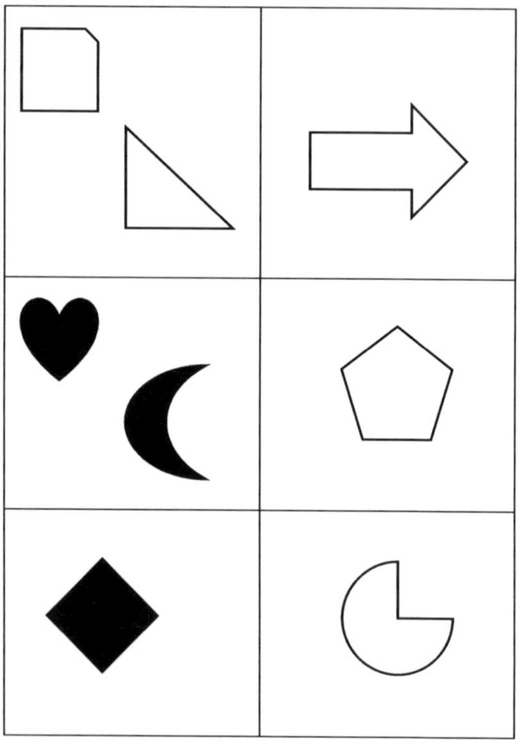

Answer 3

Following the general strategy, we should look for anything obvious that stands out. There appears to be nothing, so we can move on to the simplest box rule.

In Set A, the bottom left has a single heart which is white and has 2 sides to it. From what has been discussed thus far, there is not much else to note about this box. We can now look at the next simplest box – the middle right. This is an ideal box to compare, as it is simple and appears to be a contrast to the previous box. In this box, there is a black circle. Circles have 1 side. Notice that:

- A shape with 2 sides is white
- A shape with 1 side is black

Following the general strategy, we must now attempt to apply this rule to each of the other boxes. Try the top right. A cross has 12 sides and is white. 12 is similar to 2 in the fact that it is an even number. So perhaps all shapes with an even number of sides are white, and all shapes with an odd number of sides are black. Let us test this theory further by assessing a box with both a black and a white shape.

The top left box has a pentagon (5 sides – odd number) which is black, and a diamond (4 sides – even number) which is white. It fits! Ideally, we would love to test this theory on every single box. If you do, you will find that it applies. However, in an exam setting, you likely will not have the time. We have successfully applied this theory to 4 of the boxes, so we can be very confident that this is the correct pattern.

Let us now try the inverse of this pattern in Set B: each shape with an even number of sides is black, and each shape with an odd number of sides is white. Starting with the simplest box at the bottom left, a diamond has 4 sides (even number) and is black. That fits our theory. The box next to it has a shape with 3 sides (odd number) and is white. That also fits our theory. Congratulations, we have correctly identified the patterns in Set A and Set B! This was an example of dependent patterns, where the colour of the shape depends on the number of sides it has.

Arrangement of Shapes in a Box

Often, the shapes in each of the boxes of a set seem quite similar. If this is the case, you should immediately consider the way they are arranged.

1. **Is a specific shape always located in a specific place?**

E.g. In Set A, each box has a circle in its top right corner, whereas in Set B, each box has an arrow in its bottom left corner.

Notice here how the exact inverse does not apply, but the patterns between the boxes have an overall similarity. Therefore, if a box in the follow-up questions has a circle in its top right corner, you will know that it belongs to Set A, and any box with an arrow in its bottom left corner will belong to Set B. If a box contains both, or none, the answer will be "Neither".

2. **Is the arrangement of a shape relative to another shape?**

E.g. There is an arrow next to the circle in every box, no matter the positioning of the circle.

This kind of pattern may be present when shapes move around from box to box. For example, if the circle is on the left in one box, the right in another, down in another, middle in another, and so on. It is difficult to think that there is a constant arrangement when the shapes are always located in different places, but always consider that arrangement can be relative to the position of another shape. A shape can either constantly be adjacent to another shape (e.g. on its left, right, up, or down), or always be on a specific side of it (e.g. always on its right side).

3. **Is the arrangement of a shape dependent on any other factor?**

E.g. 1) When there is a square in the box, the black circle is located in the top right corner, whereas when there is a triangle in the box, the black circle is located in the bottom right corner.

This demonstrates the importance of comparing the location of particular shapes. You may notice that there is a black circle present in every box, and that it has 2 specific locations – top right corner and bottom right corner. You would need to identify the common factor between the boxes that contain the circle in the bottom right, as well as the common factor between the boxes that contain the circle in the top right.

E.g. 2) When the hexagon is white, the triangle is located on its right side. When the hexagon is black, the triangle is located on its left side.

This demonstrates that arrangement can be dependent on colour patterns within the box.

Example 4

There is no question associated with this example. Simply determine the pattern in each of the following sets:

Set A

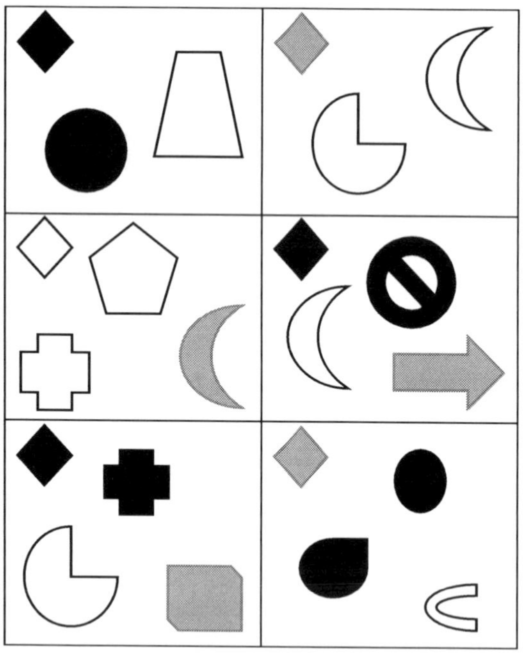

Set B

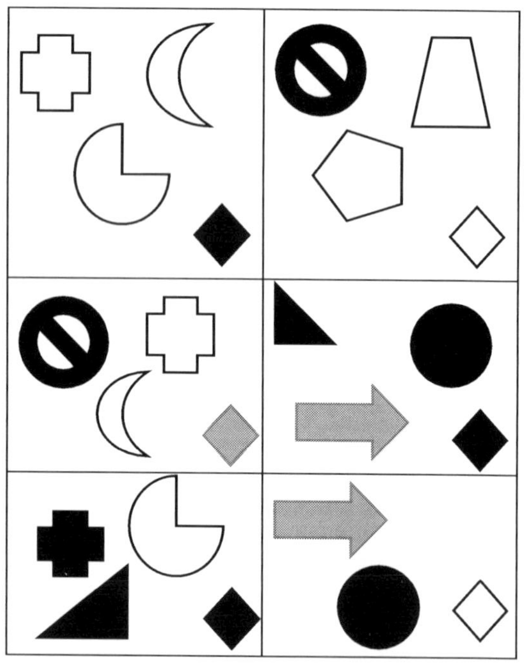

Answer 4

Let us begin again with the general strategy. You should quickly glance at both sets and see if any pattern stands out to you. In this case, there is a pattern that should be visible to some of you at just a glance. However, we will continue to practice the simplest box strategy, as that is the best way to go forwards when you cannot see any pattern.

You will notice that each box has a number of shapes – some have 4 while others have 3. We will begin by analyzing the simplest box in Set A – the top left. There is a diamond, a circle and a trapezium.

- Black shapes: diamond (4 sides) and circle (1 side)
- White shape: trapezium (4 sides)

There does not appear to be any sort of pattern with regards to the colour, as the only similarities we can see (from what we have learned thus far in the book) are the number of sides in the diamond and trapezium. These two shapes are opposite colours. Therefore, it is unlikely that colour has anything to do with the pattern, so it may be a distractor (see page 276).

Let us analyse the next simplest box to see if we can make a comparison between two boxes. The box in the top right has a diamond, a pie, and a crescent moon. What similarities can you see? The main thing that you should notice is that each box has a diamond, and the diamond is in the same location. Ignoring the colour, as we ruled that this may be a distractor, let us verify whether the location of the diamond is constant in each of the boxes. Yes, it is!

Pattern: In Set A, every single box has a diamond in the top left corner, with the colour of the diamond having no relevance at all.

Let us try to apply a similar rule for Set B. The simplest box in the bottom right corner also has a diamond which is in the bottom right, rather than the top left. Looking at the remainder of the boxes, the diamond is always in the bottom right in Set B. We have successfully identified the pattern based on arrangement!

Pattern: In Set B, every single box has a diamond in the bottom right corner, with the colour of the diamond having no relevance at all.

Number

There are various things you can count within a box to identify the relevant pattern. Some questions you can ask yourself to get started are:

1. **Are there a fixed number of shapes of a particular kind within every box?**

E.g. 1) In Set A, each box has 2 circles, whereas in Set B, each box has 3 circles.

This is a fairly straight-forward example. The next one is slightly more complex.

E.g. 2) In Set A, each box has 2 circles, whereas in Set B, each box has 3 arrows.

As previously stated, Set B and Set A will have similar patterns, but not always the inverse. In this case, the pattern is to do with the number of a shape present, but the shape is different between the sets.

2. **Do the shapes in each box have a total number of sides that is present in all of the boxes?**

E.g. 1) In Set A, each box has a total of 11 sides. Examples of this are as follows:

- Box 1: Triangle (3) + triangle (3) + circle (1) + square (4) = 11
- Box 2: Hexagon (6) + pentagon (5) = 11
- Box 3: Pentagon (5) + circle (1) + circle (1) square (4) = 11

This may be difficult to spot and it takes time to count the total number of sides in a box, but now that you know it is a possible pattern, look out for it! Besides knowing your basics, such as square, triangle, hexagon, etc., you should familiarise yourself with the table below to save you time counting during your exam.

Shape	Number of Sides
Circle	1
Heart	2
Arrow	7
Star	10
Cross	12

E.g. 2) In Set A, the sum of the sides in every box is an even number, whereas in Set B, the sum of the sides in each box is an odd number.

E.g. 3) In Set A, the sum of the sides in each box is a multiple of 2, whereas in Set B, the sum of the sides in each box is a multiple of 3.

In such an example, Set A would clearly only have an even number of sides in each box, whereas Set B would either have 3, 6, 9, 12, 15, 18, etc. number of sides in a box. Therefore, Set B has even **and** odd. You may initially find the pattern of even sides in Set A, then find that there is no such pattern in Set B. Think about multiples in this case – the number of sides may all be multiples of 3!

3. **Does each box contain a specific number of a certain angle?**

E.g. In Set A, each box has 5 right angles, whereas in set B, each box has 4 right angles.

See the table below for the number of right angles present in common shapes. Remember your odd shapes such as arrows and crosses! They each have a number of right angles in them.

Shape	Number of Right Angles
Right-angle Triangle	1
Arrow	2
Square/Rectangle	4
Cross	8
Irregular Polygons	Variable

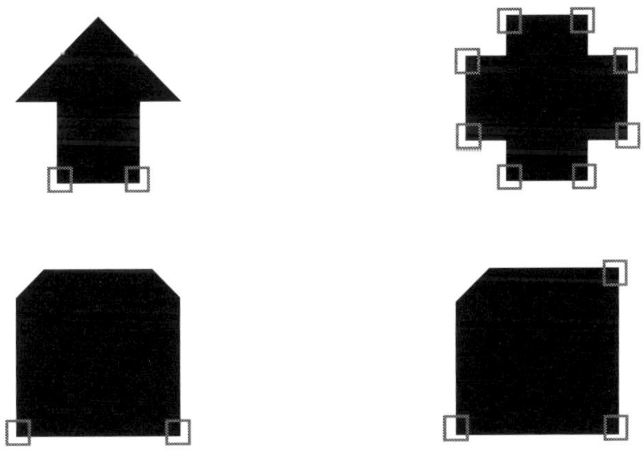

4. **Are there a specific number of diagonals, corners, or anything else in each box?**

E.g. In Set A, each box has 2 diagonal lines, whereas in Set B, each box has 4 diagonal lines.

This is an example to show that there are various different things to look out for. Rather than focusing on the bigger picture, such as number of shapes, you may have to look at finer details, such as specific aspects of each shape. For example, a star and an arrow both have diagonal lines. So, rather than counting the total number of sides, you may have look at the total number of a specific type of side, such as diagonal lines.

5. **Is there a pattern based on multiples of a number?**

E.g. 1) The number of shapes in each box in Set A is a multiple of 3, whereas the number of shapes in each box in set B is a multiple of 4.

In this example, Set A might contain boxes with 3, 6, and 9 shapes, while Set B might contain boxes with 4, 8, and 12 shapes. Multiples are more difficult to spot so you should be on the lookout for them.

E.g. 2) The sum of the sides in each box in Set A is a multiple of 4, whereas the sum of the sides in each box in Set B is a multiple of 5.

In this example, you would find that the total number of sides in each box in Set A is 4, 8, 12, 16, and so on. The total number of sides in Set B would be 5, 10, 15, 20 and so on.

It may be more difficult to notice such a relationship. The best way to do so is to first see if there is any obvious pattern, such as a large gap between the number of shapes in each box (e.g one box has 5 whereas another has 10 and another has 15 – always a large gap with nothing in between). Large gaps are more visible to the eye without needing to be counted, so if you happen to spot large gaps, you can count to check for multiples.

The most thorough way to find number patterns is to just count everything you can possibly think of, but time would not allow for such a task. It is important to note that you should not be simply counting for no reason. If there appears to be a pattern based on some numbers, and you happen to have noted some of the numbers involved, you can use these examples (such as even vs odd, multiples of numbers, etc.) to determine the bridging factor between the numbers. For example, if it is clear that there are circles in every box but the number varies between boxes, it may be worth counting how many circles are in the boxes of a set. You may find a pattern associated with the number of circles, which probably would then depend on something else present in the box. E.g. Every time there is a triangle in the box, the number of circles is a multiple of 2, whereas every time there is a square in the box, the number of circles is a multiple of 3.

6. **Is there a different numerical pattern I have not yet spotted?**

E.g. 1) In Set A, each box has a *prime number* of shapes, whereas in Set B, each box has a *composite number* of shapes.

Perhaps it has been some time since you learned about prime and composite numbers. A prime number is a number that cannot be divided by anything (besides 1 and itself) to produce a whole number. Examples include: 2, 3, 5 and 7. There are no two numbers that can be multiplied to produce any of these *prime* numbers.

A composite number is the opposite – it is possible to divide it (by other than 1 and itself) in order to produce a whole number (i.e. with no decimals). Examples include: 4, 6, 8, and 9.

- 4 / 2 = 2 (a whole number), therefore 4 is a composite number.
- 6 / 3 = 2 (a whole number), therefore 6 is a composite number.
- 8 / 2 = 4 (a whole number), therefore 8 is a composite number.
- 9 / 3 = 3 (a whole number), therefore 9 is a composite number.

Note: The number 1 is neither a prime number nor a composite number.

Prime Numbers	Composite Numbers
2, 3, 5, 7, 11, 13, 17, 19, 23, 29, 31, 37...	4, 6, 8, 9, 10, 12, 14, 15, 16, 18, 20...

E.g. 2) In Set A, the sum of the sides in each box is a prime number, whereas in set B, the sum of the sides in each box is a composite number.

This is a possibility! Learn your prime and composite numbers and consider these when you are doing your practice questions.

Example 5

There is no question associated with this example. Simply determine the pattern in each of the following sets:

Set A

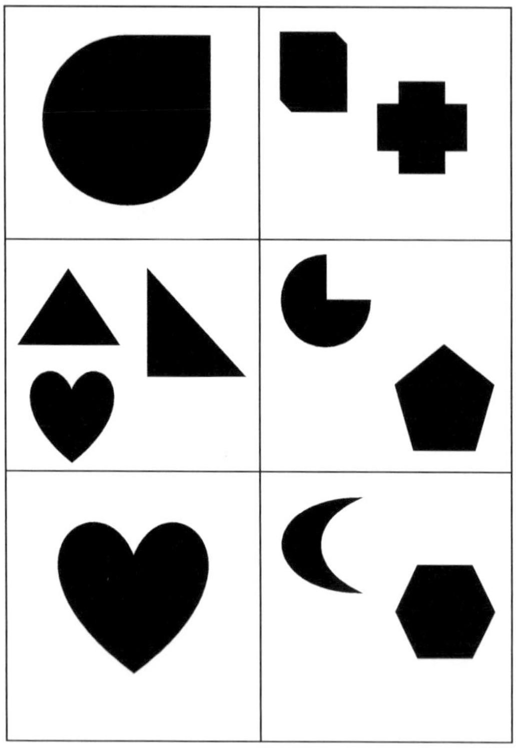

Set B

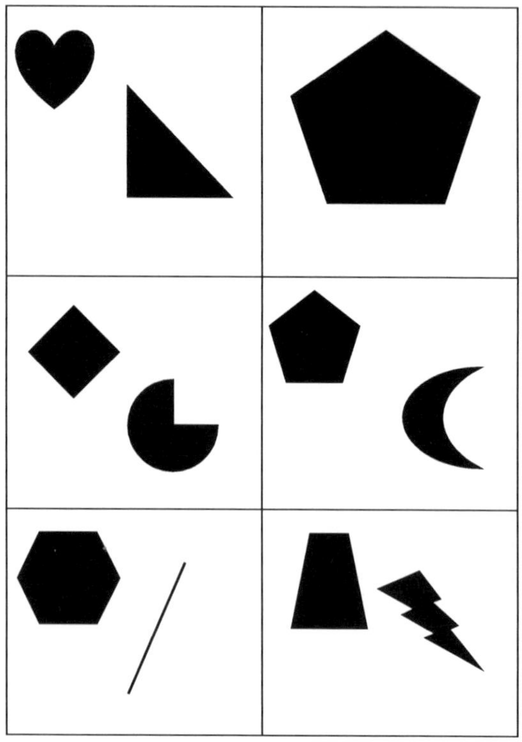

Answer 5

Following the general strategy, have a quick glance at each of the sets. There is no easily recognisable pattern. Therefore, let us start to analyse the simplest box. The top left box in Set A has a raindrop shape. When assessing for patterns in numbers, we can start with the simplest thing – number of shapes. Clearly, there is a different number of shapes in each box – either 1, 2, or 3 shapes. There appears to be no pattern here. There is also no shape that is present in every box, so it cannot be to do with the number of a particular shape in each box.

Therefore, we must delve deeper and assess the characteristics of the shapes. From the characteristics we have discussed thus far, the raindrop has the following:

- 2 sides
- 1 right angle

Let us try the next simplest box and see whether any of these apply there. The heart in the bottom left corner has the following in common:

- 2 sides

So we have already excluded the pattern of 1 right angle. Let us try the next simplest box – the bottom right. There are multiple shapes: one with 2 sides (which fits our previous theory) and one with 6 sides. This does not fit the theory of only 2 sides on each shape, which is likely an unwise theory to begin with, as most shapes will have more than 2 sides. However, we know that where there were 2 sides in a shape, there was also 2 sides in the entire box as each of those boxes only had one shape. 2 is an even number, so we might, instead, have an even number of sides in each of the boxes. In this box, 2 + 6 = 8, which satisfies this theory.

Let us check the box above it to confirm. The pie has 3 sides and the pentagon has 5. 3 + 5 = 8, also an even number! You can carry on counting and will find that this pattern holds true for all of the boxes in Set A.

It would only make sense to now try the inverse for Set B. Upon counting, you will find that the sum of the sides of each shape within an individual box in Set B is always an odd number.

Orientation

The orientation of a shape refers to the direction that it is facing. When shapes change orientation across a set, it is possible that this change is associated with the pattern. To better understand orientation, you can ask yourself the following questions:

1. **Do all of the arrows point towards a particular direction?**

E.g. 1) In Set A, each box has an arrow that points to the right, whereas in Set B, each box has an arrow that points upwards.

This kind of pattern would be very easy and straightforward. Therefore, to make it more difficult for you, the question-writers might add in various other shapes with irrelevant colours and move the position of the arrows each time. You would then have to look past all of the distractors and notice that there is an arrow in every box that always points in a particular direction.

E.g. 2) In Set A, each box has an arrow that points towards the square. In Set B, each box has an arrow that points away from the square.

In this kind of example, the square would likely move around from box to box, causing the arrow to point in various directions throughout the boxes, but it would *always* point towards the square. This is trickier to spot, as you would need to identify the relationship between the arrow and the square, rather than looking at the arrow on its own. It would be easier to spot this when comparing the two simplest squares, rather than attempting to look at each simple square individually. An example of this is shown below, although in a real question, there would be various other shapes in each box to distract you.

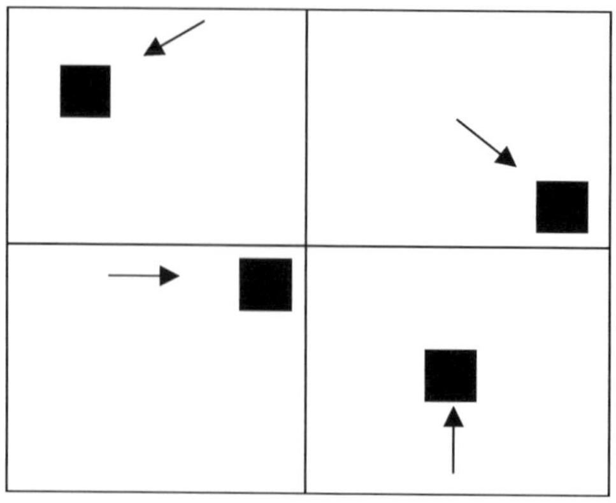

2. **Are certain shapes rotated by a particular angle, respective to the other shapes?**

E.g. In Set A, when a square is present in a box, the arrows rotate 45° to the right, but when a circle is present in a box, the arrows rotate 45° to the left.

Although there would likely be other shapes and distractive elements present in each box, the basic pattern may appear as follows:

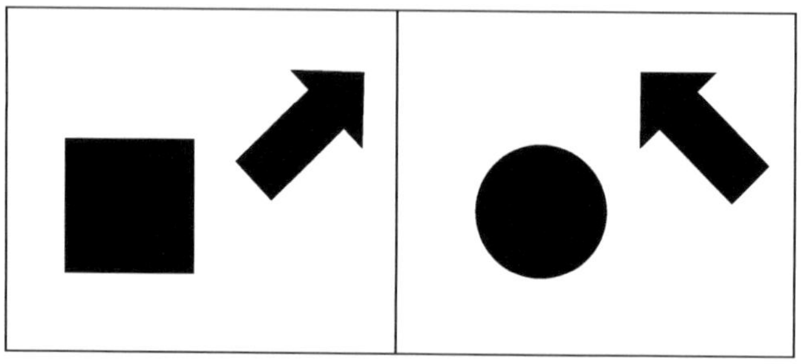

This is another example of a dependent pattern. Rotations are slightly more complex. You should not have to think about exact angles here, but notice a general pattern when shapes are rotating. This can include rotating 90°, 180°, and 270°, whereby it may be less obvious as the shape simply appears to be pointing towards the right, left, up or down of the screen.

3. **Does the orientation of a shape depend on any numerical factor?**

E.g. 1) In Set A, a box with an even number of arrows only has triangles that point downwards, whereas a box with an odd number of arrows only has triangles that point upwards.

This is another dependent relationship. The direction of the triangle depends on the number of arrows present within the box. This is something we have seen a few times now, but what if we change it up slightly?

E.g. 2) In Set A, a box with an even number of arrows only has triangles that point downwards, whereas a box with an odd number of arrows only has triangles that point to the right.

This is much more complex than the previous pattern. Usually, the dependent relationships we have looked at have demonstrated their own "inverse" within the same set (i.e. even number of arrows = downwards pointing triangles; odd number of arrows = upwards pointing triangles). However, the inverse does not apply here, as the triangles point towards the right, rather than upwards. This is much more difficult to spot, so do not worry if you cannot see this kind of pattern straight away. A simple diagram of this pattern is as follows:

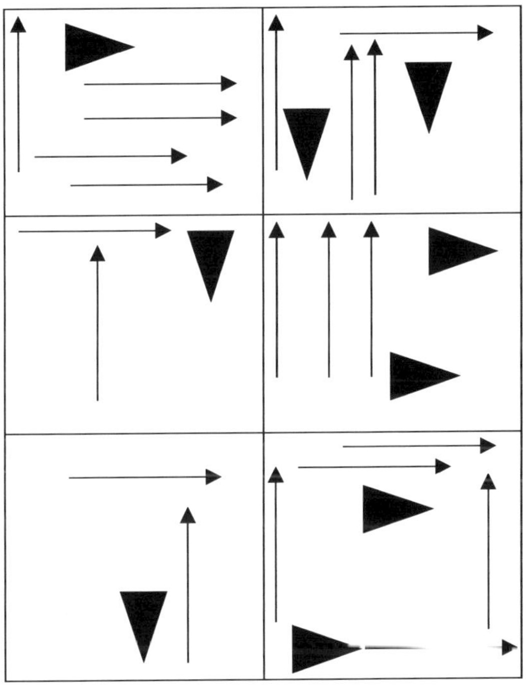

It is not hard to see that there are two directions the triangle points: right and down. In each box, there is only one direction of triangle, i.e. it never points down and to the right in a single box. However, the arrows point in two different directions within the same box. Considering this, you can try to work out the pattern. There appears to be no relationship between the direction of the arrows and the direction of the triangle, but there is a clear relationship between the number of arrows and the direction of the triangles in the box. However, it is not usually this simple. Let us look at the same pattern with a number of distractors:

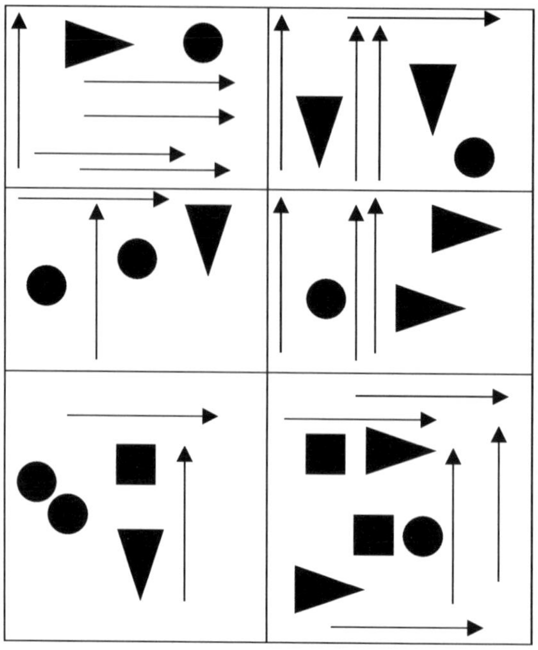

This set is the same as the above set, with random circles and squares added for distractive purposes. The relationship between the direction of the triangles and the number of arrows is the same, but it is much more difficult to spot here. Key tip: it takes time. Your brain needs to learn how to recognise patterns, and with practice, it eventually will!

4. **Is there a ratio between the number of times a shape is orientated in one direction and the number of times it is orientated in another direction?**

E.g. 1) In Set A, in a box, the number of times the arrows point upwards is always equal to the number of times they point downwards. In Set B, in a box, the number of times the arrows point upwards is double the number of times that they point downwards.

In this example, the orientation of the shape is the same between the sets – upwards and downwards. However, the ratio of up:down is different between the sets. You can expect to have various other orientations as well to distract you – such as arrows pointing left, right, diagonal in each direction, and triangles also pointing in each direction possible. If you start with the simplest square, it will be much easier to identify a pattern that is relevant to each box. The simplest square is likely to have the least number of distractors.

E.g. 2) In Set A, the number of times the triangles point towards the left is always equal to the number of times the arrows point upwards. In Set B, the number of times the triangles point towards the right is always equal to the number of times the arrows point downwards.

This is much more complex as it involves a dependent relationship between varying orientations of two different shapes. This demonstrates how many of the domains of patterns that have been discussed can appear together in one question.

5. **Are the number of shapes pointing in one direction greater or less than the number of shapes pointing in another direction?**

E.g. 1) In Set A, the number of arrows pointing towards the left is always 1 less than the number of arrows pointing towards the right.

In this example, there may be a large number of arrows pointing in all different directions. Again, if you start with the simplest box, pattern recognition will be easier. You will be able to identify the orientations that are necessary to the pattern – for example, if the simplest box has *no arrows pointing upwards*, it may be possible to ignore the orientation of the upwards pointing arrows as they may not be part of the pattern.

- *Note*: Use this suggestion with caution, as there can be patterns where the orientation is simply to do with pointing away from each other, towards each other, etc. rather than the exact direction that the arrow is pointing.

E.g. 2) In Set A, the number of triangles pointing to the right is always less than the number of triangles pointing upwards. In Set B, the number of triangles pointing to the right is always more than the number of triangles pointing upwards.

In this kind of example, if there was an equal number of triangles pointing right and left, you would know that it belongs to neither set.

6. **Is one orientation of a particular shape relative to its other orientation(s)?**

E.g. In Set A, the number of times that arrows point towards each other is always the same as the number of times that arrows point away from each other.

This example further demonstrates that orientation does not have to be in a particular direction, but can be relative to another factor, such as the other orientations of the same shape. It further takes into account numbers and ratios – the ratio of the number of times the arrows are orientated in one direction to being orientated in another direction is 1:1.

Note: Pointing towards each other means for the arrow heads to point towards each other. This is shown below:

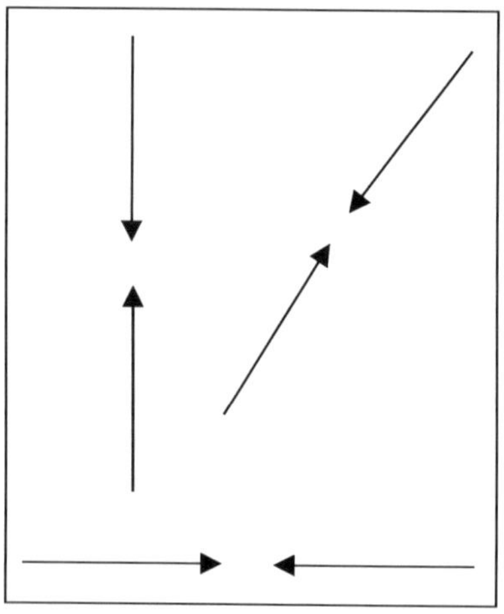

Example 6

There are no questions associated with this example. Simply determine the patterns in the following sets:

Set A

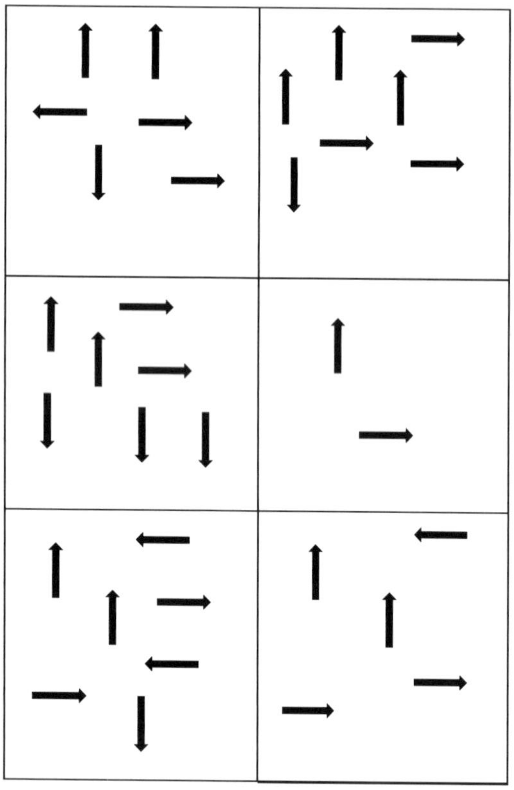

Set B

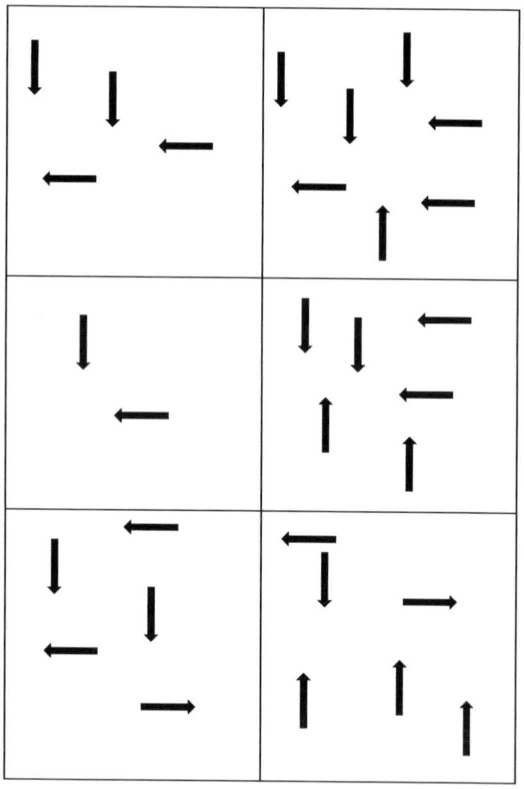

Answer 6

If we assess the various other domains of SCANOS that have been discussed thus far, we will find that none of them are useful in helping us to identify this pattern:

- S – There is only one type of shape present

- C – There is only one colour
- A – The arrows are scattered everywhere so there cannot be a pattern to do with arrangement
- N – there are slightly different numbers of arrows in each box, but perhaps not different enough to result in a pattern. This cannot exactly be excluded on a glance – you will need to count to make sure.

When there are shapes that have variable orientation, such as arrows and triangles, you should always consider orientation. Starting with the simplest box in Set A, the middle right, we find the following:

- 1 arrow pointing upwards
- 1 arrow pointing to the right

There are no arrows pointing left or upwards, so we can try to ignore any of those arrows for now. Let us check the next simplest box and compare it to the first. The bottom left box has:

- 2 arrows pointing upwards
- 2 arrows pointing to the right
- There is also 1 arrow pointing to the left – this is likely to be irrelevant as this direction was not present in the simplest box.

From the two simplest boxes, it appears that the number of arrows that point upwards is *equal* to the number of arrows pointing to the right. If you check the remaining boxes, you will find that this pattern holds true.

Now that we know there is a pattern to do with the ratio of the number of arrows pointing in different directions, we can try to identify a similar pattern in Set B. Starting from the simplest box, the middle left, we can see that there is 1 arrow pointing down and 1 arrow pointing left. If you check the remaining boxes, you will find that the number of arrows pointing downwards is always equal to the number of arrows pointing to the left.

The remaining arrows have been placed in each box to distract you. This is a prime example of how the simplest box strategy is very effective.

Symmetry

Symmetry: the perfect sense of proportion and balance noticed in objects and shapes.

Often, students ignore symmetry as a crucial factor and thus are unable to identify any related patterns. A line of symmetry is an imaginary line drawn on a shape. Across both sides of the line, the shapes are symmetrical, or are in proportion. In basic terms, you can say that across the line of symmetry, one part of the shape is a mirror image of the other part.

There are different kinds of symmetry, but for the purposes of Abstract Reasoning, we will cover a select few.

Bilateral symmetry: An object appears as a mirror image across an imaginary line of symmetry.

Example:

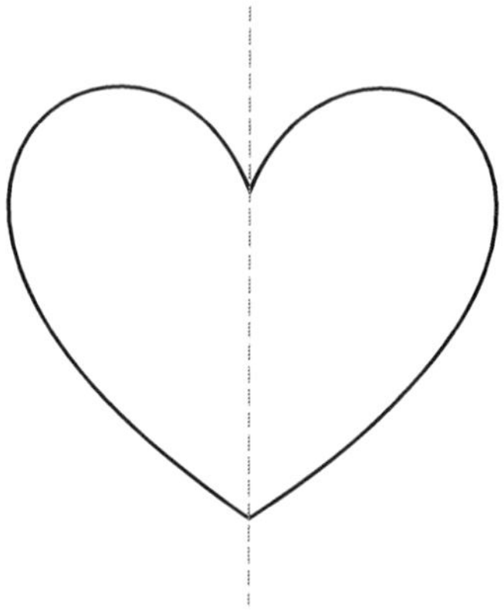

Many objects have more than one line of bilateral symmetry, although a heart has just one.

The following table demonstrates common shapes and their lines of bilateral symmetry.

Isosceles Triangle 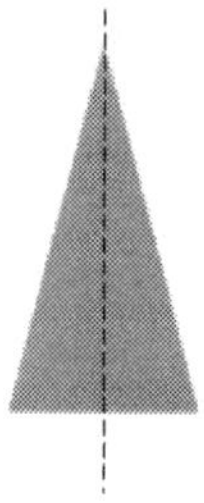 1 line of symmetry	Arrow 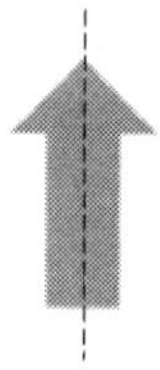 1 line of symmetry
Rectangle 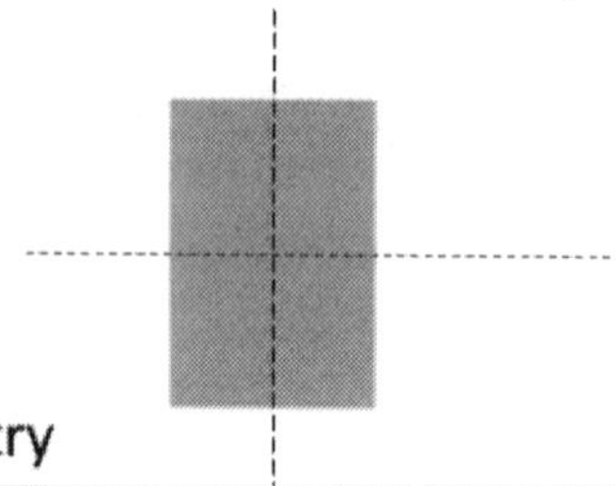 2 lines of symmetry	Triangle 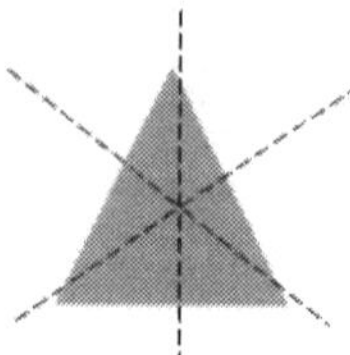 3 lines of symmetry
Cross 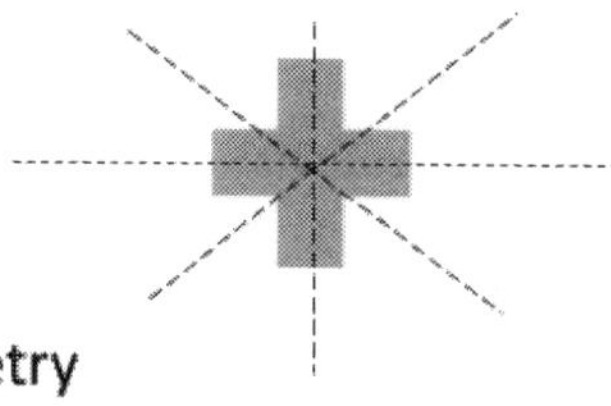 4 lines of symmetry	Square 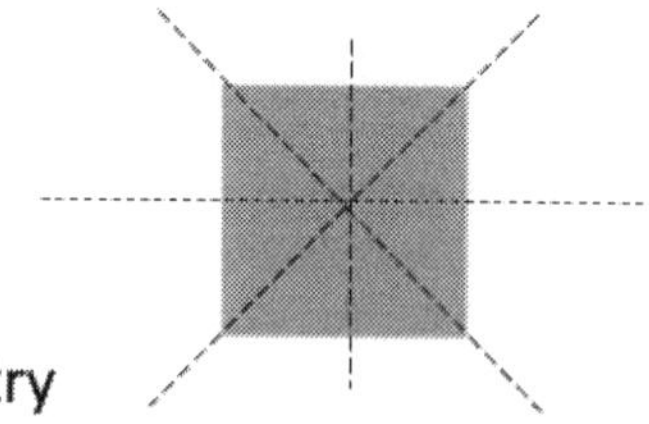 4 lines of symmetry
Regular Pentagon 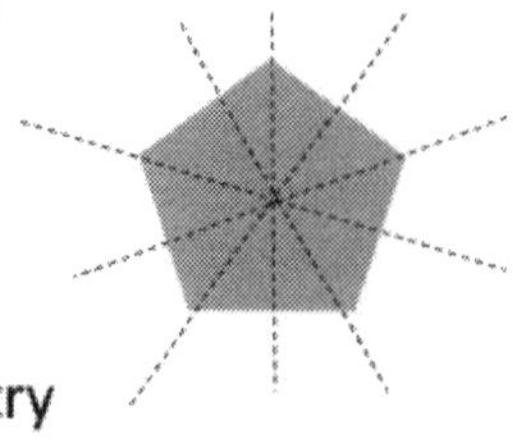 5 lines of symmetry	Regular Hexagon 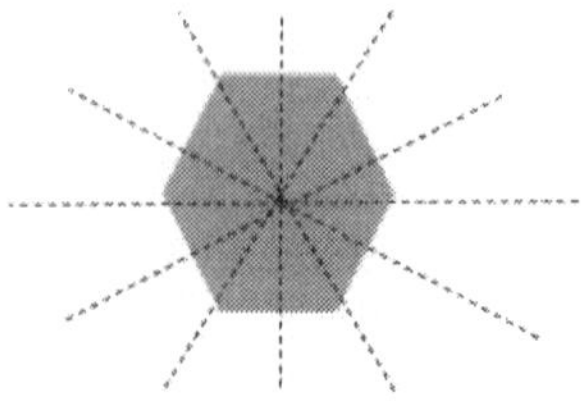 6 lines of symmetry

Rotational/Radial symmetry: The orientation of a particular shape remains the same when it is rotated in a specific direction around a point.

Order of rotational symmetry: The number of times a figure can be rotated within 360° and maintain the same orientation. E.g. The order of rotational symmetry of a square is 4, as it will have the same orientation when rotated 90°, 180°, 270° and 360° (or back to 0°).

Example:

In the diagram below, the black circle represents the corner with the starting point of the triangle. If you turn an equilateral triangle 120°, it appears exactly the same as its starting point. If you then turn it another 120°, it appears the same again. And if you turn it a final 120°, it returns to its starting point. Therefore, an equilateral triangle is said to have a rotational symmetry order of 3, as it can be turned 3 times and appear exactly the same before returning to its normal orientation.

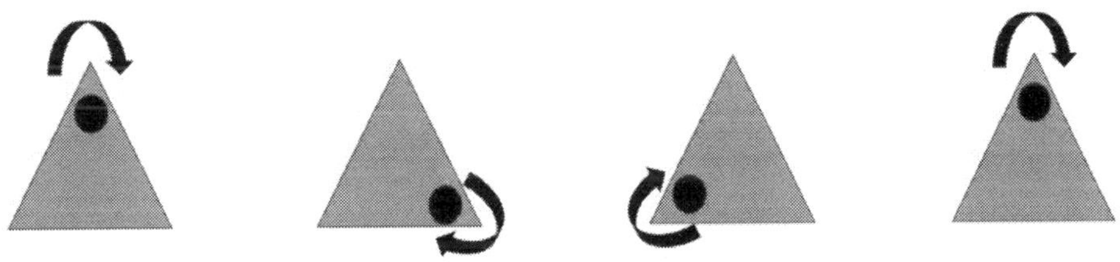

Original shape Rotated once Rotated twice Rotated three times

For regular polygons, the *order of rotational symmetry* is equal to the *number of lines of bilateral symmetry*. Remember: In order to be regular, the internal angles must all be the same. Irregular polygons have the same number of sides as their regular counterpart, but have varying internal angles. The table below demonstrates this difference. In a regular hexagon, each of the angles is the same, whereas in an irregular hexagon, there are varying angles.

Regular Hexagon	Irregular Hexagon

Degree of rotational symmetry: When rotating clockwise, the minimum number of degrees a particular shape must be rotated for the orientation of the shape to return to its original appearance. This can be calculated with the simple formula below:

$$\text{Degree of rotational symmetry} = \frac{360}{\text{total number of lines of bilateral symmetry}}$$

For example, a regular hexagon has 6 lines of bilateral symmetry, so its degree of rotational symmetry is $\frac{360}{6} = 6$

To quickly recognise symmetry patterns in your exam, familiarise yourself with the following table:

Shape	Lines of Symmetry	Rotational Symmetry Order
Hexagon	6	6
Pentagon	5	5
Square	4	4
Equilateral Triangle	3	3
Parallelogram	0	2
Rectangle	2	2
Rhombus	2	2
Isosceles Triangle	1	1

When looking for patterns involving symmetry, you can ask yourself the following questions:

1. **Do all the shapes within a box possess either bilateral or rotational symmetry?**

E.g. 1) In Set A, every shape has bilateral symmetry, whereas in Set B, none of the shapes have bilateral symmetry.

E.g. 2) In Set A, every box has 1 shape with rotational symmetry, whereas in Set B, every box has 2 shapes with rotational symmetry.

E.g. 3) In Set A, every shape has a rotational symmetry order of 3 and under, whereas in Set B, every box has a rotational symmetry order of more than 3.

Imagining the turning of a shape and counting how many turns it might take to return to original is not an easy task. Therefore, if you familiarise yourself with the previous table, you will be in a far better position to quickly tackle such a question.

2. **Does one set only have symmetrical objects?**

E.g. Every square in Set A has only symmetrical shapes, whereas every square in Set B has only asymmetrical shapes.

In this scenario, remember that irregular shapes can also have symmetry.

3. **Is the symmetry of objects dependent on the presence of other factors?**

E.g. 1) In Set A, every white shape is symmetrical, whereas every black shape has no lines of symmetry. In Set B, every black shape is symmetrical, whereas every white shape has no lines of symmetry.

This is another dependent relationship – the colour of an object depends on its symmetry.

E.g. 2) In Set A, all of the symmetrical shapes are large and the asymmetrical shapes are small, whereas in Set B, all of the symmetrical shapes are small and the asymmetrical shapes are large.

4. **Is the entire box symmetrical, rather than each shape?**

E.g. 1) In Set A, every box has a vertical line of symmetry, whereas in Set B, every box has a horizontal line of symmetry. This can be shown as follows:

Set A **Set B**

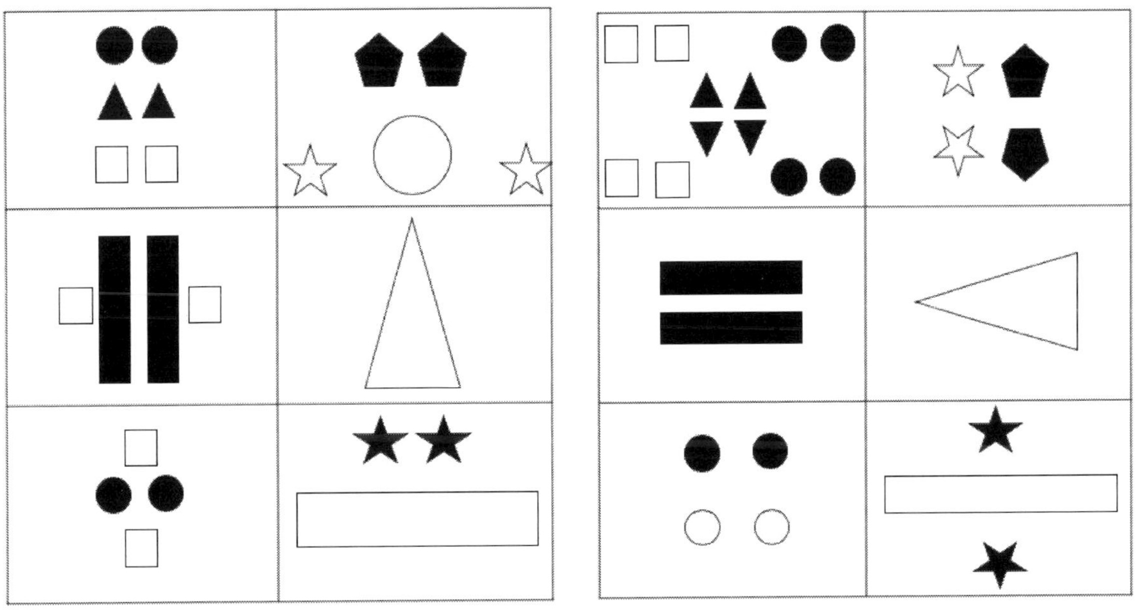

This is the kind of pattern you should be able to see at a glance. If you have never looked for such a pattern before, it can be difficult to spot. See the lines of symmetry in the reformed version below:

Set A

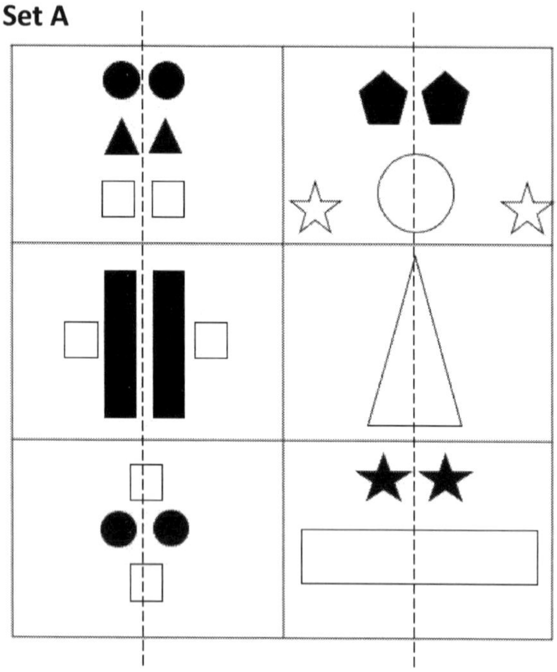

Set B

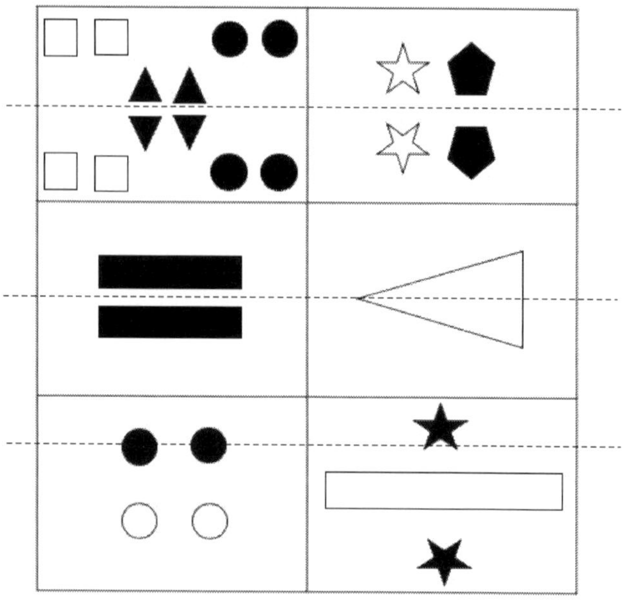

Hopefully, this variety of examples will allow you to consider the many different possibilities when assessing symmetry of shapes! There are undoubtedly more patterns, but this is to get you started.

Example 7

There is no question associated with this example. Simply determine the pattern in each of the following sets:

Set A

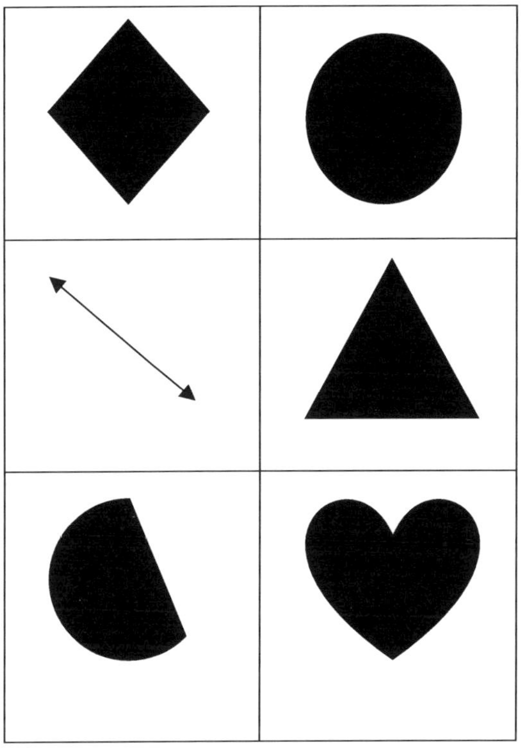

Set B

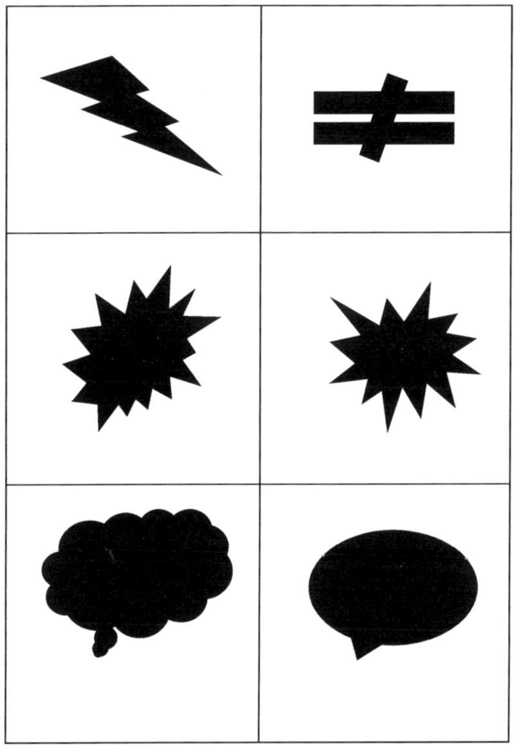

Answer 7

Following the general strategy, step back and have a quick overall glance at the two sets. There is a clear pattern that can be seen without even going on to the simplest box strategy. If you cannot see it, follow the steps using the simplest box method, analysing the characteristics of each shape. You should find that each shape in Set A has at least 1 line of symmetry, whereas there are no symmetrical shapes in Set B. There are no other patterns to be noted here.

Dependent Relationships

In dependent relationships, the working or functioning of one of the patterns is dependent on the presence of another pattern. Dependent relationships have been referred to throughout this section, and will be explained more in depth here. It is very common for a pattern to be dependent on another factor within a set, as it would be very straight forward to find the pattern without this concept. Therefore, the question-writers wish for you to maximise your abilities to solve such questions.

Example 8

There is no question associated with this example. Simply determine the pattern in each of the following sets:

Set A

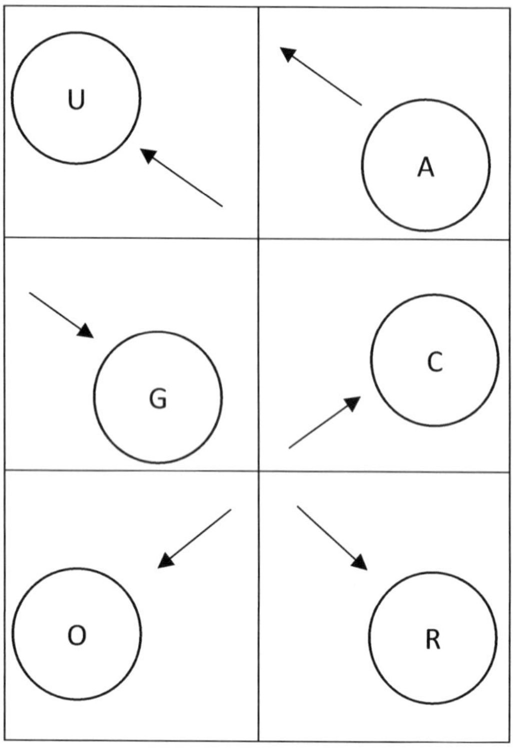

Set B

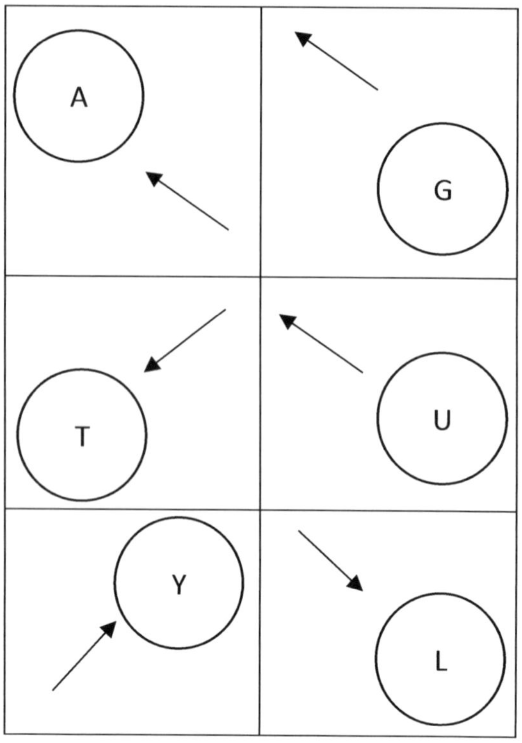

Answer 8

This is a fairly complex and comprehensive example of a question involving dependent relationships. All of the boxes look the same, so the simplest box strategy cannot be applied. Let us observe the characteristics of each box using SCANOS:

- Shape – Each box has the same shapes. No pattern here.
- Colour – There is no colour. No pattern here.
- Arrangement – There is no specific arrangement of either the circles or the arrows. It appears to be random. No pattern here.
- Number – Each box has 1 letter, 1 circle and 1 arrow. No pattern here.
- Orientation – There may be a pattern to do with orientation! See more below.
- Symmetry – The shapes are all the same, so there is not much to be said about symmetry. The letters could perhaps have some rules of symmetry, but upon inspection, some letters are symmetrical and some are asymmetrical in each set. No pattern here.

Notice that there are circles with letters and arrows, and the arrows can either point towards or away from the circle. Therefore, there is something to note about the orientation of the arrows. It is likely a dependent relationship, but it cannot depend on characteristics of the circle as each box has the same circle. Therefore, it must be dependent on the characteristics of the letter within the circle.

Set A:

- The arrow points towards: G, C, R, O, U
- The arrows point away from: A

Is there any link you can spot between the letters?

- Number of lines in each letter that arrows point towards – G has 3, C has 1, R has 3, O has 1, U has 1. Perhaps they all have an odd number of lines? But the arrow points away from the letter A, which also has 3 lines, so this cannot be the correct pattern.
- What about the characteristics of the lines? G, C, R, O, and U all have a curved line, whereas A has only straight lines. This seems to be a consistent pattern.

Pattern: In Set A, the arrows point towards letters with curved lines and point away from letters with straight lines.

If we check Set B, we will find that the inverse is true. The arrows point towards A, Y, T and L which have only straight lines, and point away from U and G which have curved lines.

Since the orientation of the arrow is dependent on the letter, this is a dependent relationship.

Distractors

The presence of distractors has previously been mentioned. A distractor is an element that has no relationship to the pattern of the set and is present simply to increase the difficulty and time taken to identify the pattern.

Example 9

There is no question associated with this example. Simply determine the pattern in each of the following sets:

Set A

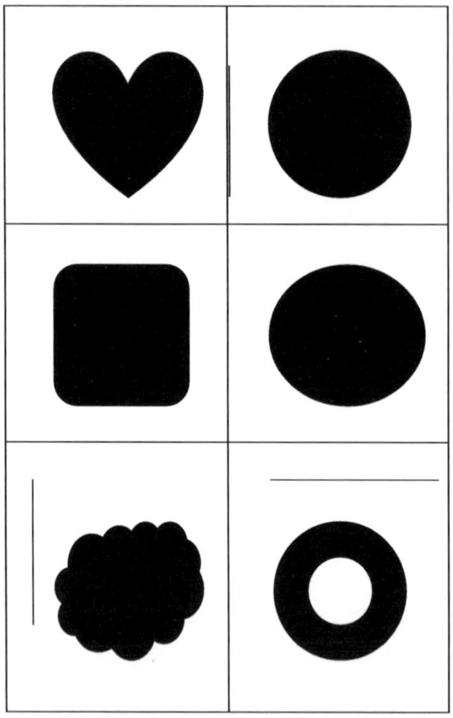

Set B

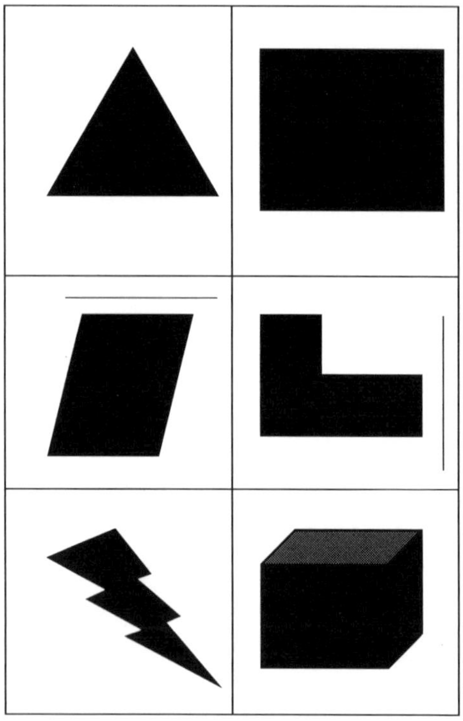

Answer 9

All of the shapes in set A have curved sides, whereas those in set B have straight sides. The extra lines within the sets have no relation to the pattern. The lines are called **distractors.** Distractors can present in many forms, with this being one of the simplest to demonstrate. Various other distractors have previously been discussed.

After learning about distractors and dependent relationships, let us examine a pattern that utilises both of these tools.

Example 10

There is no question associated with this example. Simply determine the pattern in the following set:

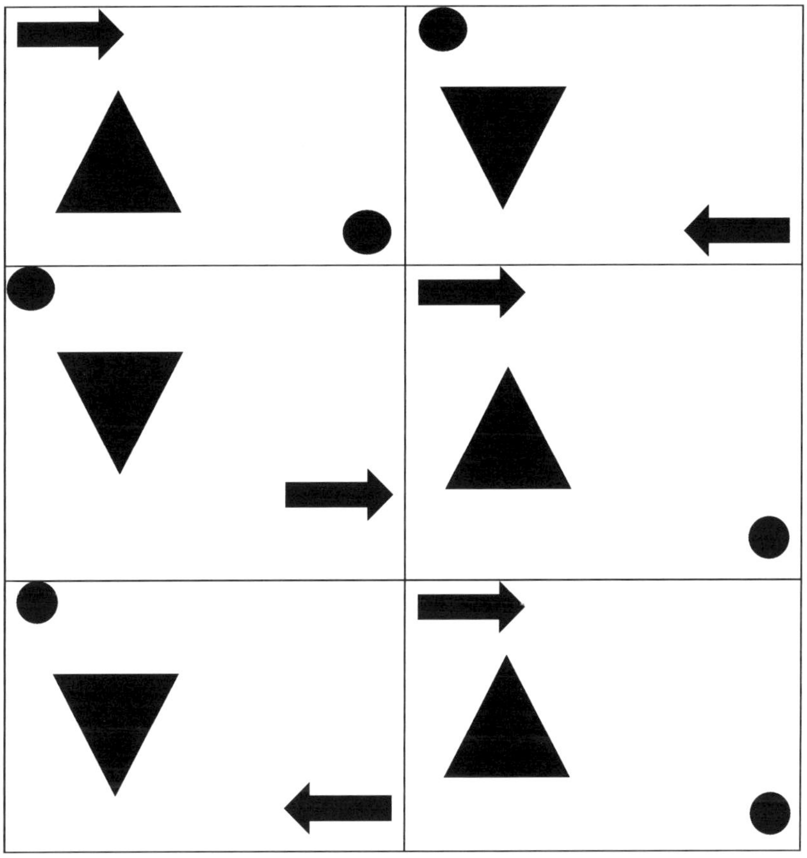

Answer 10

Certain features you should notice are:

1. There is a circle in one corner of each box – either in the bottom right or in the top left.
2. There is an arrow present in the corner of each box, opposite to the circle, facing either right or left.
3. There is a triangle present in each box which points either upwards or downwards.

Given time to further analyse these features, you will notice that usually, when a circle is in the bottom right, the arrow faces left, and when the circle is in the top left, the arrow faces left. However, in the middle box on the left, the arrow does not satisfy this pattern and it faces right.

Hence, even though it may initially seem like there is a pattern associated with the orientation of the arrows, they have nothing to do with the pattern and are thus a **distractor**.

The real pattern is solely to do with the orientation of the triangle in relation to the arrangement of the circle. Every time a circle is in the bottom right corner, the triangle faces upwards. Every time a circle is in the top left corner, the triangle faces downwards. This pattern is satisfied across each of the boxes and represents a **dependent** relationship. With time and practice, such patterns will become increasingly obvious to you and your overall efficiency in this section will increase.

Intersections

Besides SCANOS, intersections represent an essential pattern to look out for. The number of intersections in a box can be identified by counting the number of times objects cross over other objects. The simplest way to demonstrate this is with lines crossing over other lines. The diagram below shows 2 such intersections.

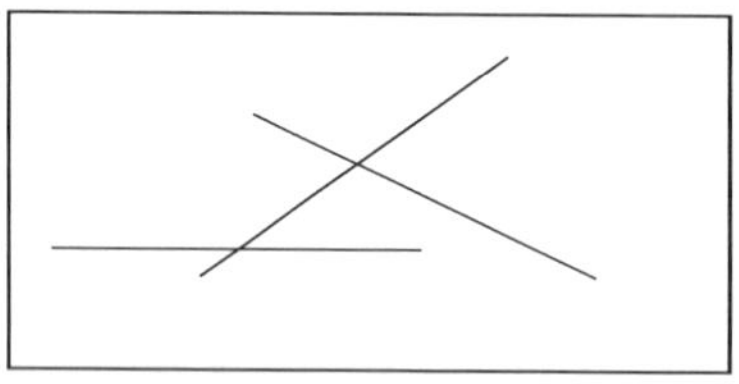

Below are some questions you can ask yourself to identify patterns involving intersections:

1. **Are there a certain number of intersections in each box?**

E.g. In Set A, each box has 4 intersections, whereas in Set B, each box has 6 intersections.

2. **Is there a pattern to the number of intersections in each box?**

E.g. In Set A, each box has an even number of intersections, whereas in Set B, each box has an odd number of intersections.

3. **Is there a dependent relationship associated with the number of intersections?**

E.g. 1) In Set A, each box with an even number of intersections has a white triangle, whereas each box with an odd number of intersections has a black triangle.

E.g. 2) In Set A, each box with an even number of intersections has an arrow pointing upwards, and each box with an odd number of intersections has an arrow pointing to the left.

E.g. 3) In Set A, each box with 2 intersections has a square in its top left corner, and each box with 3 intersections has a square in its top right corner.

E.g. 4) In Set A, each box with only symmetrical shapes has 2 intersections, while each box with only asymmetrical shapes has 1 intersection.

You can see a combination of many things that have been covered so far appearing in these examples. It seems to get more and more difficult. The sheer number of examples in each section clearly demonstrates the vast variety of patterns that can appear, thus, it is essential that you train your brain to quickly identify patterns.

Example 11

There are no questions associated with this example. Simply determine the patterns in the following sets:

Set A

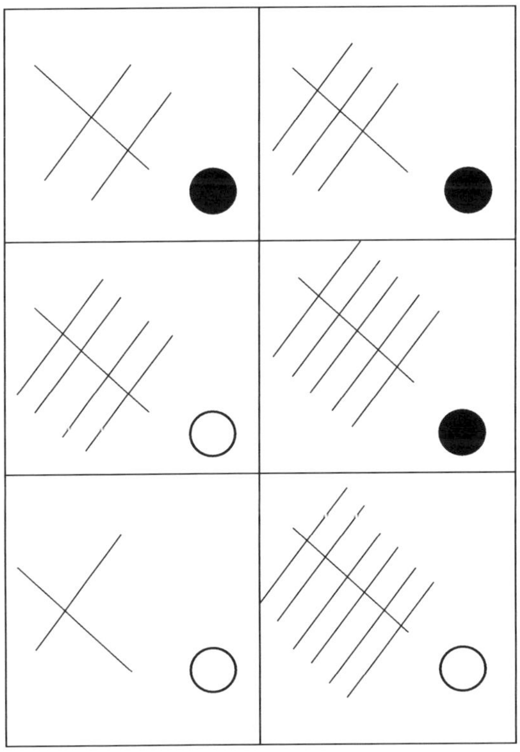

Set B

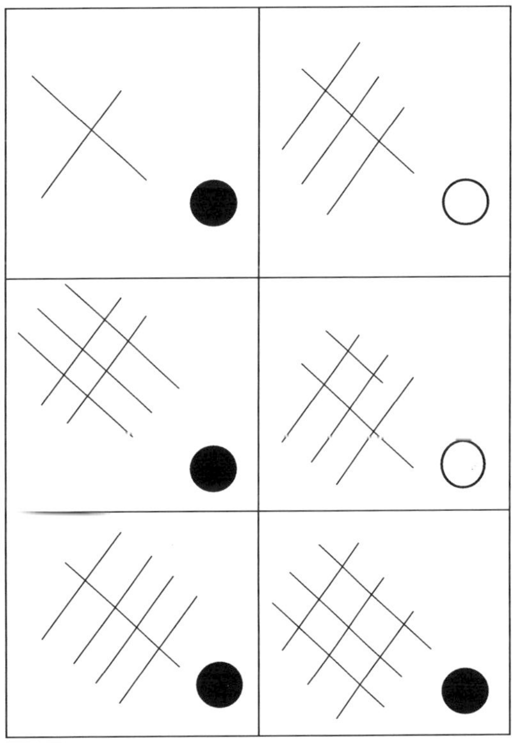

Answer 11

At first glance, we notice lines that intersect, black circles, and white circles. Starting with the simplest box in Set A at the bottom left, there are 2 lines, 1 intersection, and a white circle. The next simplest box at the top left has 3 lines, 2 intersections and 1 black circle. Look at the following table to get a better picture of everything that is going on in Set A.

Box	Number of Lines	Number of Intersections	Colour of Circle
Top left	3	2	Black
Top right	4	3	Black
Middle left	5	4	White
Middle right	6	5	Black
Bottom left	2	1	White
Bottom right	7	6	White

Number of lines

You will notice that when a circle is black, there are either 3, 4, or 6 lines. There is no evident pattern that connects these numbers. They are a mixture of odd and even numbers as well as a mixture of prime and composite numbers. They are not all multiples of any specific number, either. Further, the boxes with white circles have 5, 2, and 7 lines. These are all prime numbers, so that may have been a pattern, had it not been for the fact that there is no inverse pattern in boxes with black circles.

Number of intersections

The boxes with black circles have 2, 3 and 5 intersections, while the boxes with white circles have 4, 1, and 6 intersections. There is a more evident pattern here: When the sum of the intersections in a box is a prime number, the circle is black, but when the sum of the intersections in a box is *not* a prime number, the circle is white.

- *Note*: "Not prime" is essentially the same as "composite" but also accounts for the number 1, which is not a composite or a prime number.

The inverse of this pattern applies to Set B: When the sum of the intersections in a box is a prime number, the circle is white, but when the sum of the intersections in a box is *not* a prime number, the circle is black.

This example demonstrates how intersections can have dependent relationships. To tackle this type of pattern:

1. Find each box with similar characteristics (such as the same colour of circle) and count the number of intersections in each of those boxes.
2. Determine a pattern between the number of intersections.
3. Count the number of intersections in the opposing group (within the same set) and determine whether the inverse of the pattern applies. If it does not, see whether there is a different overall pattern.

Overlaps

Although this has not yet been discussed, it is very common for shapes to overlap in Abstract Reasoning. For the purposes of this book, we will refer to 2 shapes overlapping once as "1 overlap". Example of 1 overlap:

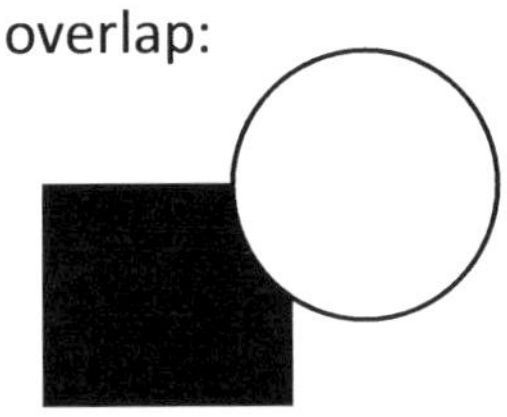

1. **Are there a certain number of overlaps in each box in a set?**

E.g. 1) In Set A, each box has 1 overlap, whereas in Set B, each box has 3 overlaps.

E.g. 2) In Set A, each box has an even number of overlaps, whereas in Set B, each box has an odd number of overlaps.

E.g. 3) In Set A, the squares always have 3 overlapping objects, whereas in Set B, the circles always have 3 overlapping objects.

2. **Is there a specific type of shape that is always overlapped?**

E.g. 1) In Set A, shapes only overlap (cover part of) a triangle, whereas in Set B, shapes only overlap (cover part of) a square.

This would mean that in Set A, only triangles are allowed to be partly hidden behind other shapes. If a circle is hidden behind another shape, or overlapped by another shape, the box it is in cannot belong to Set A.

E.g. 2) In Set A, black shapes are always overlapped, whereas in Set B, white shapes are always overlapped.

3. **Is there a specific place that the overlap occurs?**

E.g. In Set A, the square is always overlapped in its bottom right corner, whereas in Set B, the square is always overlapped in its top right corner.

4. **Is there a dependent relationship involving overlaps?**

E.g. 1) In Set A, when the square is overlapped in its bottom right corner, the circle is black, whereas when the square is overlapped in its top right corner, the circle is white.

E.g. 2) In Set A, when there are 2 overlaps in a box, the triangle points upwards, whereas when there is 1 overlap in a box, the triangle points downwards.

These examples show multiple domains of patterns – dependent relationships, overlaps, orientation, colour, and numbers. Do not be surprised if patterns with multiple domains are more difficult to spot, as they will come with practice!

Example 12

There are no questions associated with this example. Simply determine the patterns in the following sets:

Set A

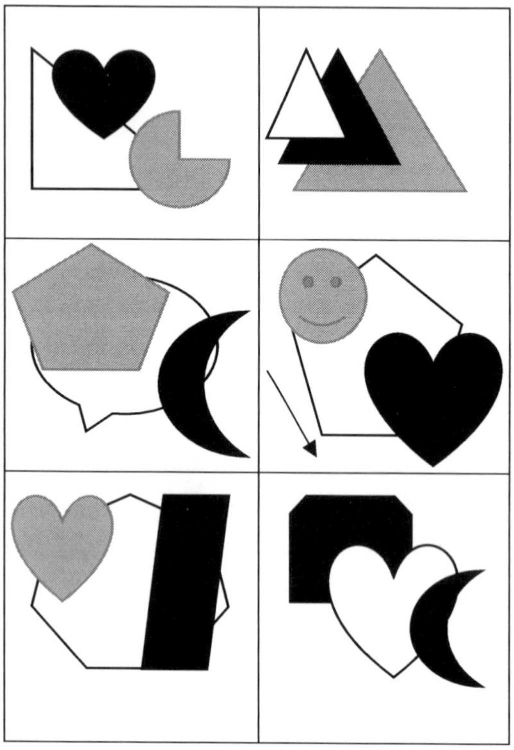

Set B

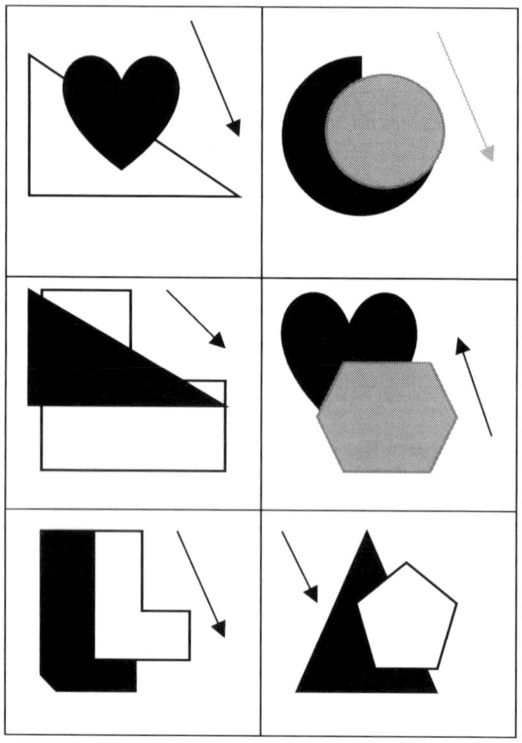

Answer 12

Following the general strategy, there is nothing particularly obvious that stands out except for the fact that there are overlaps present. The simplest box appears to be the top left box in Set B. There is 1 overlap present. The arrows appear to be distractors, as there are a number of arrows present in Set B, and only 1 in Set A, so there is unlikely to be a relationship that is based on a single arrow in Set A.

Checking the remaining boxes in Set B, they all seem to have only 1 overlap. In Set A, there appear to be 2 overlaps present in each box.

This is a fairly straight-forward example of patterns involving overlaps, but as demonstrated with the written examples, there are bound to be far more complex patterns.

Connecting Shapes

Sometimes, sets will present with shapes that are connected via lines. You must examine the characteristics of the lines connecting the shapes, and the shapes themselves. You have learned many techniques for analysing characteristics thus far, so let us begin!

See the following example:

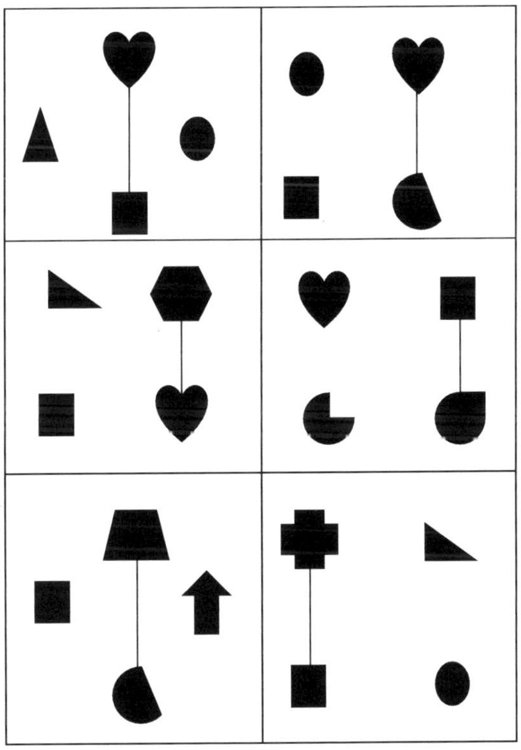

The connecting lines:

- Are always straight, vertical lines.
- There is only one connecting line per box.
- The lines are arranged in different locations in each box – sometimes to the right, sometimes left, and sometimes in the middle.

The shapes being connected:

- Are always black, like all the other shapes.

- Only connect to one shape – do not connect to multiple shapes.
- All appear to have symmetry – but some shapes that are not connected also have symmetry.
- Both curved and straight lines exist in the shapes being connected.
    - Potential pattern – is a curved shape always connected to a straight shape? No, because the bottom right box has connected shapes with only straight lines, and the top right box has two connected shapes with curved lines.
- The number of lines in each connected shape is always **even** – this is constant through all of the boxes.
    - 2 lines: heart, raindrop, semicircle
    - 4 lines: square, trapezium
    - 6 lines: hexagon
    - 12 lines: cross

Therefore, the pattern is that the lines only connect shapes with an even number of sides. The positioning of the lines seems to have no relevance, nor do the extra shapes in each box.

Example 13

There are no questions associated with this example. Simply determine the patterns in the following sets:

Set A

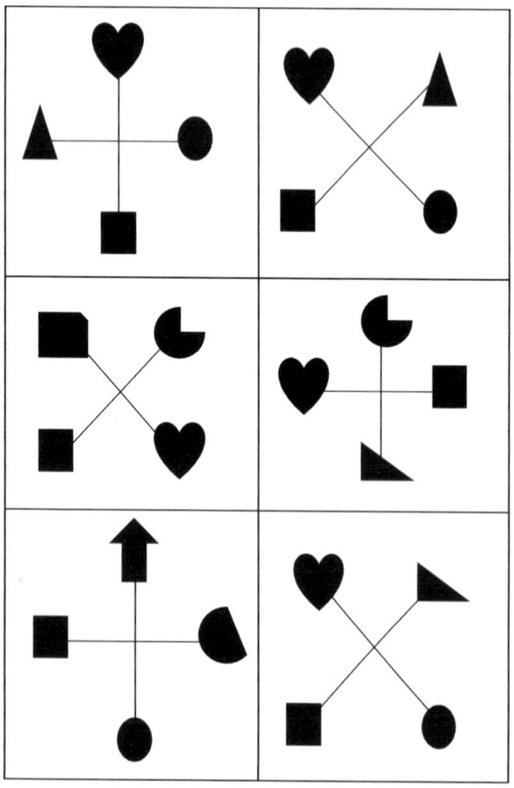

Set B

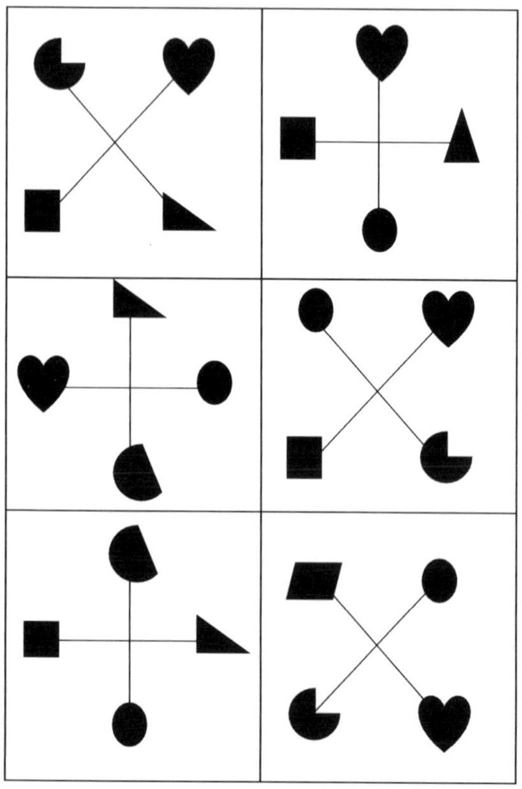

Answer 13

Since all the boxes have the same number of shapes, the simplest box strategy is not possible.

Characteristics of the lines:

- Diagonal lines which form an X shape
- Vertical and horizontal combination of lines which form a + shape

Note: these "shapes" are not relevant, but just a method of categorizing the types of line crossovers that occur.

Characteristics of the shapes in "+ line" boxes:

- Top left box:
    - Heart (2 lines) connected to square (4 lines)
    - Triangle (3 lines) connected to circle (1 line)
- Middle right box:
    - Pie (3 lines) connected to triangle (3 lines)
    - Heart (2 lines) connected to square (4 lines)
- Bottom left box: 7
    - Arrow (7 lines) connected to circle (1 line)
    - Square (4 lines) connected to semicircle (2 lines)

This pattern is very tricky, as it changes within the "+ line" boxes themselves. It appears that a shape with an even number of lines is always connected to a shape with an even number of lines, whereas a shape with an odd number of lines is always connected to a shape with an odd number of lines. Further, both even and odd shapes are always present within each box.

Characteristics of the shapes in the "X line" boxes:

- Top right box:
    - Triangle (3 lines) connected to square (4 lines)
    - Heart (2 lines) connected to circle (1 line)
- Middle left box:
    - Irregular pentagon (5 lines) connected to heart (2 lines)
    - Pie (3 lines) connected to square (4 lines)
- Bottom right box:
    - Heart (2 lines) connected to circle (1 line)
    - Triangle (3 lines) connected to square (4 lines)

It appears that "X line" boxes always have a mismatch – a shape with an even number of lines is always connected to a shape with an odd number of lines.

So the overall pattern in Set A is as follows:

- In boxes with + lines, a shape with an even number of lines must connect to another shape with an even number of lines, while a shape with an odd number of lines must connect to another shape with an odd number of lines.
- In boxes with X lines, a shape with an even number of lines must connect to a shape with an odd number of lines.

The pattern is the inverse for Set B, where X lines have mismatched connections (i.e. even + odd) and + lines have matched connections (i.e. even+even and odd+odd).

This example was fairly difficult, as your exam questions may be. In this case, shapes are connected only based on the number of lines they have. You should be aware of other characteristics to look out for, including colour, symmetry, arrangement, overlaps, and so on!

Now that we have discussed various different strategies for answering Type 1 questions, try the question below.

Example 14

A

B

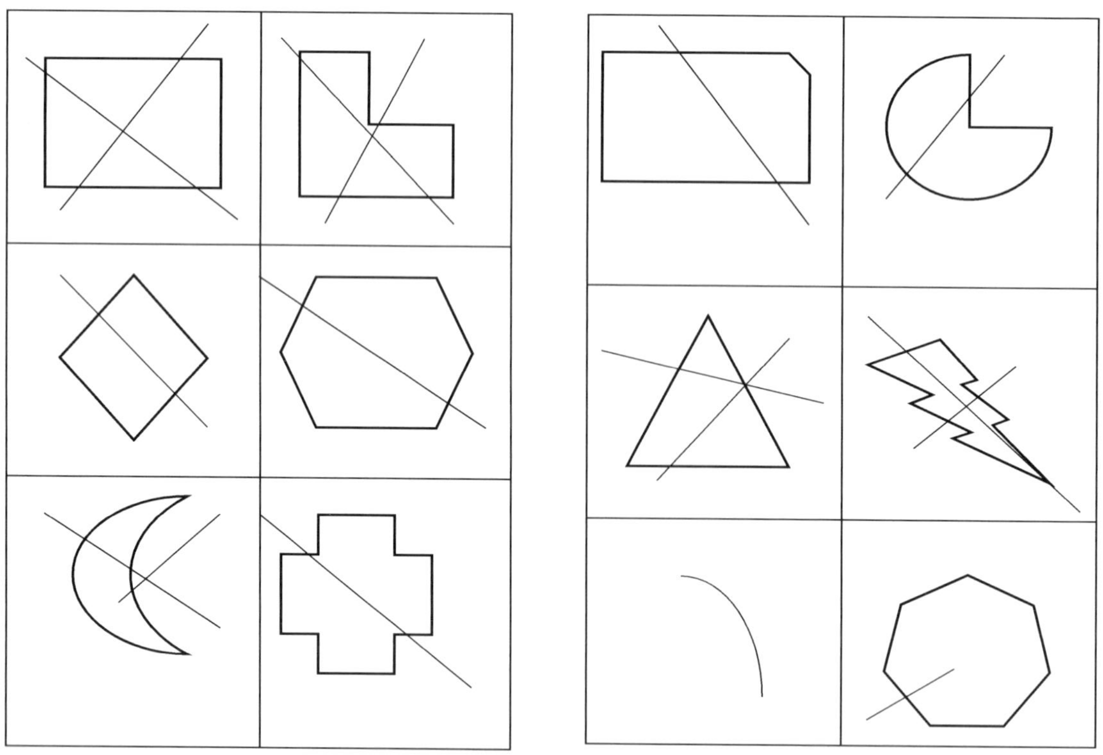

Determine whether the test shapes (1-5) belong to set A, set B or neither.

1 2 3 4 5

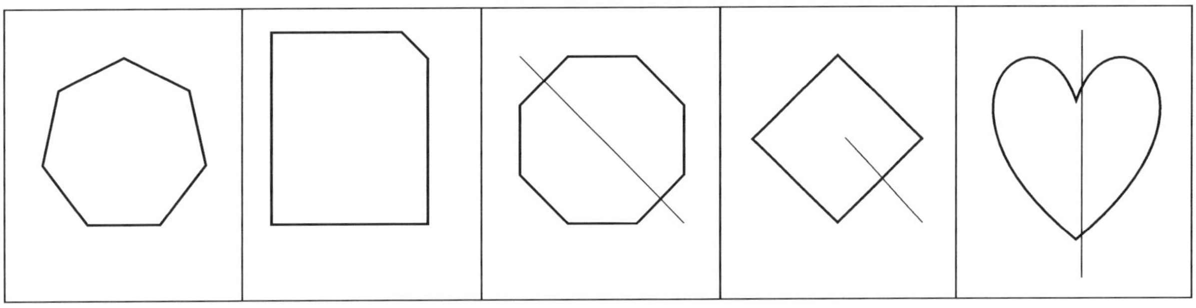

1	2	3	4	5
A. Set A	A. Set A	A. Set A	A. Set A	A. Set A
B. Set B	B. Set B	B. Set B	B. Set B	B. Set B
C. Neither	C. Neither	C. Neither	C. Neither	C. Neither

Answer 14

Let us analyse Set A using SCANOS

S – There is 1 shape in each box – nothing particular to note about the shape pattern.
C – No colour element involved.
A – There is only 1 shape in each box – nothing to note about arrangement.
N – Number of sides and intersections in each box

- Top left: 4 sides, 4 intersections
- Top right: 6 sides, 4 intersections
- Middle left: 4 sides, 2 intersections
- Middle right: 6 sides, 2 intersections
- Bottom left: 2 sides, 3 intersections
- Bottom right: 12 sides, 2 intersections

O – Orientation is not relevant here.
S – The shapes all appear to have at least 1 line of symmetry.

Although it may have initially appeared that there must be a pattern based on the number of intersections in each box, likely "always an even number of intersections", the bottom left box does not satisfy this. However, the number of sides is consistently even in each box, therefore, this is the pattern.

Further, in Set B, there is no intersection in the bottom left box. The inverse pattern applies in Set B: each box/shape has an odd number of sides.

Therefore, the intersecting lines are present as a distractor, and the pattern is solely based on the number of sides (even or odd) in each shape/box.

Using these patterns, the answers are as follows:

1. The correct answer is B. This shape has 7 sides.
2. The correct answer is B. This shape has 5 sides.
3. The correct answer is A. This shape has 8 sides.
4. The correct answer is A. This shape has 4 sides.
5. The correct answer is A. This shape has 2 sides.

Type 2 Questions: Series

The majority of questions in Abstract Reasoning are Type 1 – an example being the previous question shown. Type 2 questions will always make their appearance, but far less frequently than the first type. In this question type, you will be given a series of shapes, normally 3 or 4, and will be required to assess the sequence of changes, or the differences between the shapes, rather than the similarities. This will allow you to decipher which shape is next in the series by applying the pattern rules demonstrated.

Each question is only worth 1 mark, compared to Type 1 questions that have 5 marks each, therefore you should spend far less time on this type of question – ideally, no more than 15 seconds. The strict time limit makes these questions much more difficult, although given endless time to solve, they are not too tricky.

A very straight-forward example is shown below. See if you can identify the pattern, then answer the question.

Example 15

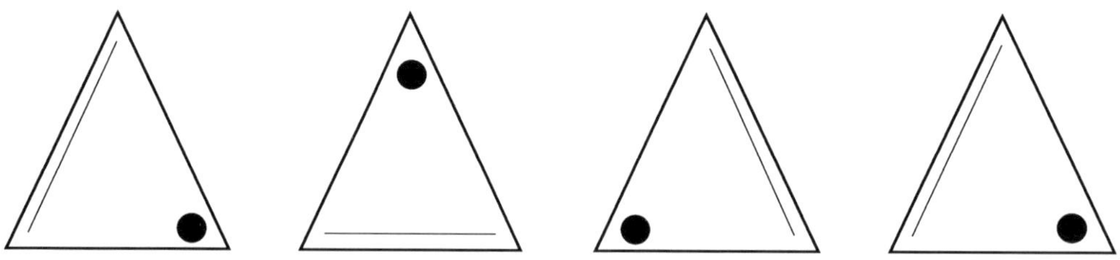

Which of the shapes satisfies the above given sequence?

A.

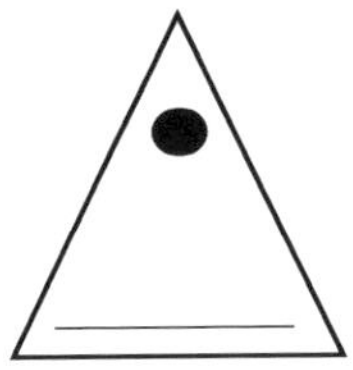

B.

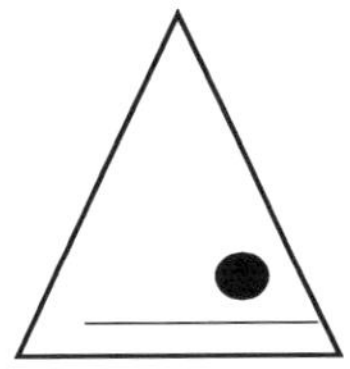

C.

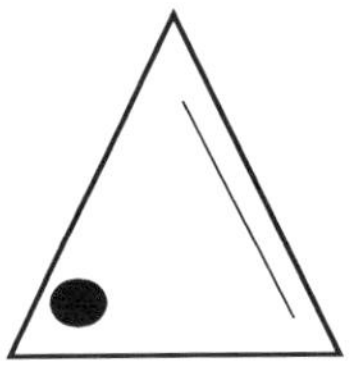

D.

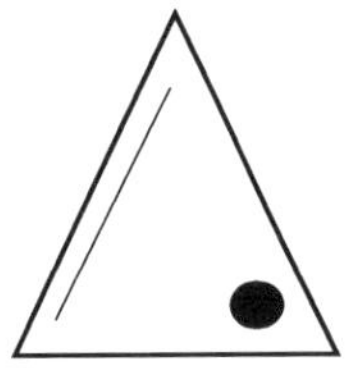

Answer 15

The correct answer is A.

The circle moves one place in an anti-clockwise direction with each subsequent shape in the series. The line also follows the exact same pattern.

The Conveyer Belt Strategy

Imagine the initial shape is travelling along a conveyer belt, with a specific pattern being applied at each stage along the belt to alter the shape. The conveyer belt does its job for 3 or 4 stages, then requires some external input. Your job is to determine the appearance of the shape at the next stage of the conveyer belt, given the pattern that has been applied in the previous number of stages. This pattern will not change.

To identify the pattern, follow these steps:

1. Look at the overall picture and determine what appears to be changing – whether there is some sort of movement, change in colour, change in size, change in number, etc.
2. Start with the first and second stages of the conveyer belt, or the second and third, or third and fourth.
    - You cannot skip stages and look at the second and fourth, for example. Each stage occurs in sequence to the last, so you will be unable to identify the pattern if you skip stages.
3. Select one shape or aspect (that you determined in step 1) that changes between the two stages you are comparing. Identify the pattern of change.

- Usually, there is not only one thing that is changing. You should not try to look at everything that changes all at once. If you select only one aspect, it will be much easier to answer the question. Sometimes, there is only one pattern (although multiple changes may be present as distractors, or may be following the same pattern), so it is not worth your limited 15 seconds to continue to assess for further patterns *unless* you are unable to decide on an answer with the first pattern alone.

4. Move on to the next stage in the sequence. Does the pattern hold? Or is it slightly different than you thought?
5. Compare the final stage. Confirm that the pattern holds true.
6. Look at the answer options and eliminate any answer that does not satisfy the pattern. If there is only one option left, great! You have the answer. If there are multiple options left, there must be another pattern.
7. In this case, follow steps 1-5 for a different shape or aspect that changes between the stages, eliminating any answer that does not follow the pattern of change. You should have your answer after two patterns. If you do not, simply guess the answer from the remaining options, as you cannot afford to spend much longer on this question type – it is only worth 1 mark out of 55, and the entire Abstract Reasoning test is 13 minutes long!

Common Patterns

A series of movements

This was demonstrated in the example above – a shape or line moves a certain number of places in a specific direction along each stage of the conveyer belt.

E.g. 1) The line moves one place clockwise along each stage, while the circle moves one place anti-clockwise along each stage.

E.g. 2) The line moves one place anti-clockwise along each stage, while the circle moves 2 places anti-clockwise along each stage.

E.g. 3) The circle moves one place clockwise along each stage, while the line moves clockwise along each stage by one place extra than the previous stage (1 place from the first stage to the second stage, 2 places from the second stage to the third, 3 places from the third stage to the fourth).

We have demonstrated how movements can be clockwise or anti-clockwise, but they can also be up and down, left and right, diagonal in any direction, or a series of movements in each stage, such as 1 place down and 2 places to the right. Consider the following example:

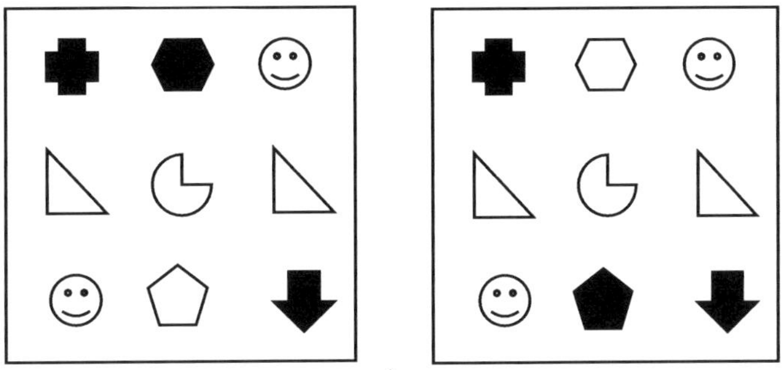

Every placement of every shape remains the same between the two images. The changes are as noted:

- The hexagon in the middle row changes from black to white.
- The pentagon in the middle changes from white to black.

The next stage in the series is not shown, so the pattern cannot be confirmed, but it is likely to be either:

- The black colour in the middle row shifts 1 place upwards in each stage.
  Note: When something cannot go any more places in one direction, it will restart on the opposite end. In this case, if the black colour cannot move any further up from the hexagon, it restarts at the bottom.
- The black colour shifts 2 places downwards in each stage.

A series of rotations

Rather than the same object or colour simply moving, it would appear different due to a change in orientation.

E.g. 1) The arrow rotates 45° clockwise along each stage.

E.g. 2) The black arrow rotates 45° clockwise along each stage, while the grey arrow rotates 45° anti-clockwise along each stage.

E.g. 3) The triangle rotates an *extra* 90° along each stage (i.e. rotates 90° from the first stage to the second, then 180° from the second to the third, then 270° from the third to the fourth).

This third example demonstrates a pattern that is more difficult to spot, as there is a pattern within a pattern – the triangle is rotating, but the rotation is not a set number between each stage, rather there is a pattern to the rotation.

A series of numerical changes

E.g. 1) The sum of the number of sides in a box doubles along each stage

In this example, the sum of the sides might start at 1 (a circle), then is 2, then is 4, then is 8.

E.g. 2) The number of shapes in the box increases by 3 along each stage.

E.g. 3) The number of intersections halves along each stage.

E.g. 4) The number of coloured shapes increases by 2 along each stage.

E.g. 5) The number of lines increases by 2 along each stage, while the number of intersections decreases by 1.

A series of curvature changes

E.g. 1) Along each stage, the middle shape in the box alternates between having straight edges only, and having curved edges.

In this example, the first box might have a square as the middle shape, then the next has a crescent moon, the third has a hexagon, and the fourth has a circle. When looking at the answers, you would immediately eliminate any option that has a curved shape in the middle, as the next stage should have a straight-lined shape in the middle.

E.g. 2) The large shape in each stage alternates between having straight edges only and having curved edges.

E.g. 3) The curved shapes in the box alternate between black and white along the stages.

This is quite a difficult pattern as not only are the colours changing, but they are changing based on a particular pattern between different shapes (curvature). If the shapes between the boxes change too, and the only similarity is the curvature, this pattern becomes difficult to identify. An example of this pattern is shown below:

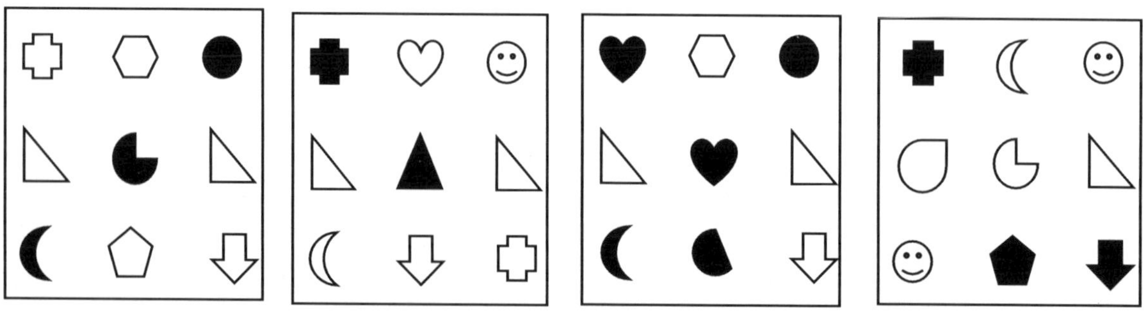

At first glance, this pattern is very confusing.

Let us follow the step-by-step approach.

You can see that in the first stage, all of the curved shapes are black, whereas in the second stage, two straight-edged shapes are black. The colour of the straight-edged shapes is a distractor. If you look closely, the curved-edged shapes in the second stage are all white, whereas in the third stage they are all black. It is easier to spot the black shapes than the white shapes, as the solid colour stands out much more. However, you must watch out for distractors.

Example 16

There is no question associated with this example. Simply determine the pattern in the following series:

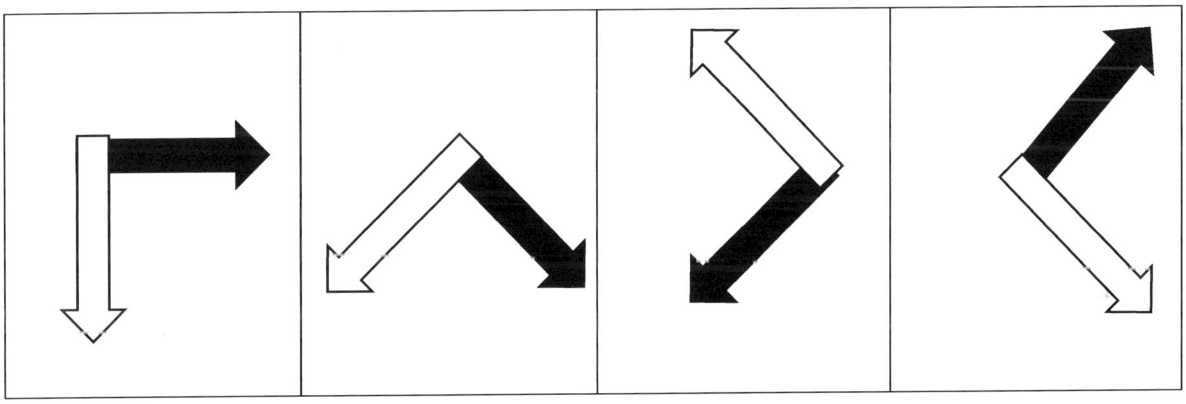

Answer 16

Following the strategy, let us compare the first and second boxes, looking at only one aspect that changes. Starting with the black arrow (for no particular reason, feel free to start with the white!) we can see that it appears to rotate about 45° clockwise. In the next stage, it appears to rotate a further 90° clockwise, and in the final stage it appears to rotate an additional 180° clockwise. The pattern seems to be that the degree of rotation doubles along each stage.

To answer an associated question, you would look for the option with a black arrow that appears to have rotated a further 360° from the fourth stage in the series, so it should be in the exact same place as it is in the fourth stage. If you have multiple answer options that appear like this, there would likely be a different pattern involved, associated with the white arrow. Therefore, following the strategy outlined previously, you would need to go back to the conveyer belt and assess the pattern of changes that the white arrow undergoes along the stages.

This pattern may not be very straight-forward, and like with any difficult or time-consuming question, you can always flag, make your best guess, and go.

Type 3 Questions: Relationships

This is another type of question that makes a minimal number of appearances, but will undoubtedly come up. You are presented with an image on the left which is directly related to an image on its right, connected by the words "is to". There is then a second image on the bottom left, and you must apply the pattern that links the top two images together in order to determine the image that will appear on the bottom right. You have roughly 15 seconds, as there is only one mark for this type of question. An example of this is shown below.

Example 17

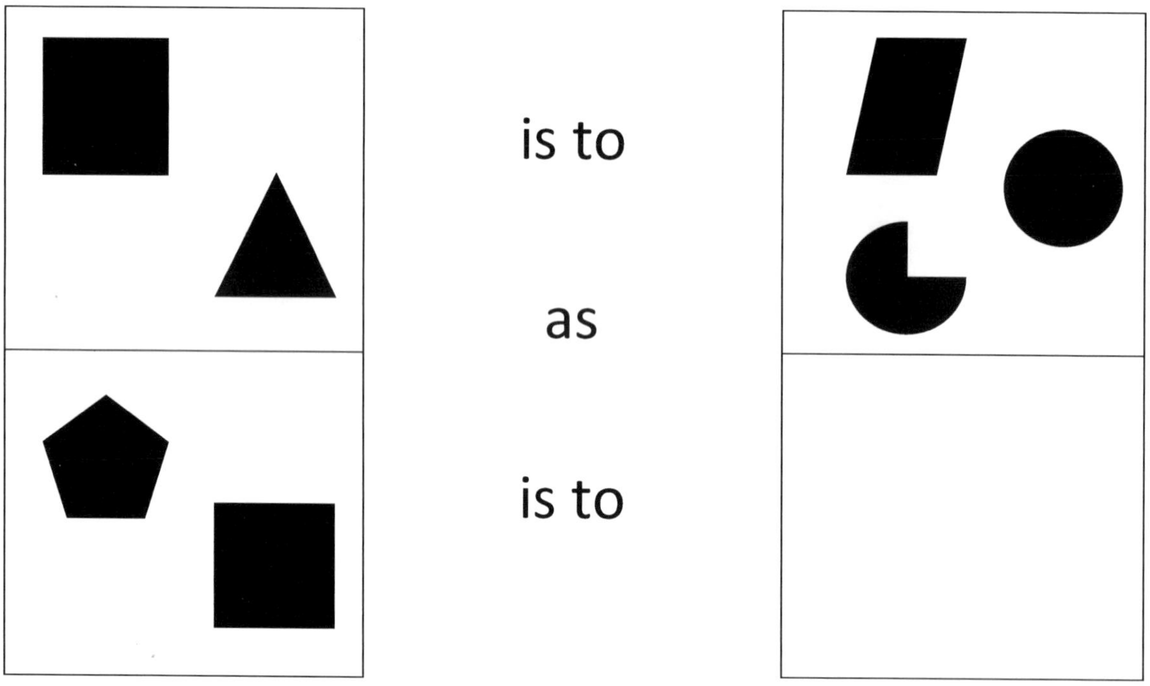

Which figure completes the statement?

A. B. C. D.

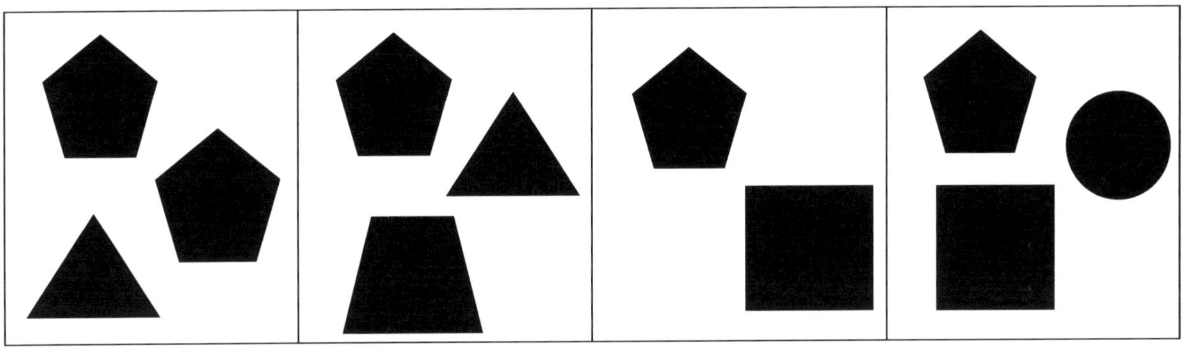

Strategy

Before answering this question, let us determine the strategy that should be used to maximise efficiency.

The best part about this type of question is the lack of distractors – you only have 2 images that you can use to identify a pattern, therefore, adding any distractors would be very cruel, although possible.

This question type is similar to Type 3, as you must identify the pattern behind the "change" that occurs from left side to right side, and apply that pattern to determine your answer. The strategy you can utilise is as follows:

1. Take a glance at both sides to see if there is any obvious change you notice – look out for all of the characteristics you have learned, such as size, shape, number, colour, etc.
2. Select one aspect that appears to be changing and verify the change between the boxes. Identify any further characteristics of the change.
3. Apply that change to the box underneath, using the answer options to confirm. If the same pattern that you have identified in the top column is applicable to any of the answer options that fit into the bottom column, that is your answer.
4. If you are unable to select an answer based on this single pattern, you can:
    - Assess which aspects have *not* changed between the boxes, i.e. the immobile aspects. If this immobile aspect happens to change in any of the answer options, you can immediately eliminate it.
        - For example, if there is no change in colour between the boxes, but one of the answer options has a change of colour, that option is immediately eliminated.
    - Assess for a second pattern.

Answer 17

Using the strategy above, at a quick glance, we can see the following features:

- Change in number of shapes.
- Change in the types of shapes, so there is a likely change in the total number of lines.
- No change in colour, symmetry, size, arrangement, or orientation.

Let us focus on one of these aspects: number of shapes. This is quick and easy to work with. There are 2 shapes in the first box and 3 shapes in the second. The box underneath also has 2 shapes, so its missing box should have 3 shapes. This immediately allows us to eliminate option C which only has 2 shapes.

- *Note:* This exact number does not have to follow! If the box underneath had 4 shapes, perhaps its missing box would have 5 (i.e. 5 is 1 more than 4, as 3 is 1 more than 2).

We are unable to decide between options A, B and D based on number of shapes alone, so we need to identify another pattern. Count the number of sides – there are 7 sides in the first box and 8 sides in the second. 8 is 1 more than 7, so we would expect the bottom column to also hold this same pattern. The pattern underneath has 9 sides in total, so the missing box should have 10 sides. Rather than counting all of the sides in each of A, B and D, look to see if there is anything obvious. Option D has the exact same shapes, with an additional circle. We know that a circle has 1 side, so we can safely select this option.

This may seem difficult so let us explore this type of question in further detail.

Common Patterns

Rotations

E.g. 1) The shapes around the edges of the box rotate 1 space clockwise, while the middle shape remains the same.

This may appear as follows:

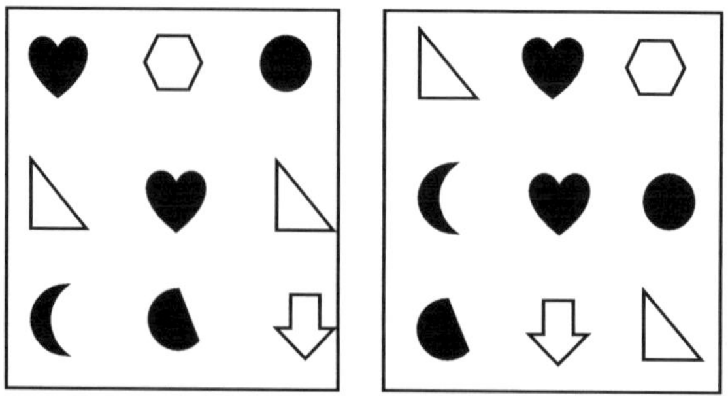

Recognising the immobile and unchanged middle shape would allow you to eliminate any answer options that do not have a solid black heart in the middle.

E.g. 2) The shapes around the edges of the box rotate 1 space clockwise, while the middle shape changes colour.

This may appear as follows:

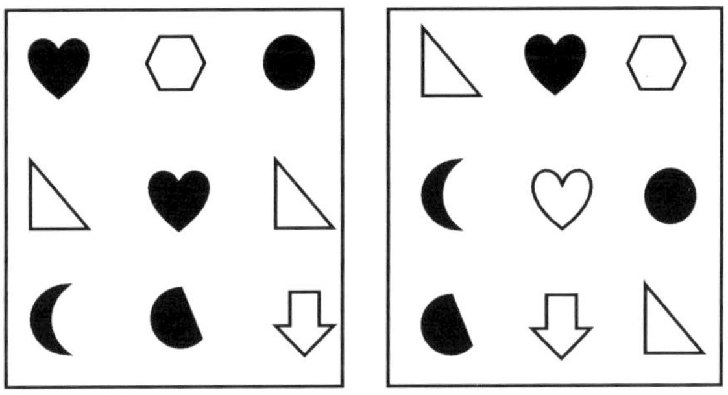

E.g. 3) The entire box rotates 90° clockwise.

This may appear as follows:

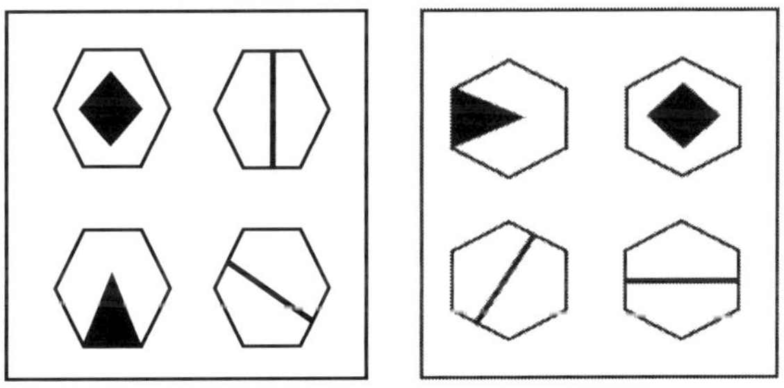

This rotation may be difficult to picture. If you are struggling, try to draw out the diagram, or print out this page, and turn the page 90° clockwise. It should now look exactly like the second image. In the UCAT, you will not have the luxury of printing out any pages, so the best way to identify rotation is by focusing on one aspect at a time. For example, the movement of shapes. No hexagon has stayed in its original position, so we can assume that the hexagons may have each rotated 90° around the box. However, the patterns within the hexagons have also adjusted from their original orientations. Look at the bottom left corner, with a wedge-shaped coloured area. In the second box, this coloured area is coming from the left of the hexagon, rather than from the bottom. To obtain such a change, it must have rotated 90° clockwise. You will notice that you can apply this same strategy to each of the hexagons to assess the degree of rotation, although some are more difficult to notice than others.

Having noticed that the shapes both move one place clockwise, and the patterns within them rotate 90° clockwise, you can either select answer options based on these two individual points, or realise that this means the entire box has rotated.

Intersections

E.g. The number of intersections in the first box is 2 less than the number of intersections in the second box.

Numbers

E.g. 1) The number of sides in the second box is 3 times greater than the number of sides in the first box.

E.g. 2) The number of corners in the first box is 1 less than the number of corners in the second box.

The number of corners will not necessarily be the same as the number of sides, as some shapes do not have corners – e.g. a circle. Make sure you account for this.

E.g. 3) The number of diagonal lines in the first box is 3 more than the number of diagonal lines in the second box.

E.g. 4) The number of straight lines in the first box is the same as the number of curved lines in the second box.

Colour

E.g. 1) The coloured shapes all move clockwise from one box to the next, while the uncoloured shapes are immobile.

E.g. 2) There are double the number of coloured shapes in the second box as there are in the first box.

Size

E.g. 1) From the first box to the next, the large shapes become small and the small shapes become large.

E.g. 2) From the first box to the next, the number of large shapes increases by 1.

E.g. 3) From the first box to the next, the large shapes all change colour, i.e. the black ones become white and the white ones become black.

Note: As always, there are many other patterns and features to look out for! These are some examples that should give you an idea of what might come up. Look out for patterns that you see and write them in a notebook. You can refer this notebook if you ever get stuck.

Type 4 Questions: Set Selection

This question type is very similar to Type 1 questions. However, you will not be asked to decide between Set A and Set B for each of 5 given boxes. Instead, you will be given Set A and Set B, followed by a series of 5 questions that each have 4 boxes to choose from. In each of the questions, you will be asked one of the following:

- Which of the following test shapes belongs in Set A?
- Which of the following test shapes belongs in Set B?

Strategy

The same basic strategy applies as for Type 1 questions.

1. Move your head back and get a good overall view of the two sets.
2. If you are unable to see a pattern, select the simplest box and follow the simplest box strategy.
3. Answer each of the questions. There is only one correct answer, so when you find it, do not check any more of the boxes – you will be wasting precious seconds!

Example 18

Note: There are only 2 questions associated with this example for demonstrative purposes. In the UCAT, there would be 5 associated questions.

A

B

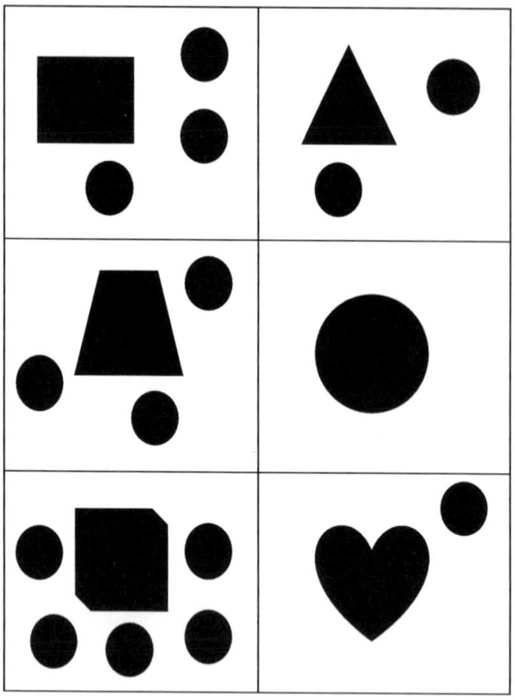

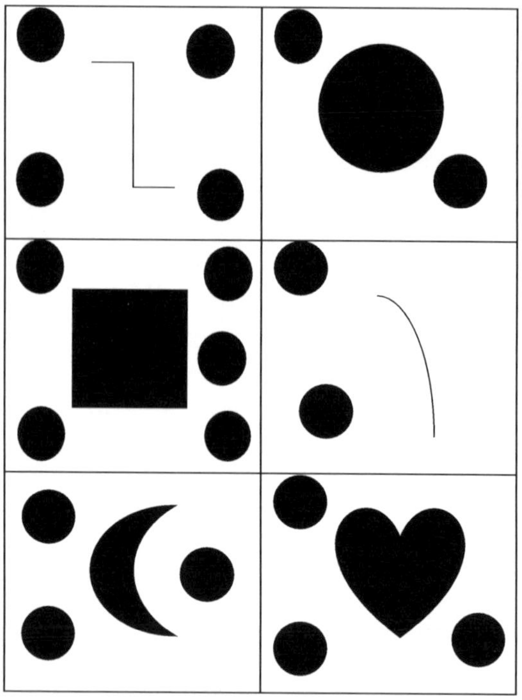

1. **Which of the following test shapes belongs in Set A?**

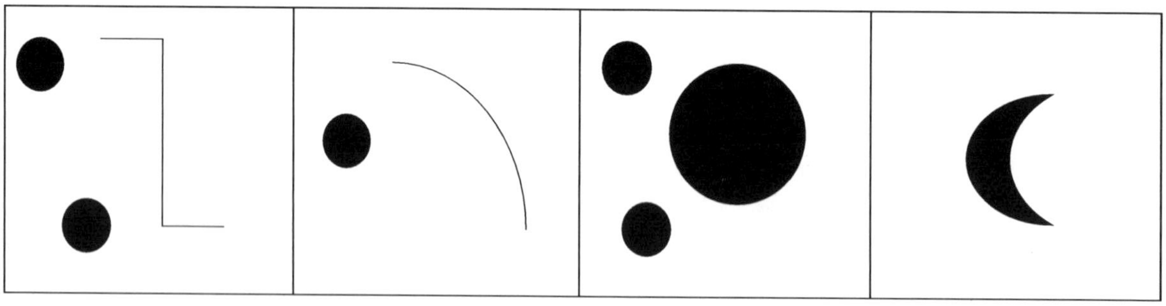

A. B. C. D.

2. **Which of the following test shapes belongs in Set B?**

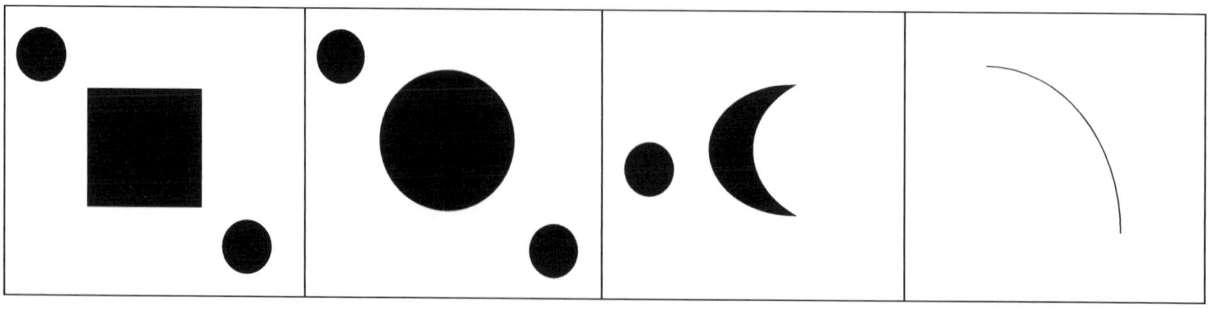

A. B. C. D.

Answer 18

Following the strategy, if you look at the sets from a distance, you will see that there are large and small shapes. The simplest box in the Set A is the middle right box. Let us identify the characteristics of this box in order to determine the pattern:

- S – Large in size. Only 1 circle present – no other shapes.
- C – Irrelevant as all boxes are the same colour.
- A – Irrelevant as there is no specific arrangement in this box.
- N – A circle only has 1 side.
- O – Orientation does not apply to a circle with a single colour.
- S – Has infinite lines of symmetry. Symmetry is probably irrelevant as all shapes appear to have symmetry.

So, from this we can note that there is a single black circle with 1 side. It is hard to spot a pattern with this alone, so let us compare the next simplest box (the bottom right) using the same characteristics.

- 1 large heart, 1 small circle.
- Heart has 2 sides, circle has 1 side.

It is still difficult to identify a pattern here, although you may have some ideas. Let us look at the next simplest box – the top right:

- 1 triangle, 2 small circles.
- Triangle has 3 sides, circles have 1 side each.

After going through all of these, the pattern should start to become more evident. It appears that the number of small circles present is always 1 less than the total number of sides in the large shape.

- Large circle has 1 side. 1 - 0 = 0, so 0 small circles are present
- Large heart has 2 sides. 2 - 1 = 1, so 1 small circle is present.
- Large triangle has 3 sides. 3 - 1 = 2, so 2 small circles are present.

You can confirm this with any of the other squares.

To identify the pattern in Set B, we will look for something similar. Analysing the simplest square (top right), the large shape has 1 side, and there are 2 small circles. It appears that the rule in Set B is the inverse of Set A – the number of small circles is always 1 *more* than the total number of sides in the large shape.

Using the patterns identified, the answers are as follows:

1. The correct answer is A. The large shape has 3 sides, and there are 2 small circles present.
2. The correct answer is B. The large shape has 1 side, and there are 2 small circles.

Important Things to Remember

1. It is impossible and fairly pointless to try to cover every type of pattern that might possibly appear in Abstract Reasoning. Hopefully, the strategies you have learned through this section and the examples that have been demonstrated will give you an excellent understanding of how to answer the four types of questions. The rest of it will be practice and training your brain to identify patterns quickly.
2. Abstract Reasoning is hard to being with. You can start your practice untimed to give yourself a chance to work through all of the strategies and identify the relevant patterns. Once you become more comfortable with pattern recognition, you can start doing questions in timed conditions. However, do not spend too long in the untimed stage, as you need to push your brain to identify patterns quickly.
3. When you do practice questions, keep a notebook and write down every pattern that comes up. You should build a bank of patterns throughout your weeks of revision. Whenever you are stuck on a question, you can refer to the bank to determine whether any of the patterns you have written down might fit. If not, then add the new one to your bank once you figure out the answer.
    - If you do *thousands* of questions, you will find that the same 60 or so patterns are repeated throughout! So, the more you do, the easier it will get, as you will begin to recognise the patterns that appear.
4. Make a note of all of the distractors that appear. This will allow you to recognise distractors in future patterns to increase your efficiency at recognising patterns.
5. On exam day, in the minute before your Abstract Reasoning section, try to write down as many patterns as you can remember. This will help jog your memory and provide you with a reference point if you are stuck during the test. To prepare for this minute, practice writing out the patterns you can remember in the minute before your mock tests at home.
6. Do not waste your time on the hardest questions. As with every section, the question-writers like to waste your time with extremely difficult questions. Often, when the beginning questions are difficult, students are afraid to flag as they have not yet answered anything. However, these questions are there on purpose to waste your time! Do not be afraid to guess and flag.
7. Do not worry if you are struggling with identifying patterns. There are a lot of very challenging and time-consuming patterns. In the beginning weeks of your revision, you are not expected to be able to identify all of these within a number of seconds. Allow yourself room for improvement over the weeks, and hopefully, the more

difficult patterns will get easier for you. On average, students see the biggest improvement in Abstract Reasoning from their initial mock test to their final score.

Abstract Reasoning Mock Test

Note: This test is not correctly representative of an Abstract Reasoning UCAT test with regards to number and variety of questions.

- To ensure that you have sufficient exposure to each question type, there is a greater mixture of question types than expected.
- There are 61 questions, rather than 55. Thus, you should spend 14 minutes and 30 seconds on this test if you wish to time yourself.
- Type 4 questions have 2 associated questions, rather than 5. This will give you exposure to a greater variety of questions and patterns, as it allows for more Type 4 sets.
- The Abstract Reasoning portion of the complete mock test at the end of the book is fully representative of the UCAT exam with regards to type and variety of questions.

The test starts on the next page.

Question 1

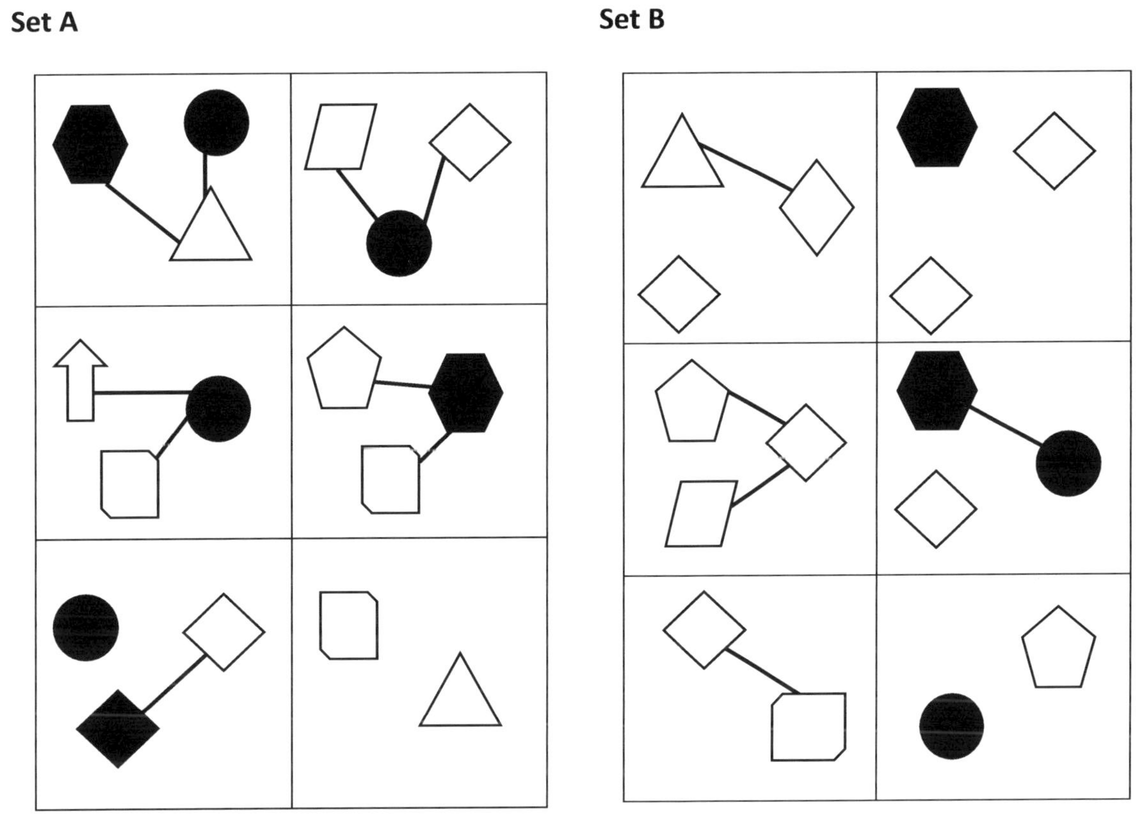

Determine whether the test shapes belong to Set A, Set B or neither.

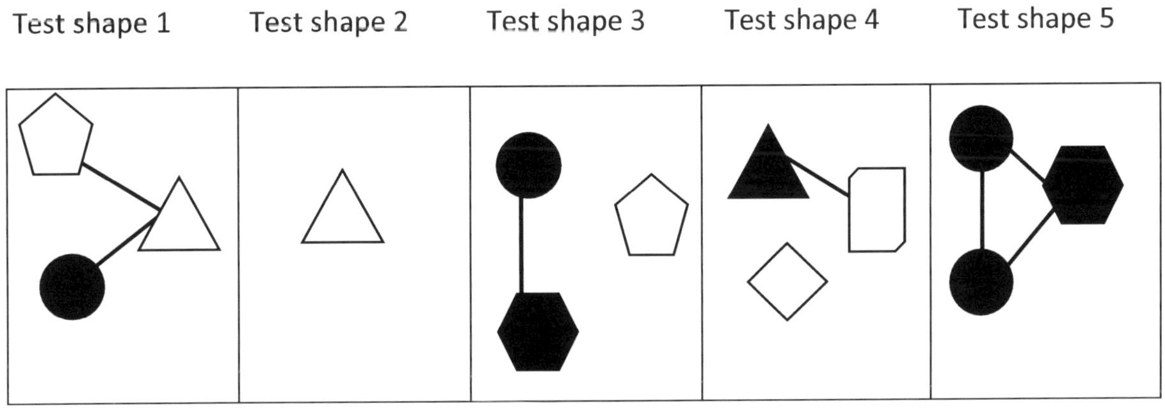

Test shape 1	Test shape 2	Test shape 3	Test shape 4	Test shape 5
D. Set A	D. Set A	D. Set A	D. Set A	D. Set A
E. Set B	E. Set B	E. Set B	E. Set B	E. Set B
F. Neither	F. Neither	F. Neither	F. Neither	F. Neither

Question 2

Set A

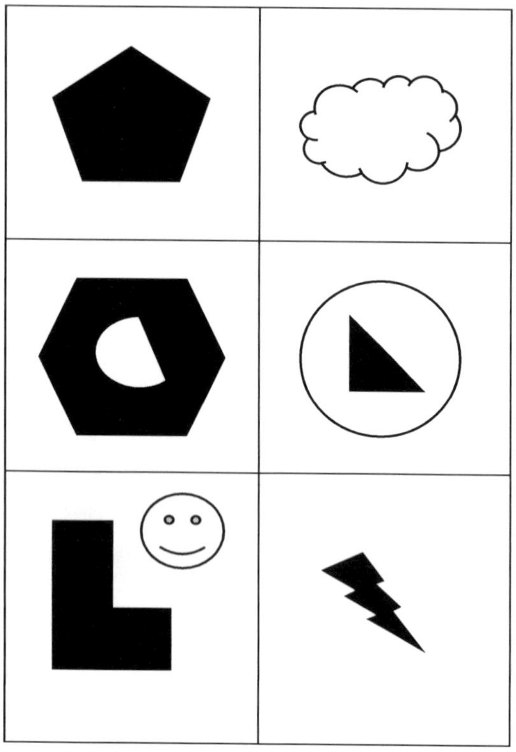

Set B

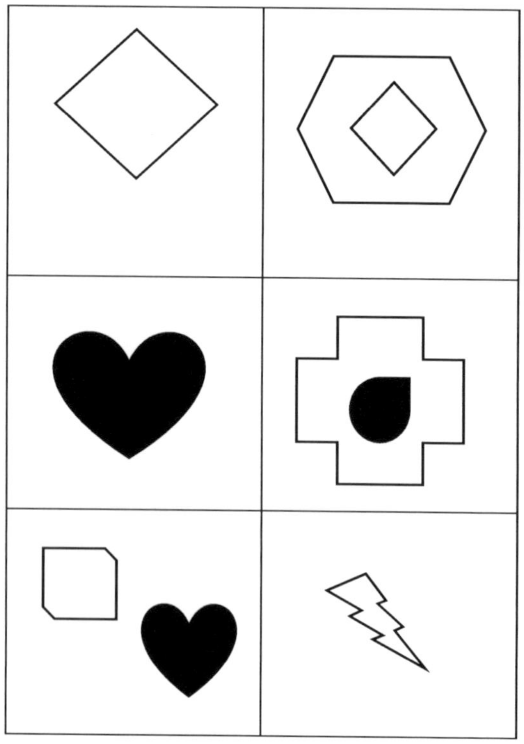

Determine whether the test shapes belong to Set A, Set B or neither.

Test shape 6	Test shape 7	Test shape 8	Test shape 9	Test shape 10

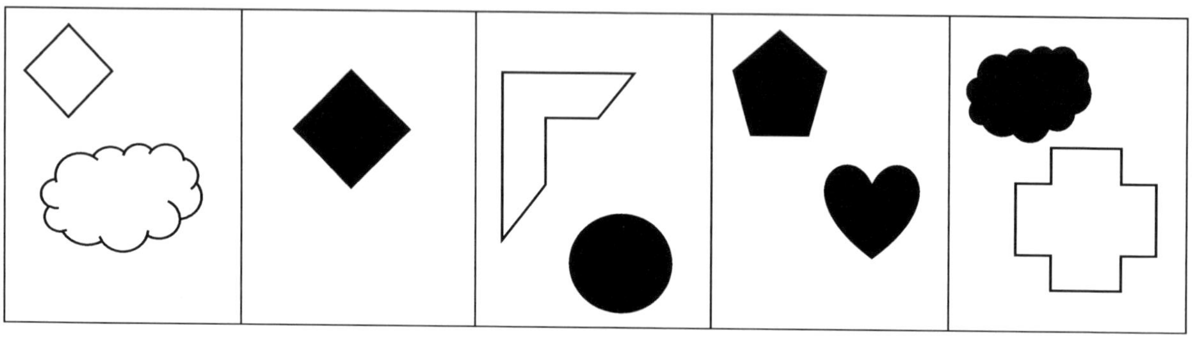

Test shape 6	Test shape 7	Test shape 8	Test shape 9	Test shape 10
A. Set A	A. Set A	A. Set A	A. Set A	A. Set A
B. Set B	B. Set B	B. Set B	B. Set B	B. Set B
C. Neither	C. Neither	C. Neither	C. Neither	C. Neither

Question 3

Set A

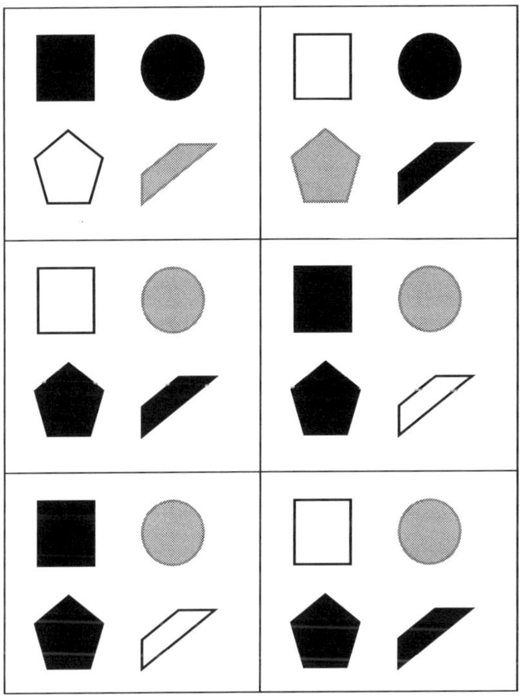

Set B

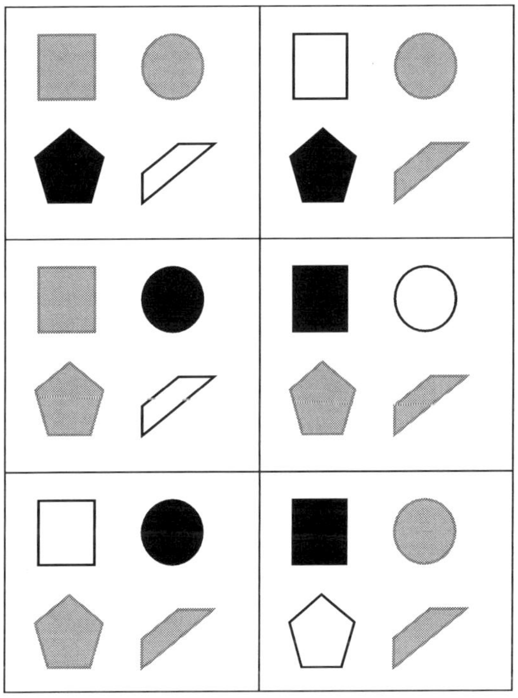

Determine whether the test shapes belong to Set A, Set B or neither.

Test shape 11	Test shape 12	Test shape 13	Test shape 14	Test shape 15

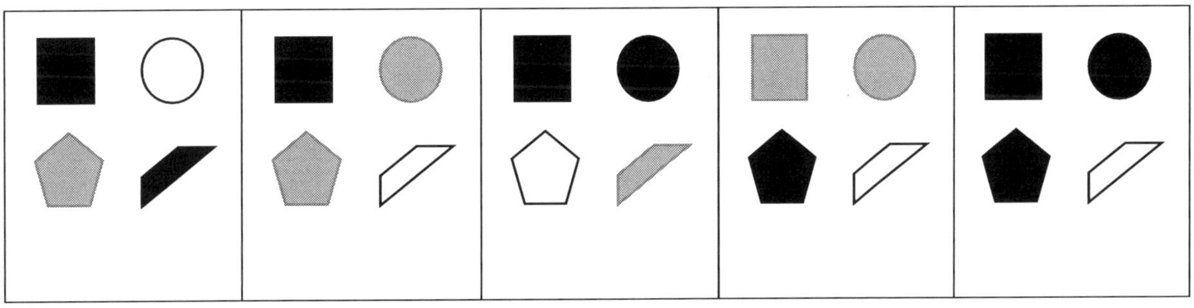

Test shape 11	Test shape 12	Test shape 13	Test shape 14	Test shape 15
A. Set A	A. Set A	A. Set A	A. Set A	A. Set A
B. Set B	B. Set B	B. Set B	B. Set B	B. Set B
C. Neither	C. Neither	C. Neither	C. Neither	C. Neither

Question 4

Set A

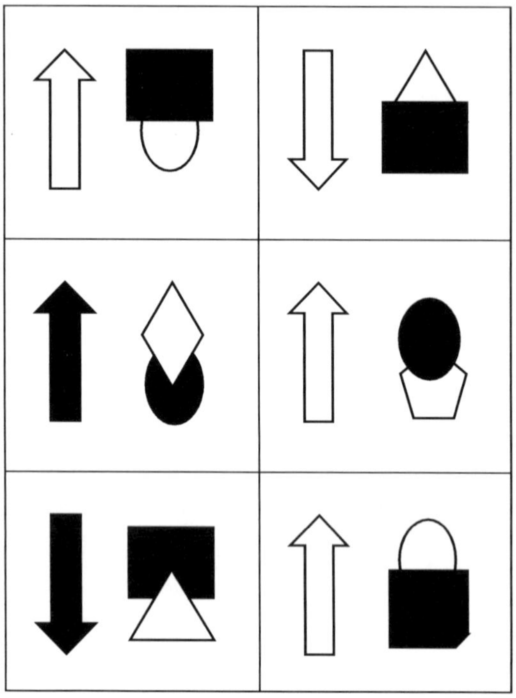

Set B

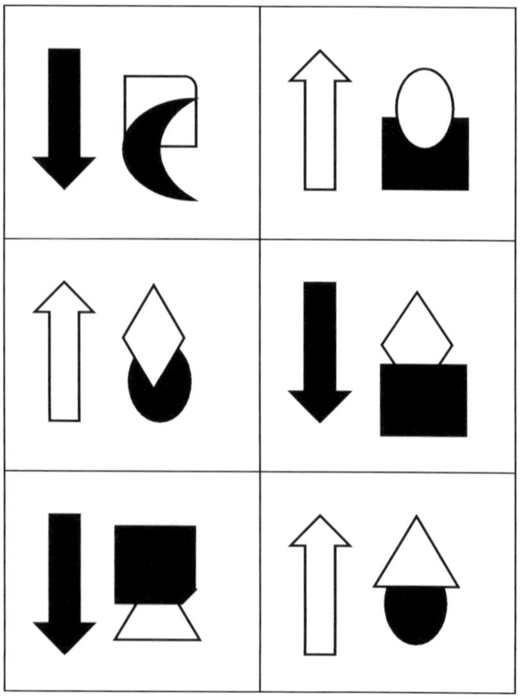

Determine whether the test shapes belong to Set A, Set B or neither.

Test shape 16	Test shape 17	Test shape 18	Test shape 19	Test shape 20

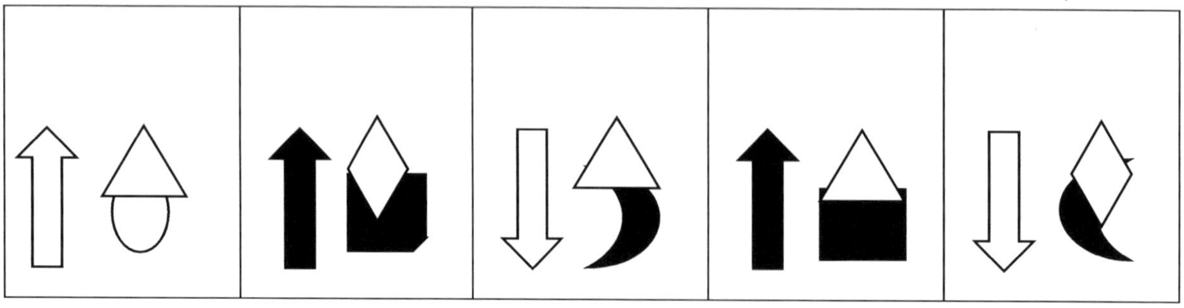

A. Set A B. Set B C. Neither	A. Set A B. Set B C. Neither	A. Set A B. Set B C. Neither	A. Set A B. Set B C. Neither	A. Set A B. Set B C. Neither

Question 5

Set A

2	8
5	S
C	3

Set B

Y	7
4	A
L	1

Determine whether the test shapes belong to Set A, Set B or neither.

Test shape 21	Test shape 22	Test shape 23	Test shape 24	Test shape 25
9	T	I	O	U

Test shape 21	Test shape 22	Test shape 23	Test shape 24	Test shape 25
A. Set A	A. Set A	A. Set A	A. Set A	A. Set A
B. Set B	B. Set B	B. Set B	B. Set B	B. Set B
C. Neither	C. Neither	C. Neither	C. Neither	C. Neither

Question 6

Set A

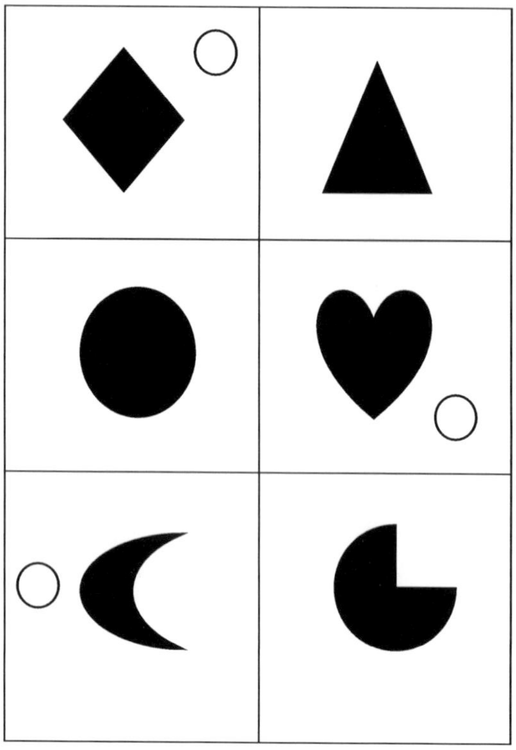

Set B

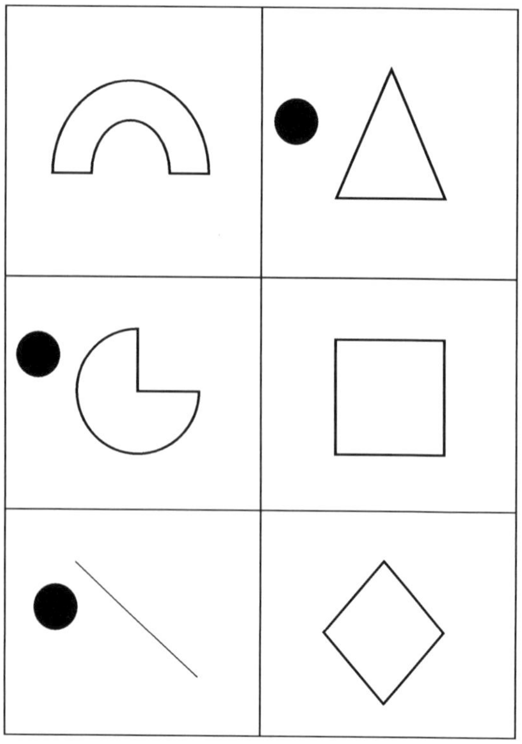

Determine whether the test shapes belong to Set A, Set B or neither.

Test shape 26 | Test shape 27 | Test shape 28 | Test shape 29 | Test shape 30

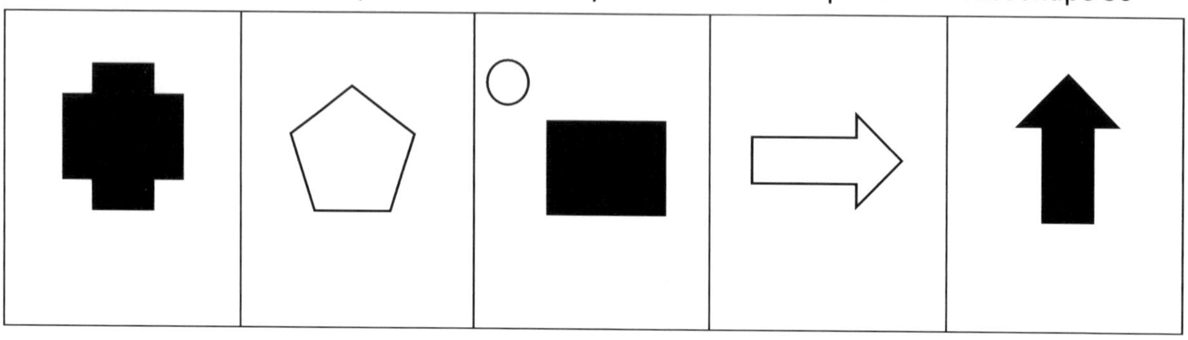

Test shape 26	Test shape 27	Test shape 28	Test shape 29	Test shape 30
A. Set A	A. Set A	A. Set A	A. Set A	A. Set A
B. Set B	B. Set B	B. Set B	B. Set B	B. Set B
C. Neither	C. Neither	C. Neither	C. Neither	C. Neither

Question 7

Set A

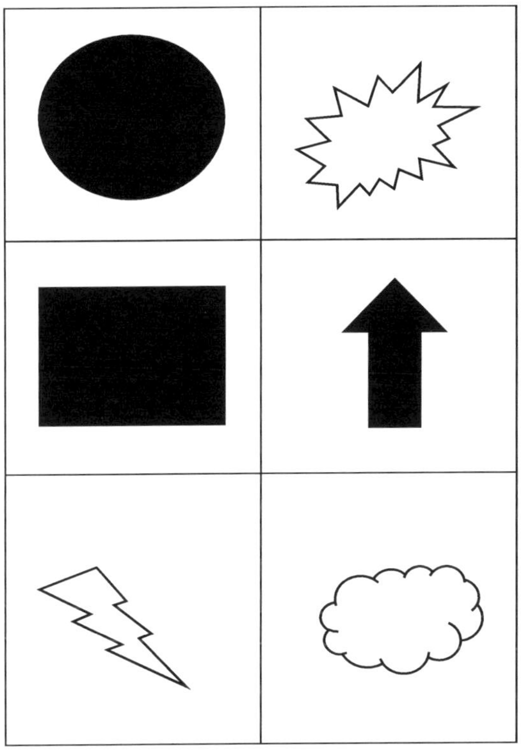

Set B

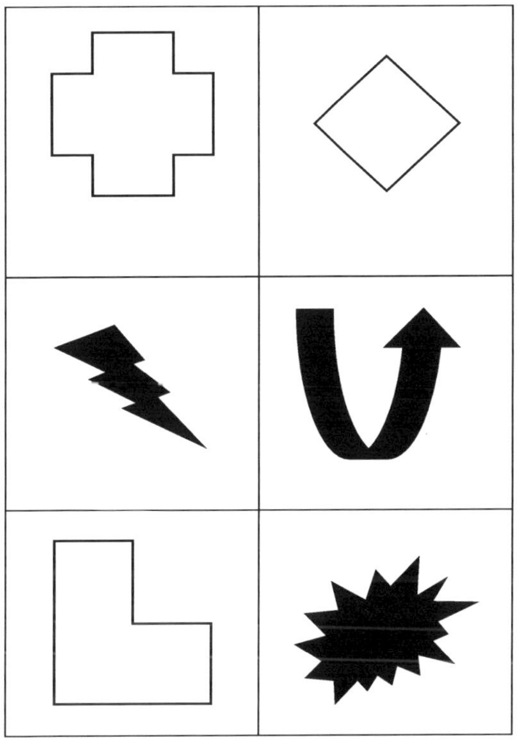

Determine whether the test shapes belong to Set A, Set B or neither.

Test shape 31	Test shape 32	Test shape 33	Test shape 34	Test shape 35

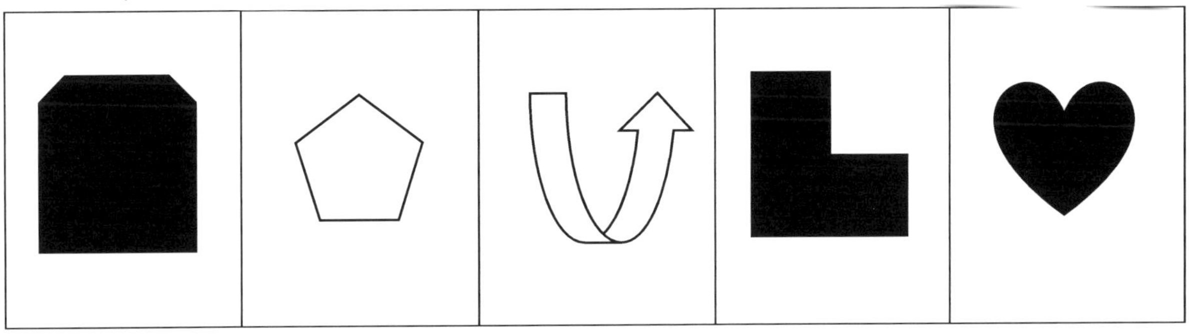

Test shape 31	Test shape 32	Test shape 33	Test shape 34	Test shape 35
A. Set A	A. Set A	A. Set A	A. Set A	A. Set A
B. Set B	B. Set B	B. Set B	B. Set B	B. Set B
C. Neither	C. Neither	C. Neither	C. Neither	C. Neither

Question 8

Set A

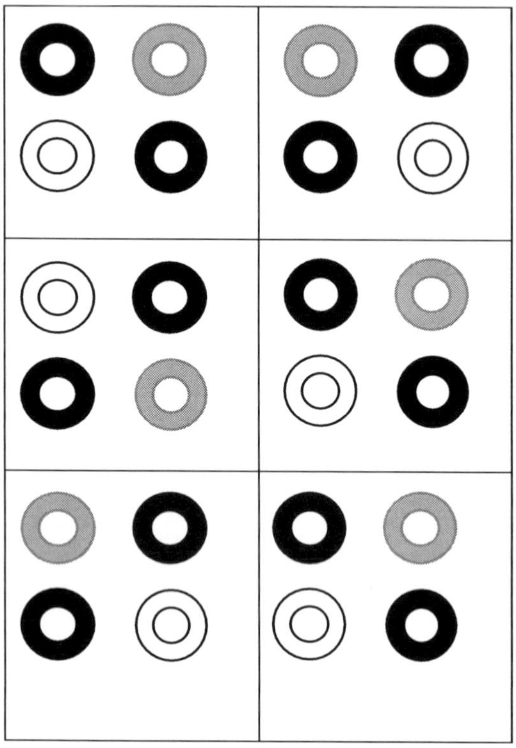

Set B

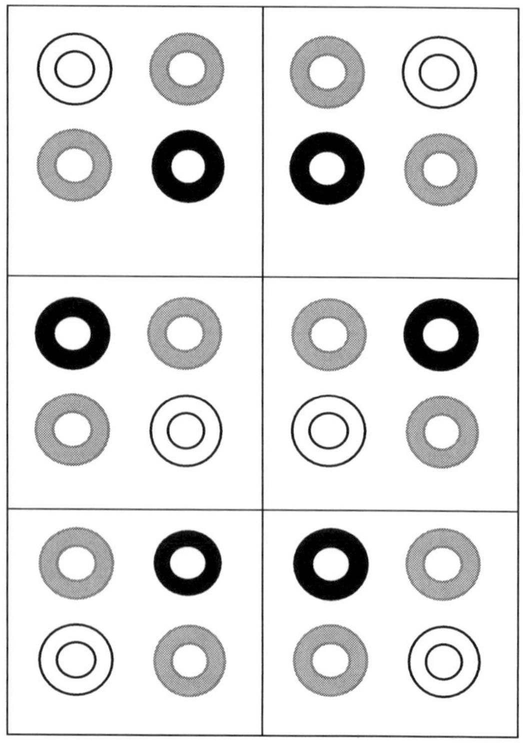

Determine whether the test shapes belong to Set A, Set B or neither.

Test shape 36 | Test shape 37 | Test shape 38 | Test shape 39 | Test shape 40

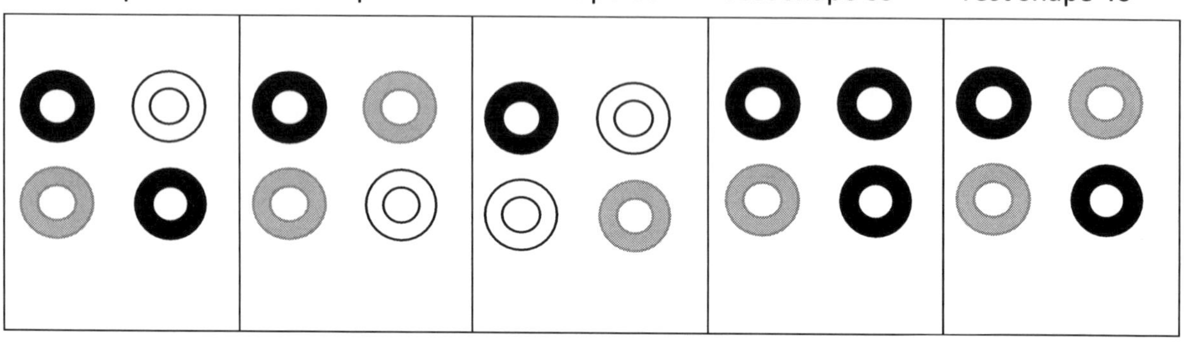

Test shape 36:
A. Set A
B. Set B
C. Neither

Test shape 37:
A. Set A
B. Set B
C. Neither

Test shape 38:
A. Set A
B. Set B
C. Neither

Test shape 39:
A. Set A
B. Set B
C. Neither

Test shape 40:
A. Set A
B. Set B
C. Neither

Question 9

Set A

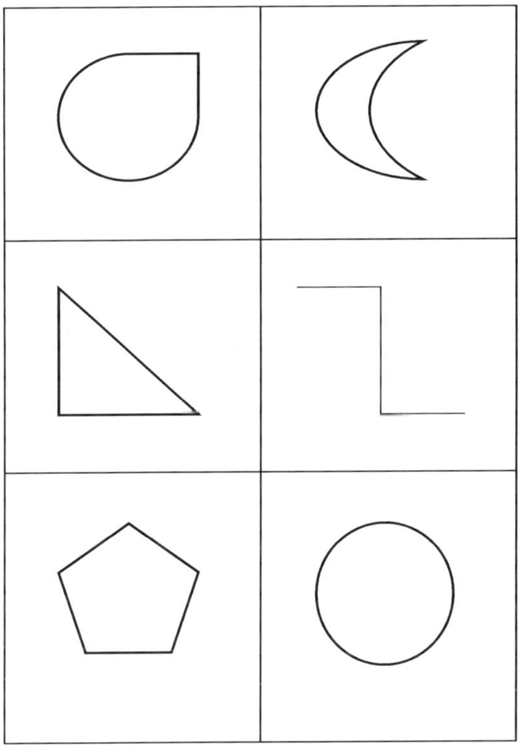

Set B

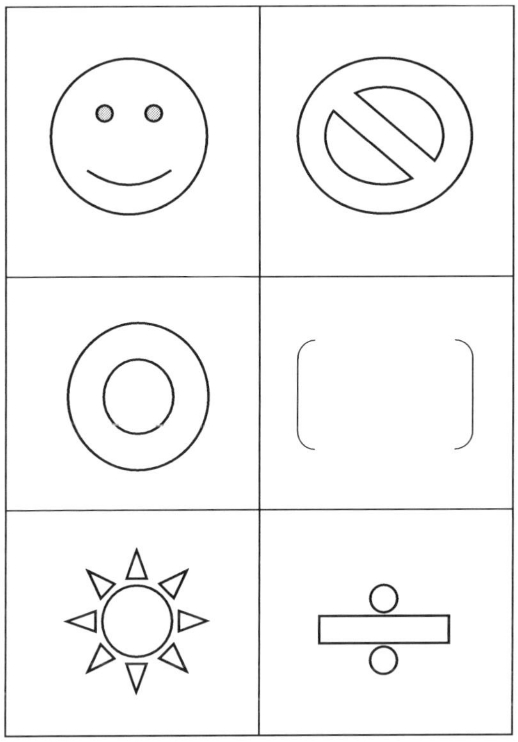

41. Which of the following test shapes belongs to Set A?

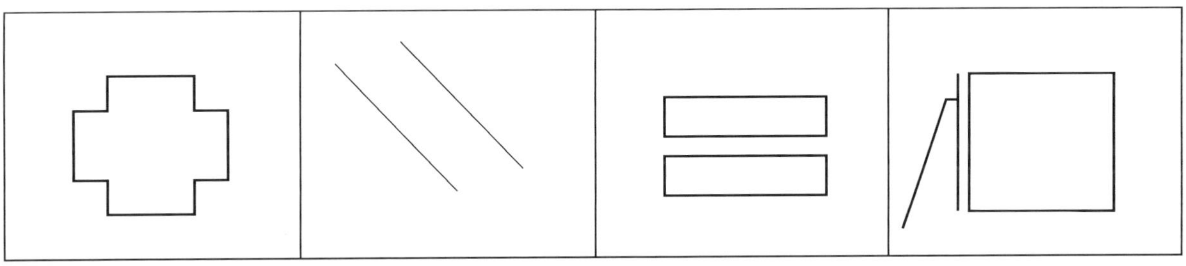

A. **B.** **C.** **D.**

42. Which of the following test shapes belongs to Set B?

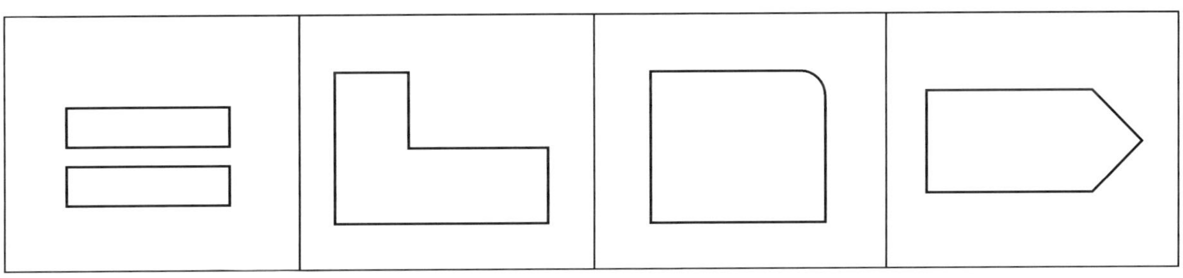

A. **B.** **C.** **D.**

Question 10

Set A **Set B**

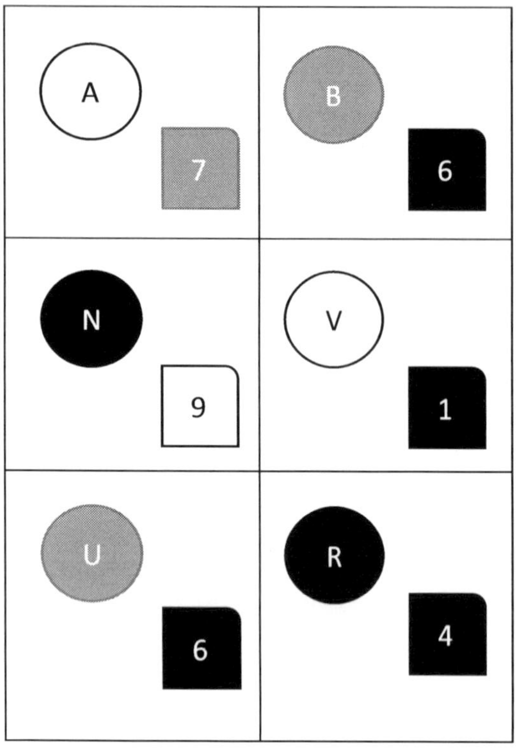

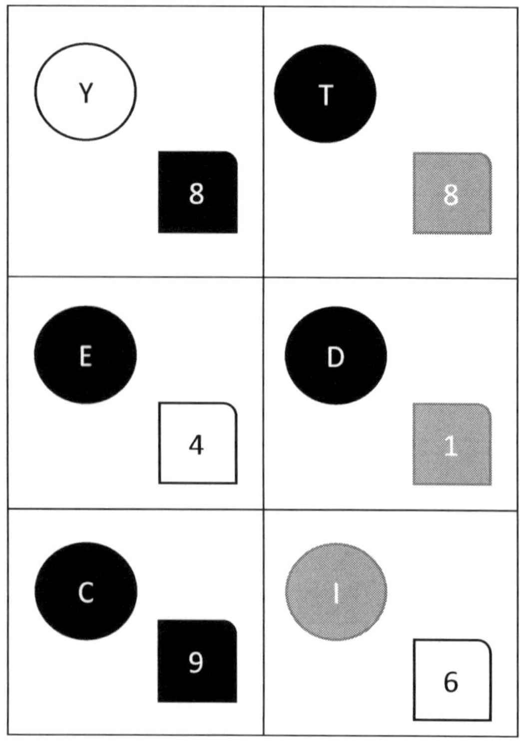

43. Which of the following test shapes belongs to Set A?

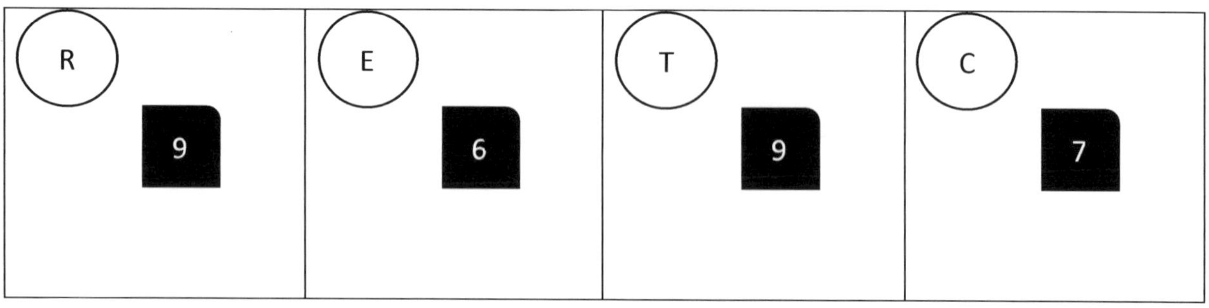

A. **B.** **C.** **D.**

44. Which of the following test shapes belongs to Set B?

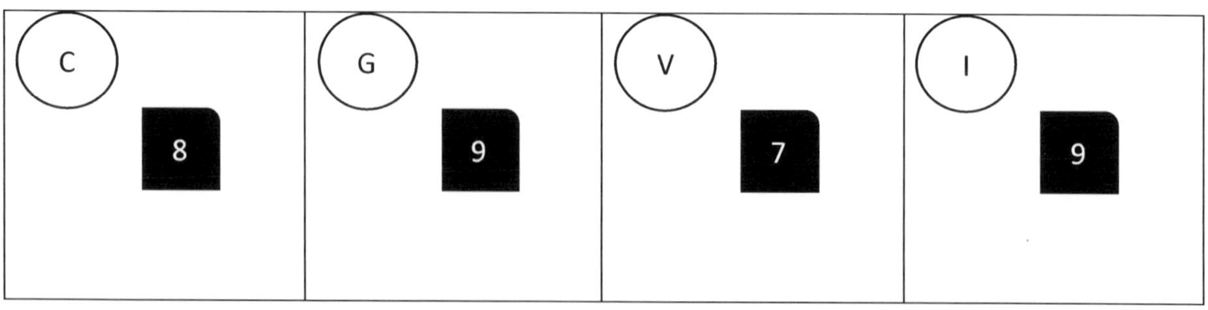

A. **B.** **C.** **D.**

Question 11

Set A

Set B

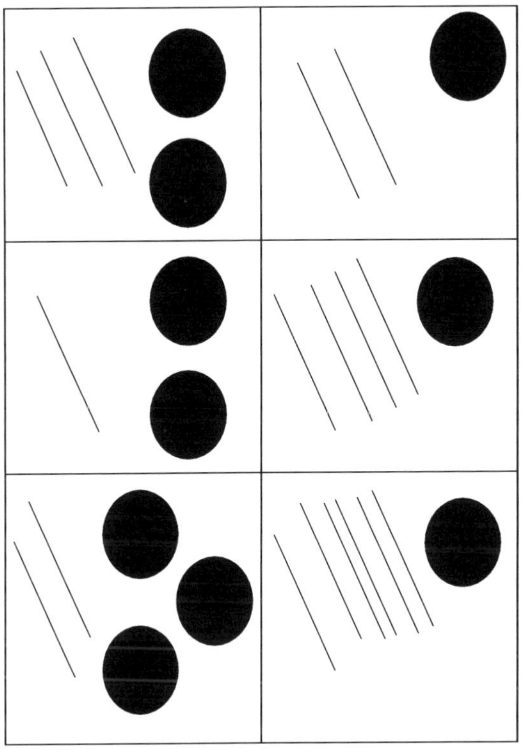

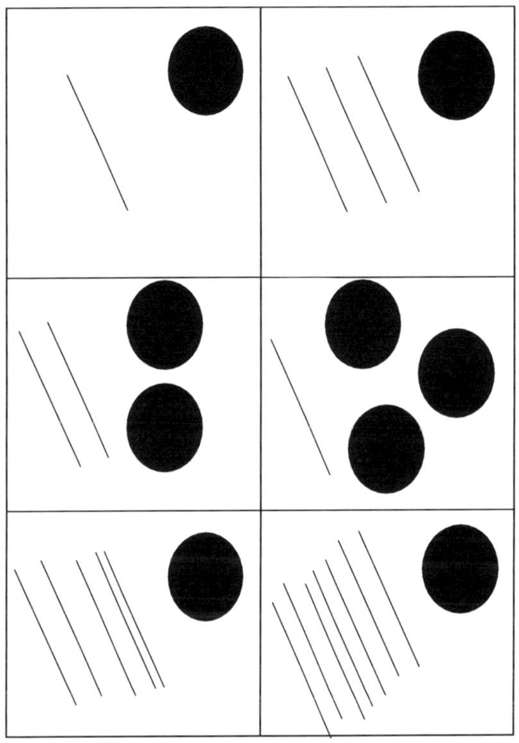

45. Which of the following test shapes belongs to Set A?

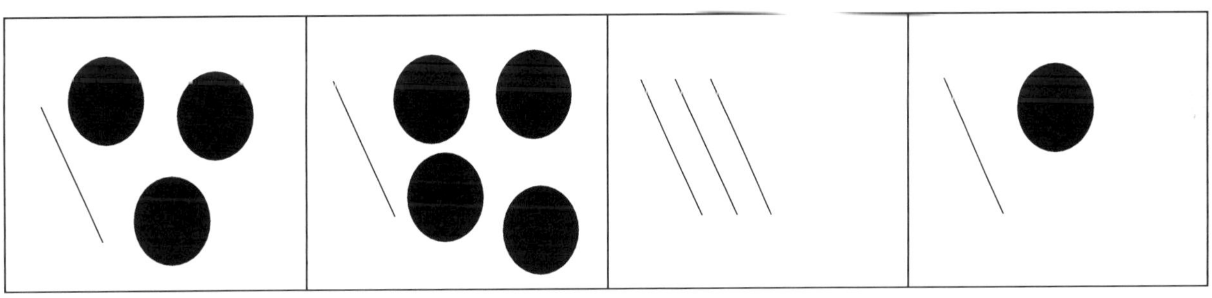

A. **B.** **C.** **D.**

46. Which of the following test shapes belongs to Set B?

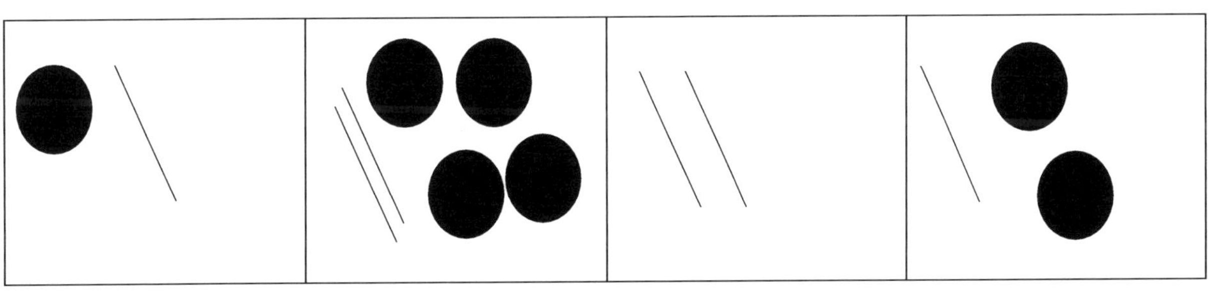

A. **B.** **C.** **D.**

Question 12

Set A

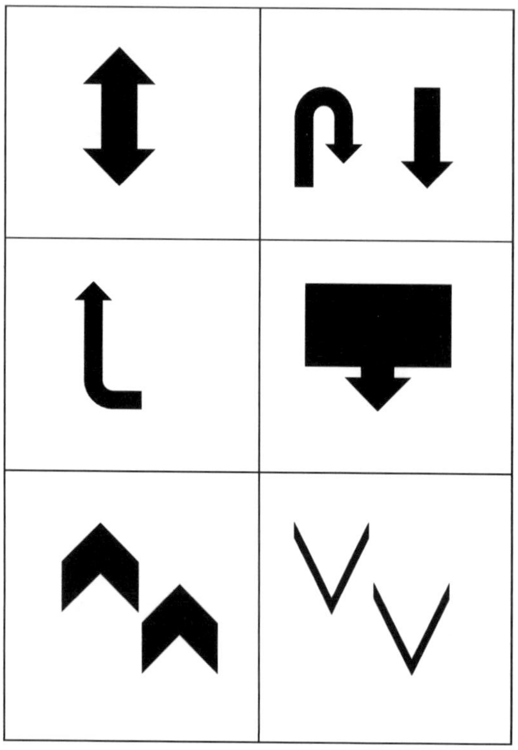

Set B

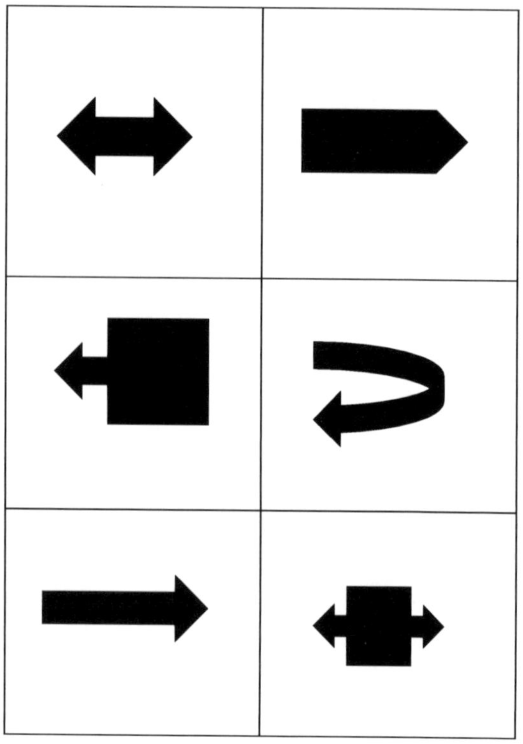

47. Which of the following test shapes belongs to Set A?

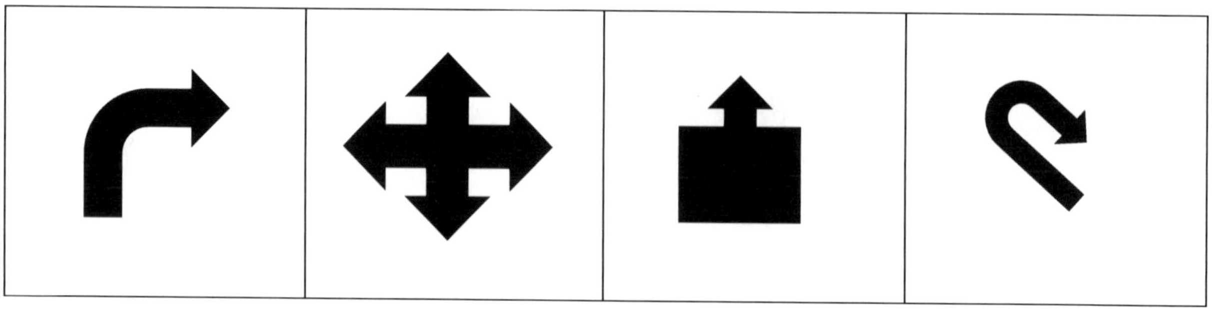

A. **B.** **C.** **D.**

48. Which of the following test shapes belongs to Set B?

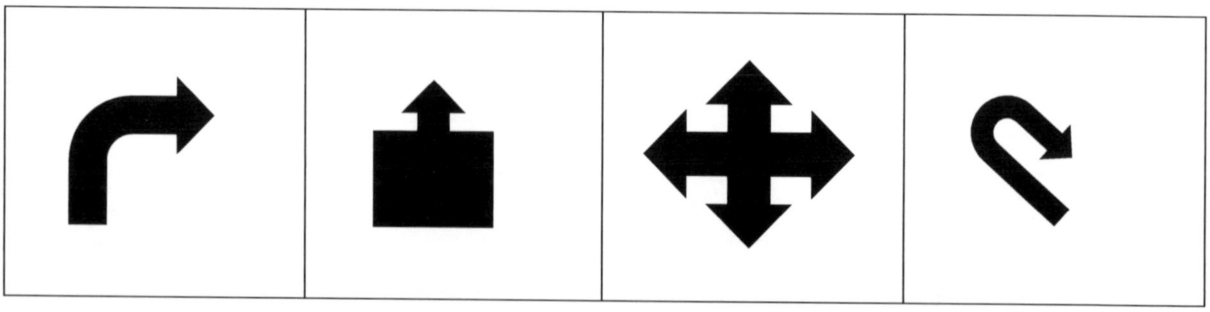

A. **B.** **C.** **D.**

Question 13

Set A **Set B**

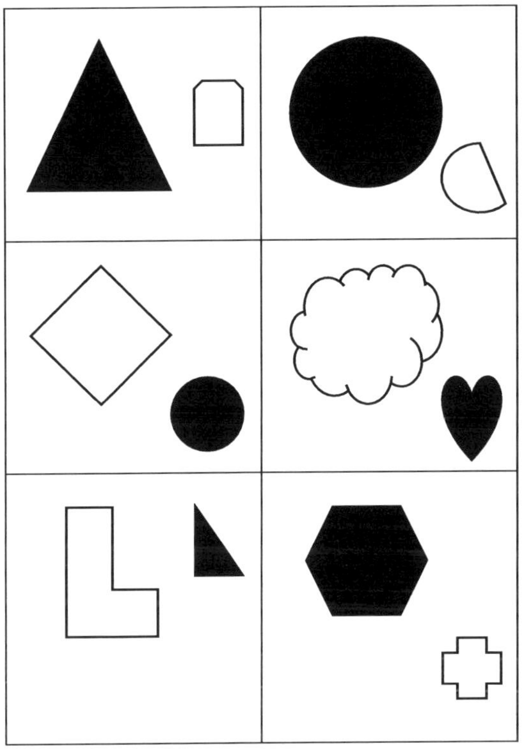

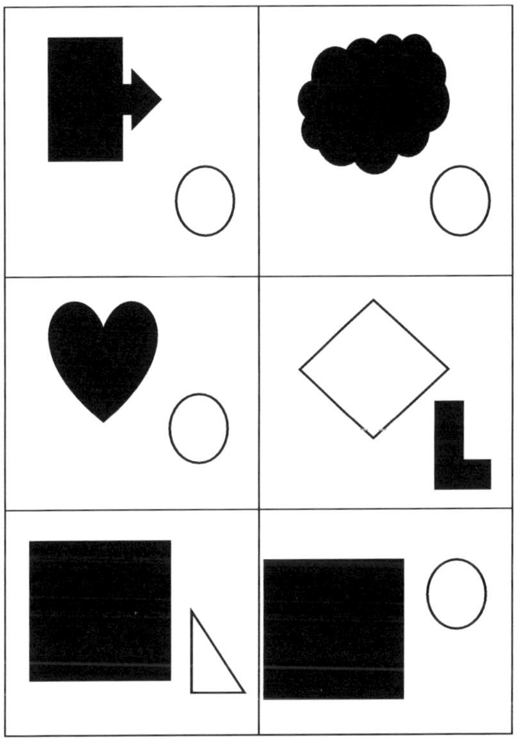

49. Which of the following test shapes belongs to Set A?

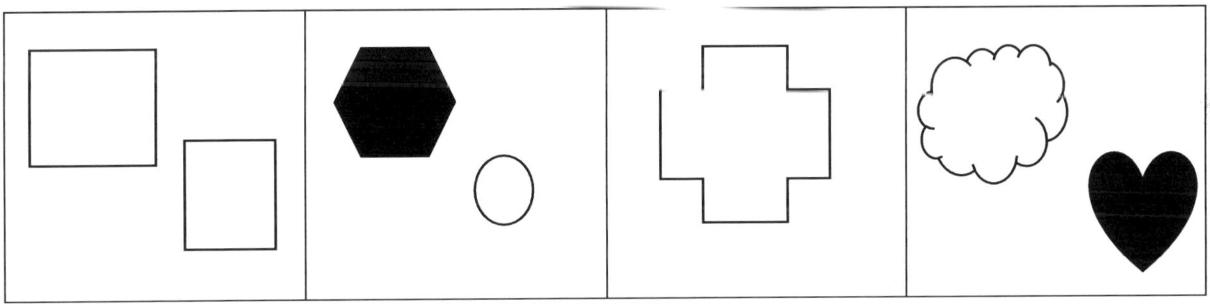

A. **B.** **C.** **D.**

50. Which of the following test shapes belongs to Set B?

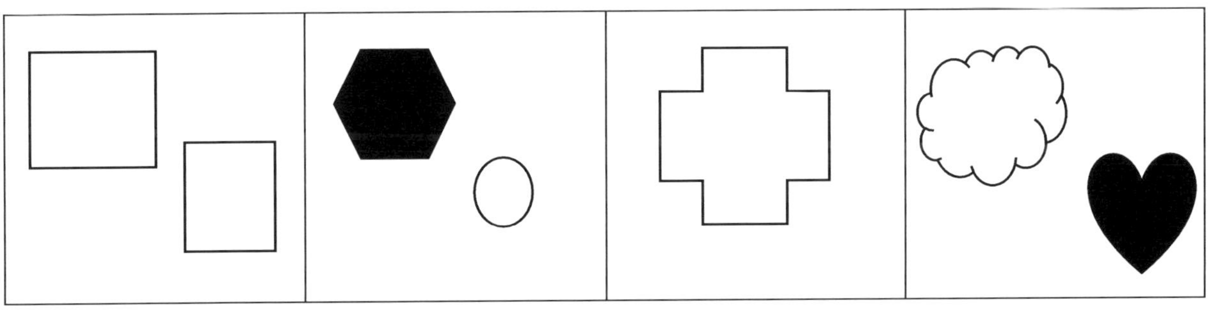

A. **B.** **C.** **D.**

Question 14

Set A

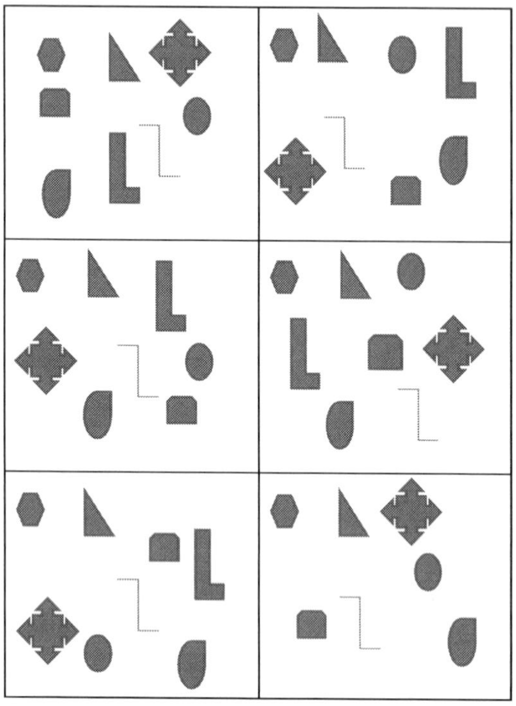

Set B

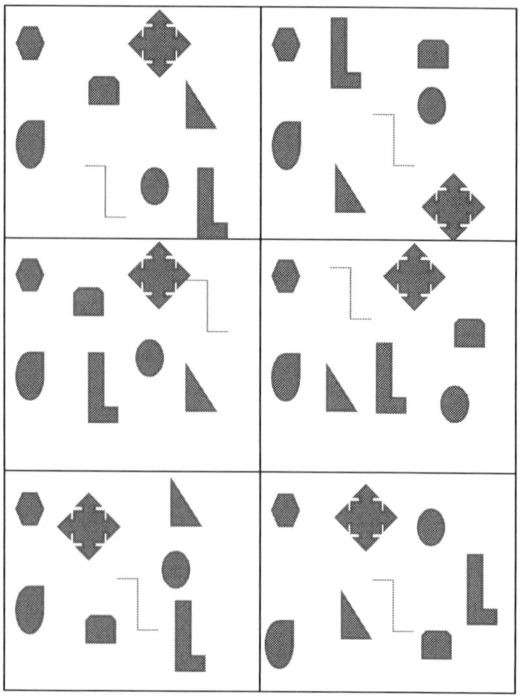

51. Which of the following test shapes belongs to Set A?

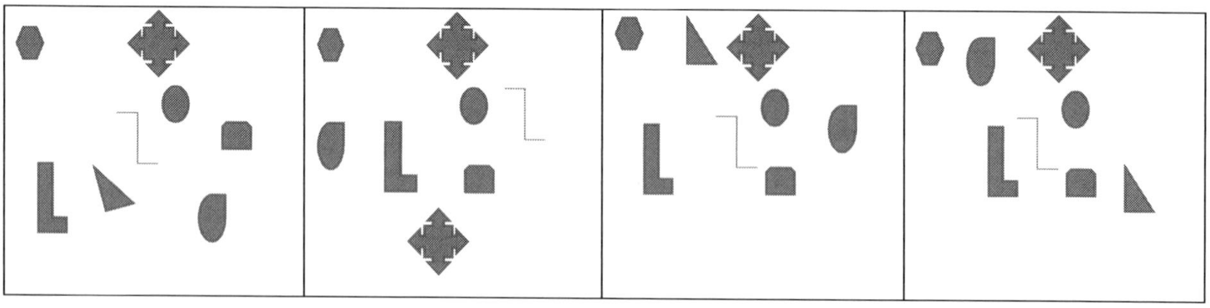

A. **B.** **C.** **D.**

52. Which of the following test shapes belongs to Set B?

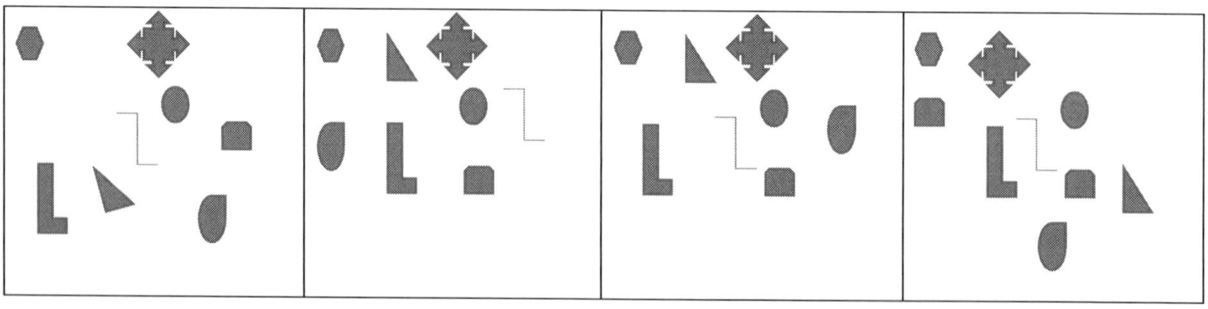

A. **B.** **C.** **D.**

Question 15

Set A

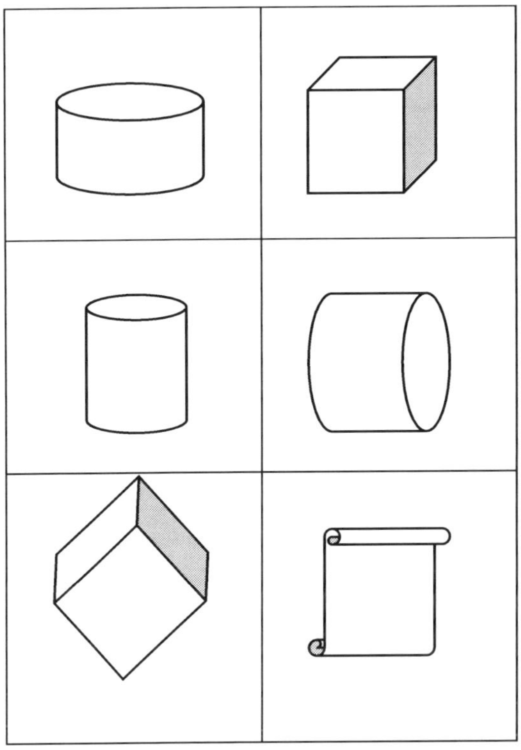

Set B

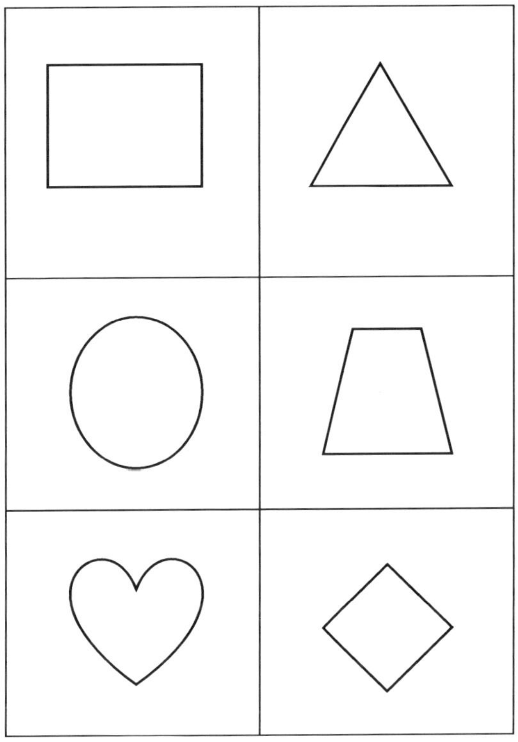

53. Which of the following test shapes belongs to Set A?

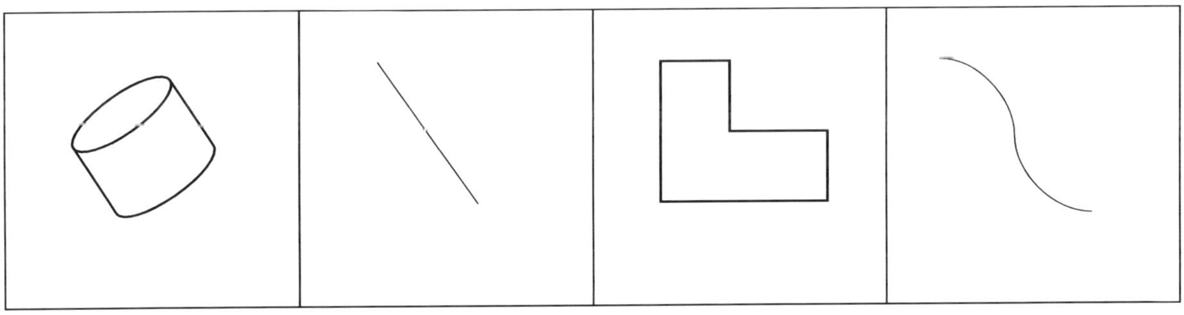

A. **B.** **C.** **D.**

54. Which of the following test shapes belongs to Set B?

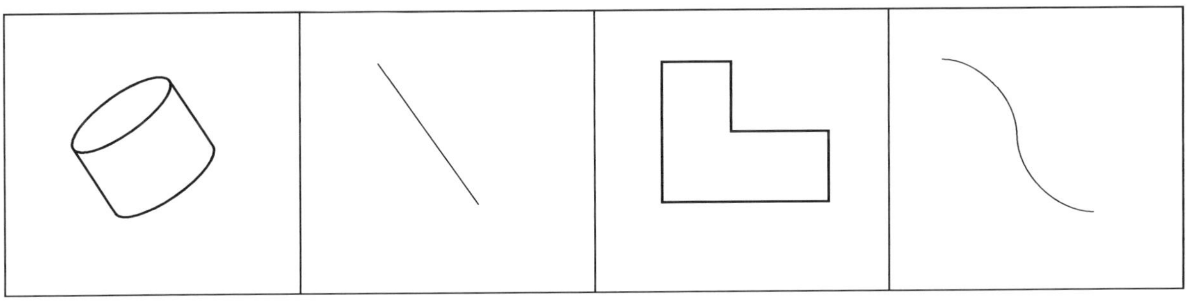

A. **B.** **C.** **D.**

55.

A	N	V	L

Which figure completes the series?

O	R	J	S
A.	**B.**	**C.**	**D.**

56.

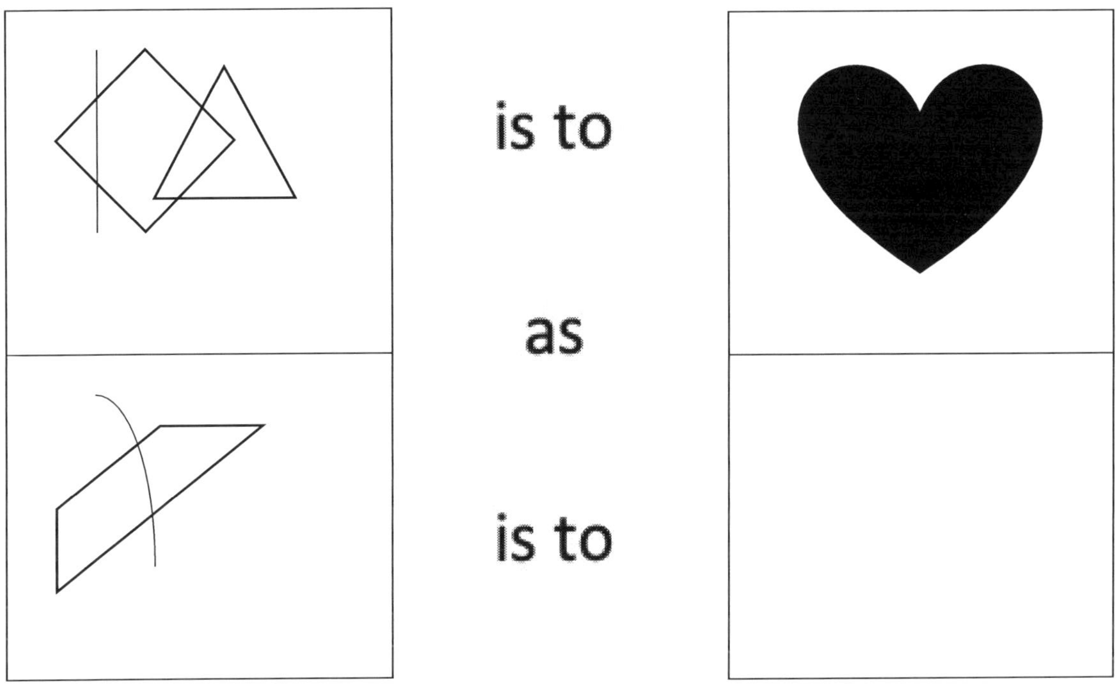

Which figure completes the statement?

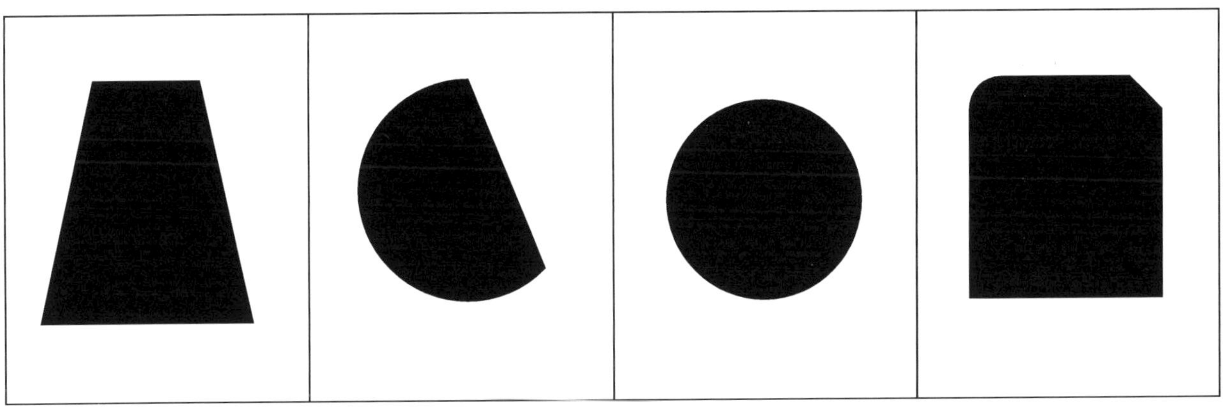

A. **B.** **C.** **D.**

57.

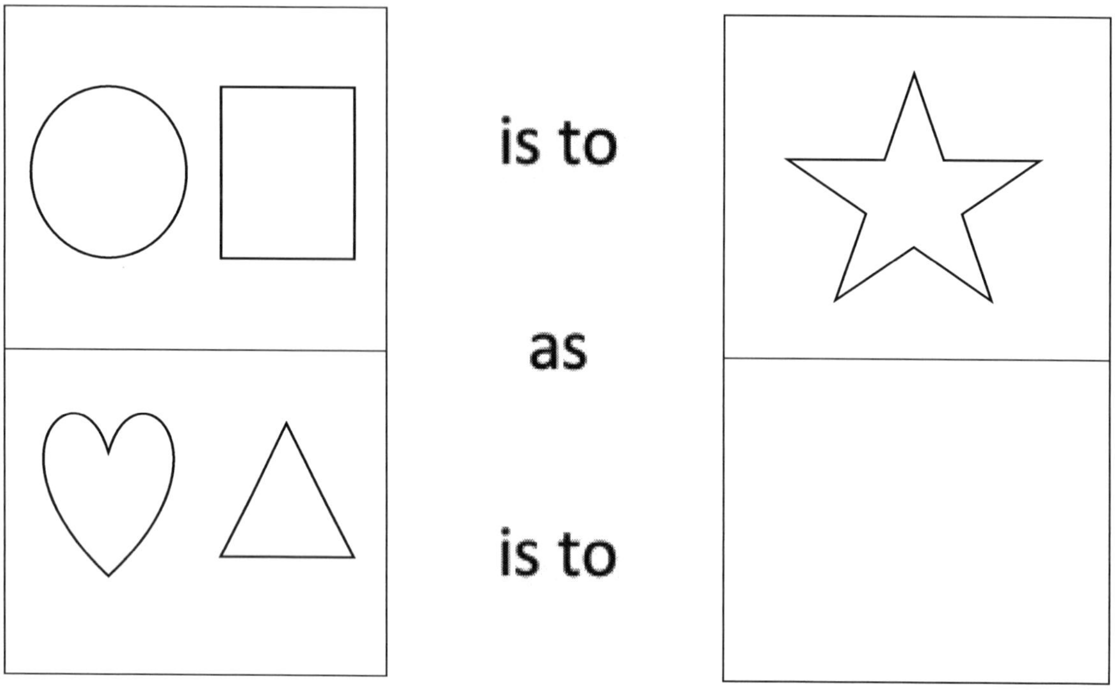

Which figure completes the statement?

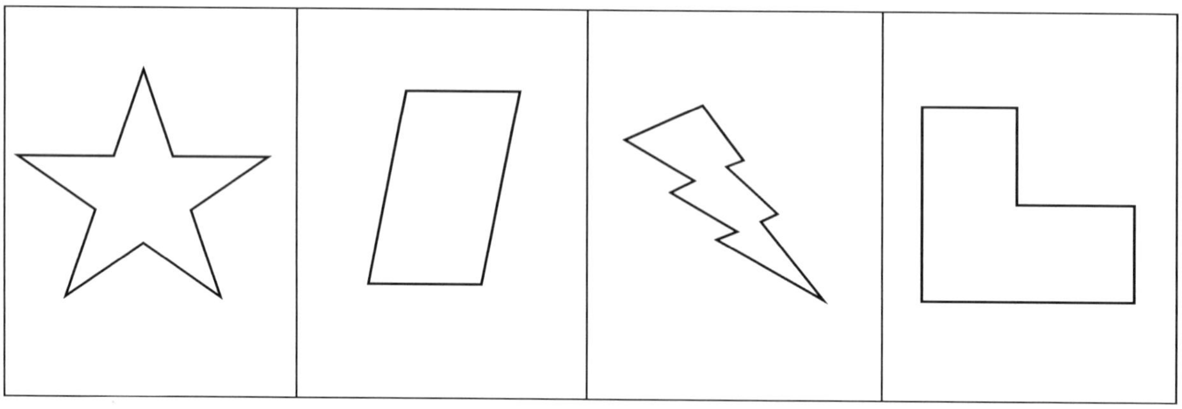

A. **B.** **C.** **D.**

58.

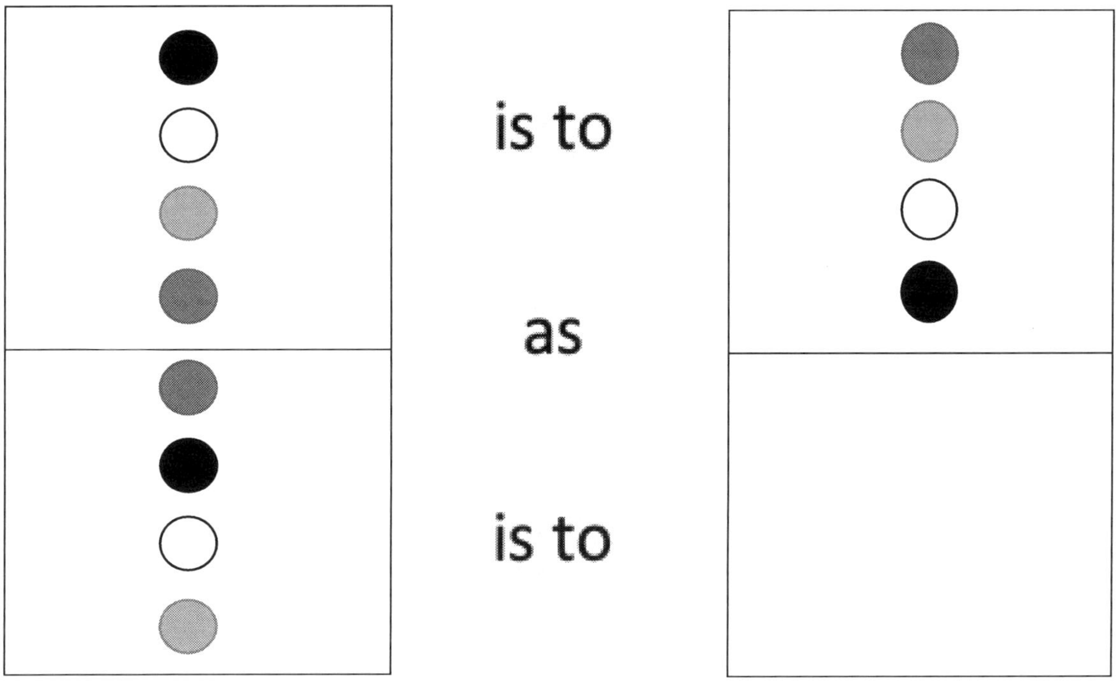

Which figure completes the statement?

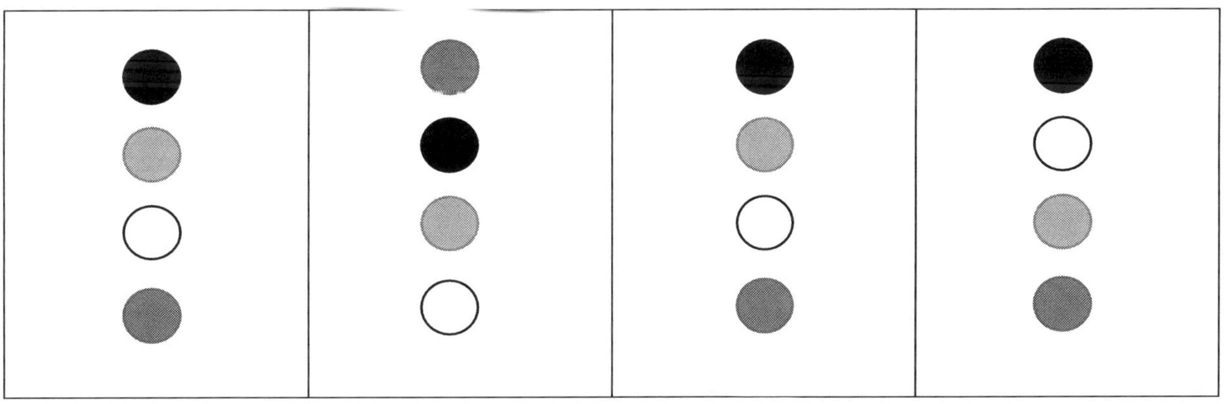

A. **B.** **C.** **D.**

59.

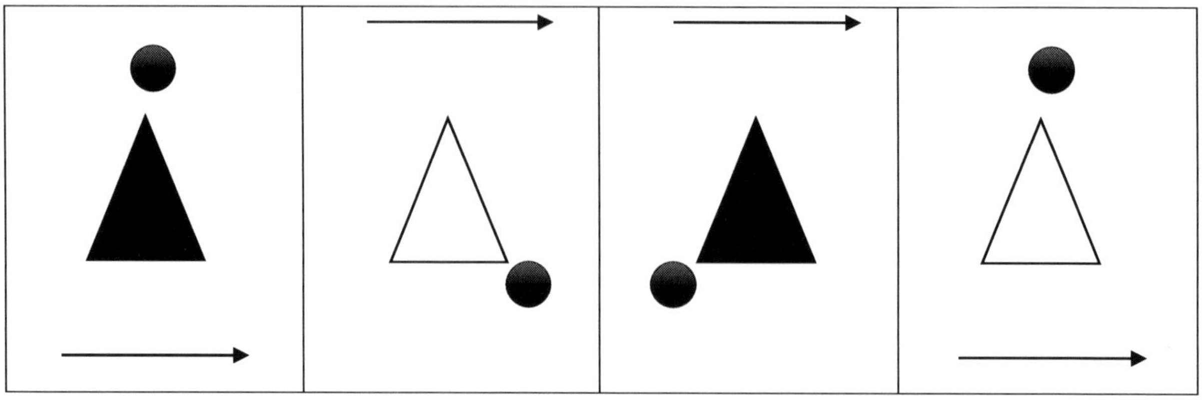

Which figure completes the series?

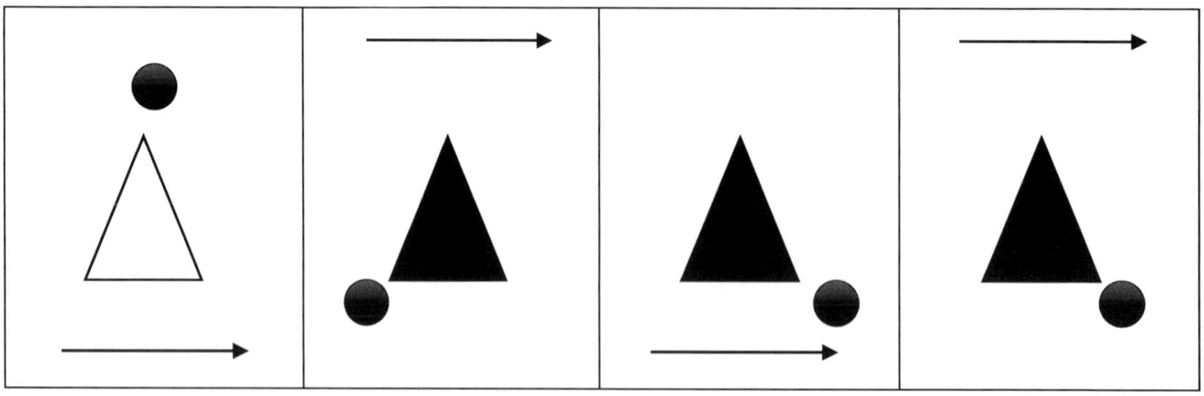

A. B. C. D.

60.

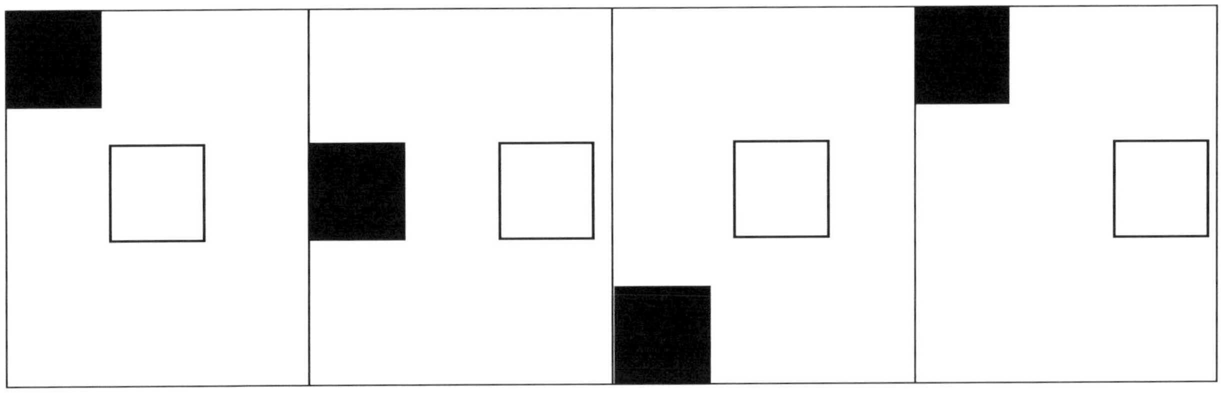

Which figure completes the series?

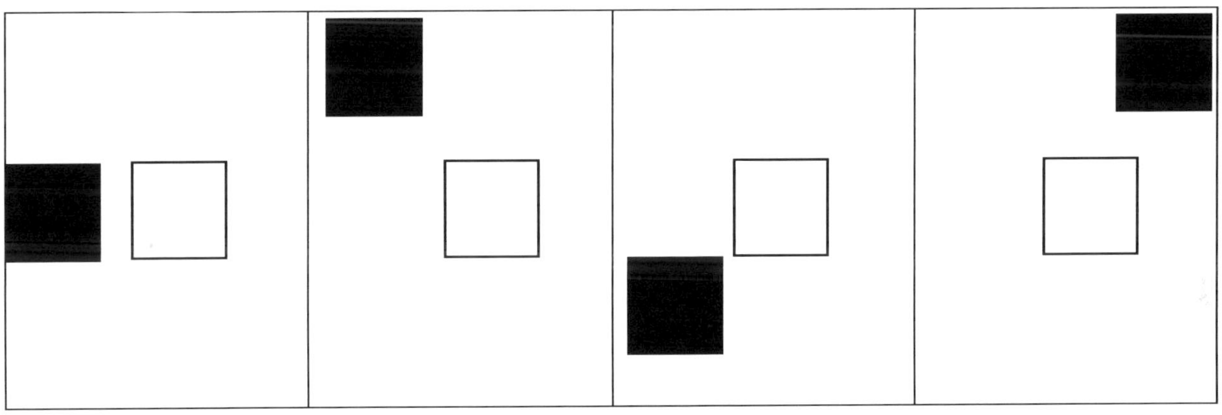

A. **B.** **C.** **D.**

61.

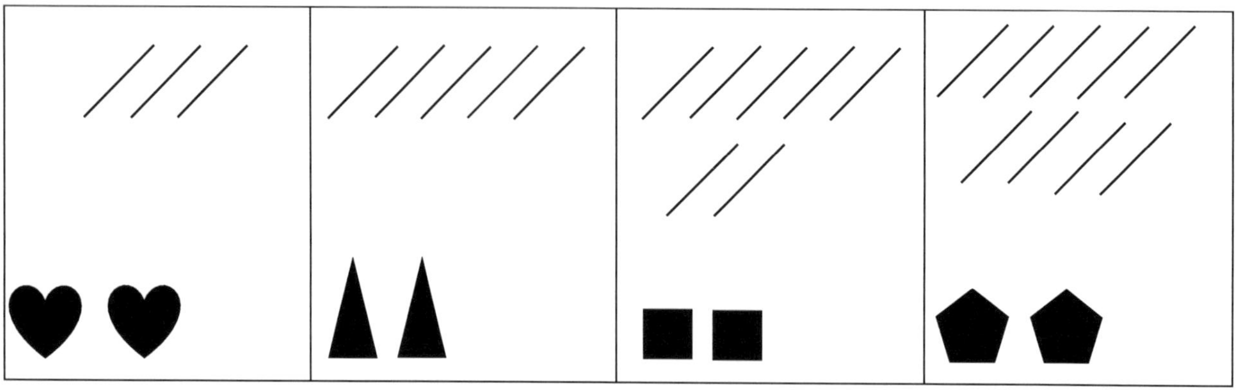

Which figure completes the series?

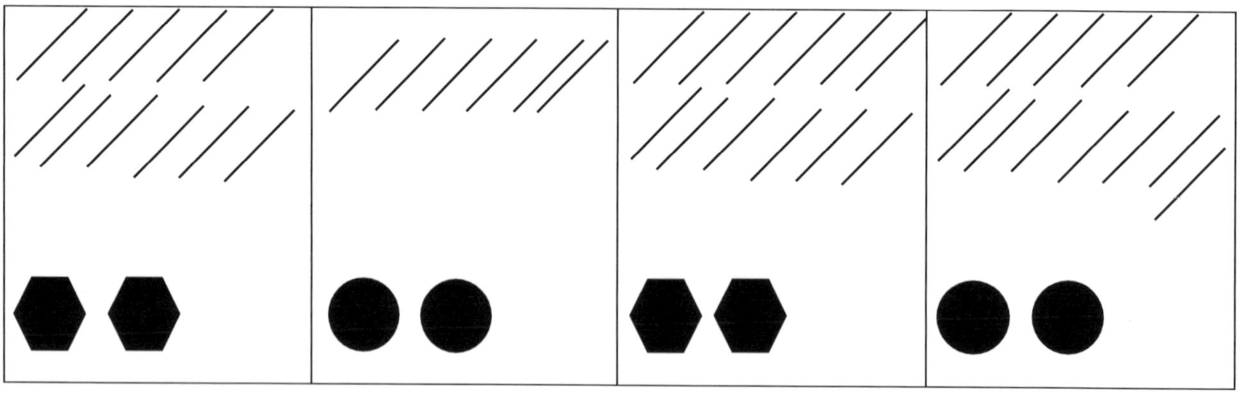

A. B. C. D.

Abstract Reasoning Answers

Question 1

Pattern:

- Set A: Shapes of opposite colour are connected by a solid line.
- Set B: Shapes of the same colour are connected by a solid line.
- *Note*: It is worth checking whether there is a specific type of shape being connected each time. In this case there is not, and the pattern is only associated with the colour of the shape and the solid line.

Answers:

Test shape 1. The correct answer is C.
Test shape 2. The correct answer is C.
Test shape 3. The correct answer is B.
Test shape 4. The correct answer is A.
Test shape 5. The correct answer is B.

Question 2

Pattern:

- Set A: Black shapes are made up of straight edges, white shapes are made of curved edges.
- Set B: Black shapes are made up of curved edges, white shapes are made of straight edges.

Answers:

Test shape 6. The correct answer is C.
Test shape 7. The correct answer is A.
Test shape 8. The correct answer is B.
Test shape 9. The correct answer is C.
Test shape 10. The correct answer is B.

Question 3

Pattern:

- Set A: Each box has 2 adjacent black shapes.
- Set B: Each box has 2 adjacent grey shapes.

- *Note:* There is no simplest box here, as all of the boxes have the exact same shapes. When you look from a distance, you may be able to notice that black is the more dominant colour in Set A while grey is the more dominant colour in Set B. You can then observe the patterns revolving around these colours.

Answers:

Test shape 11. The correct answer is C.
Test shape 12. The correct answer is C.
Test shape 13. The correct answer is A.
Test shape 14. The correct answer is B.
Test shape 15. The correct answer is C.

Question 4

Pattern:

- Set A: The overlapping figure is black when the arrow is white, and the overlapping figure is white when the arrow is black.
- Set B: The overlapping figure and the arrow always have the same colour.

Answers:

Test shape 16. The correct answer is C.
Test shape 17. The correct answer is A.
Test shape 18. The correct answer is B.
Test shape 19. The correct answer is A.
Test shape 20. The correct answer is B.

Question 5

Pattern:

- Set A: All the characters in this set contain curved edges.
- Set B: All the characters in this set contain straight edges.
- *Note:* If you see letters and/or numbers in a set, attempt to view them as abstract shapes and observe the same characteristics as you normally would – the number of edges, the number of right angles, curved/straight lines, etc.

Answers:

Test shape 21. The correct answer is A.
Test shape 22. The correct answer is B.
Test shape 23. The correct answer is B.
Test shape 24. The correct answer is A.

Test shape 25. The correct answer is A.

Question 6

Pattern:

- Set A: All solid figures are black. If the figure contains an even number of sides, it has a white circle adjacent to it.
- Set B: All solid figures are white. If the figure contains an odd number of sides, it has a black circle adjacent to it.

Answers:

Test shape 26. The correct answer is C.
Test shape 27. The correct answer is C.
Test shape 28. The correct answer is A.
Test shape 29. The correct answer is C.
Test shape 30. The correct answer is C.

Question 7

Pattern:

- Set A: All symmetrical figures are black, and all asymmetrical figures are white.
- Set B: All symmetrical figures are white, and all asymmetrical figures are black.

Answers:

Test shape 31. The correct answer is A.
Test shape 32. The correct answer is B.
Test shape 33. The correct answer is A.
Test shape 34. The correct answer is A.
Test shape 34. The correct answer is A.

Question 8

Pattern:

- Set A: Starting from any figure, in an anticlockwise order, the sequence of colours is: black, grey, black, white. The colours move around but the sequence does not change.
- Set B: Starting from any figure, in an anticlockwise order, the sequence of colours is: white, grey, black, grey.

Answers:

Test shape 36. The correct answer is A.

Test shape 37. The correct answer is B.

Test shape 38. The correct answer is C.

Test shape 39. The correct answer is C.

Test shape 40. The correct answer is C.

Question 9

Pattern:

- Set A: Each of the figures has a continuous outline, i.e. if they were to be drawn, it would not be necessary to lift the pen to complete the drawing.
- Set B: Each of the figures do *not* have a continuous outline, i.e. if they were to be drawn, it *would* be necessary to lift the pen to complete the drawing.
- *Note:* This is a difficult pattern, and likely one that you would have to flag and skip in the exam.

Answers:

41. The correct answer is A.
42. The correct answer is A.

Question 10

Pattern:

- Set A: When the letter has only straight lines, the number is odd. When the letter has curved lines, the number is even.
- Set B: When the letter has only straight lines, the number is even. When the letter has only curved lines, the number is odd.
- *Note:* The shapes and colours are distractors. There is a wide disparity in colour between the different boxes – some with grey and black, some white and grey, some white and black, some black and black, and so on. Because of this large disparity, it is unlikely that colour is a pattern, as the pattern would be far too complex to present as such. Further, when there are two elements within a box, such as a number and a letter, there is likely a dependent relationship between them.

Answers:

43. The correct answer is C.
44. The correct answer is B.

Question 11

Pattern:

- Set A: The sum total of the number of lines and circles is an odd number.
- Set B: The sum total of the number of lines and circles is an even number.
- *Note:* As the number of lines and circles clearly and evidently changes between the boxes, it is likely that the pattern has to do with numbers.
- *Tip*: Count in twos or threes to increase your speed and save precious seconds.

Answers:

45. The correct answer is B.
46. The correct answer is B.

Question 12

Pattern:

- Set A: All the arrows point either upwards or downwards.
- Set B: All the arrows point either toward the left or the right.
- *Note:* When you see arrows, you should immediately think of their orientation.

Answers:

47. The correct answer is C.
48. The correct answer is A.

Question 13

Pattern:

- Set A: The black figure has a fewer number of sides than the white figure.
- Set B: The white figure has a fewer number of sides than the black figure.

Answers:

49. The correct answer is D.
50. The correct answer is B.

Question 14

Pattern:

- Set A: The hexagon and the triangle are adjacent in every box.
- Set B: The hexagon and the raindrop are adjacent in every box.
- *Note:* This question may be extremely time consuming, or you may be lucky and happen to notice the pattern quickly. If it is taking too long, flag, guess and go!

Answers:

51. The correct answer is C.
52. The correct answer is B.

Question 15

Pattern:

- Set A: All boxes contain 3 dimensional figures.
- Set B: All boxes contain 2 dimensional figures.

Answers:

53. The correct answer is A.
54. The correct answer is C.

Single Questions

55. The correct answer is A. Across the series, the pattern transitions between being symmetrical and asymmetrical.
56. The correct answer is C. The number of sides of the figure on the right-hand side is half the number of intersections of the figures on the left-hand side. *Note:* The presence of intersections or overlaps should always strike as a potential key characteristic of the box.
57. The correct answer is A. The number of sides on the right-hand side is double the total number of sides on the left-hand side.
58. The correct answer is B. The black and blue circles swap positions and the grey and white circles swap positions. *Note:* You can also say that the outermost circles swap positions and the inner most swap as well. However, this would require a grey circle to be at the top in one of the answers, and this is nowhere to be found.
59. The correct answer is C. The triangle changes colour in every box. The circle moves clockwise by one point along the triangle. The arrow is always under the triangle when the circle is on top, and on top of the triangle when the circle is below. *Note:* The arrow may be less noticeable, but will help you differentiate between C and D.
60. The correct answer is A. The black square moves down the left side of the box, from the top corner to the middle to the bottom and back to the top corner. The white square alternates between being in the middle and on the right.
61. The correct answer is A. The shapes increase in number of sides each time (2, then 3, then 4, then 5). The number of lines is always 1 less than the total number of sides of the shapes in the box.

SECTION 5

Situational Judgement Test

INTRODUCTION

The Situational Judgement Test is the final section of the UCAT. It consists of 69 questions that are to be completed in 26 minutes. This gives roughly 37 seconds per question. This section is designed to test your professional judgement in clinical and non-clinical settings based on governing principles for doctors and medical students. Each scenario that you are presented with will have a key theme taken from Good Medical Practice by GMC. No knowledge of medicine is required to answer these questions.

This section of the UCAT is scored separately to the rest. Band 1 is given to the highest achievers, and Band 4 to the lowest. Many students struggle to study for the Situational Judgement Test, as questions often seem to have the wrong answers. Hence, this is the only section of the UCAT where partial marks may be awarded, as the correct response can have an element of subjectivity. Therefore, rather than teaching fool-proof strategies for answering each question, the main focus of this section is to help you identify key themes and how they can apply to real-world scenarios. Nevertheless, we have included some brilliant strategies that will help you answer each type of question, but it is important to note that strategies cannot always be relied upon due to the element of subjectivity.

Logistics of the Situational Judgement Test

Before you get started, you must understand the logistics of how the questions work in the Situational Judgement Test.

1. Each question in a scenario is independent of all of the other questions. When determining how to answer a question, you do not need to bear in mind your answers to any of the previous questions.
2. You can use each answer option once, more than once, or not at all. For example, you may be given 4 actions in a scenario that are all "A very appropriate thing to do".
3. Each question will describe one action (appropriateness questions) or one consideration before taking action (importance questions). Do not assume that this is the *only* action taken or *only* consideration that will be made. It can be "very appropriate" or "very important" without being the complete set of actions required in response to a scenario.
4. The answers have a degree of subjectivity, thus, partial marks can be awarded for answers that are close to the correct answer. There is no further information given on the awarding of partial marks.
5. This is not a personality test, and it can be studied for. Although not perfect, there are structured systems for answering the questions based on medical principles. These strategies are discussed throughout the book.
6. You should not answer the questions based on how you would react yourself. Rather, you should decide what the best action would be for the character in the scenario, given information about who they are, i.e. a medical student, a doctor, a dentist, or a dental student.
7. Some scenarios are in non-medical settings, but you still need to apply the medical principles of professionalism and integrity and respond accordingly. A doctor or a dentist is never "off work" in terms of the rules that govern them by the GMC and GDC respectively

Key Themes

The table below lists the key themes that will present in scenarios you are given. You must train yourself to recognise these themes and answer each question based on its overlying theme. These themes are discussed in more detail on page 349.

Qualities	Principles	Skills
Empathy	Confidentiality	Conflict resolution
Compassion	Consent	Prioritisation
Honesty and Integrity	Professionalism	Leadership and Teamwork
Respect and dignity	Patient safety	Dealing with pressure
Patient-centredness and altruism	Due diligence	Decision Making
Dedication and commitment	4 pillars of medical ethics	Communication skills

Note: Aside from the written content of this section, ensure that you try all of the questions at the end, as many themes are explained in further detail through the questions.

Reading List

It would also be wise to conduct your own further reading on these topics. Below is a small list of useful resources.

1. Good Medical Practice by GMC
2. Outcomes for Graduates by GMC
3. GDC Standards for the Dental Team

General Strategy

Some general steps that need to be applied to each type of question are:

1. Ensure that you have a good understanding of the scenario prior to answering the questions. Do not skim read like you would in Verbal Reasoning.
2. Pick out the key relevant details from the scenario, such as the major problem and the theme overlying this problem.
3. Understand the position or job role of the character in question, as this will help shape your response.

The following table summarises the roles of characters that may appear in this test. You must understand each character's limitations and answer the questions based on this knowledge.

	Can	Cannot
Medical Students	- Mainly observational role - Able to perform some basic clinic skills with the approval of their supervisor - Not necessary to be observed during history taking, examinations, and clinic skills - Able to view records of patients in the location of their clinical placement	- Cannot prescribe - Cannot make any decisions about patient care - Cannot perform any clinical skills without permission from a supervisor - Cannot act beyond their own limits. - Must abide by the governing principles of the GMC
Junior Doctors	- Able to prescribe - Able to perform clinical skills and make decisions about patient care within the limitations of their expertise - Can request investigations - Can diagnose patients - Can propose treatment plans	- Cannot make extremely complex decisions about patient care - Cannot make specialist decisions about patient care - Must abide by the governing principles of the GMC
Consultants	- Make the overall decisions about patient care - Make any specialist decisions about patient care - Have the highest level of responsibility for their patients	- Cannot break any rules due to their seniority. - Must abide by the governing principles of the GMC
Dental Students	- Can perform basic clinical procedures under general supervision, i.e. regular checks - Can write prescriptions, but these must be checked and signed by a dentist	- Cannot treat patients without a treatment plan from the tutor - Must abide by the governing principles of the GDC
Dentists	- Can perform all relevant clinical procedures independently	- Cannot perform specialist clinical procedures unless trained - Must abide by the governing principles of the GDC

Types of Questions

There are two main types of questions in the Situational Judgement Test, with the latter type presenting in two different formats. Each of these question types will be discussed in detail in the upcoming pages.

1. Importance Questions
2. Appropriateness Questions
   a. Format 1 (most common)
   b. Format 2 (least common)

Importance Questions

In this type of question, you will be provided with a scenario, but not given any action in response to the scenario. You will instead be given various considerations that can be made prior to taking action, and are required to judge the importance of each consideration. These are ranked on a scale of "Very important" to "Not important at all".

The following table defines the answer options given in this style of question.

Importance	Definition
A. Very important	Something vital to consider in order to resolve the main problem. If it is not considered, problem-solving will be hindered.
B. Important	Important but not essential. It can help in solving the main problem, but ignoring it will not hinder problem-solving.
C. Of minor importance	Does not affect the main problem if this is considered – i.e. no harm or benefit will occur from this. May help solve a minor problem.
D. Not important at all	Something you would definitely not take into consideration, as it may cause harm or hinder the resolution of the main problem.

To better understand this, let us break down what each scenario and question set consists of:

1. A main problem with an associated theme
2. Potentially other minor problem(s)
3. The primary goal: always to resolve the **main** problem
4. Considerations that support the primary goal: important
5. Considerations that deter the primary goal: not important

Let us use the example of patient safety. If a scenario outlines that a patient may be at risk of harm, and also outlines that a medical student is running late for placement – there are two problems.

- Theme of the major problem: Patient safety
- Theme of the minor problem (running late): Professionalism.

In this kind of scenario, there will be a number of considerations that can be made. The primary goal is to ensure the safety of the patient who is in danger, as patient safety is far more important than being on time for placement.

- Any consideration that will help remove the danger from this patient (i.e. support the resolution of the main problem) will be considered important.
- Any consideration that will come in the way of solving this safety concern will be unimportant.
- If a consideration will help to resolve the timeliness issue of the student, but not impact the issue of patient safety, it may be considered of minor importance.

Importance Questions: Strategy

When given a statement following a scenario, consider the following questions:

- What is the main problem? What theme or category does it fall under?
- If I consider this statement, will it help resolve the main problem?
- If I consider this statement, will it hinder me from resolving the main problem?
- If I ignore this statement, will I be hindered from resolving the main problem?
- Are there any minor problems that considering this statement may help me resolve?

These questions can be formulated into a strategy for solving importance questions. The flow chart below outlines a general approach that can be followed for each question. The main problem must first be defined, then you can go through this flow chart for each "consideration" or question.

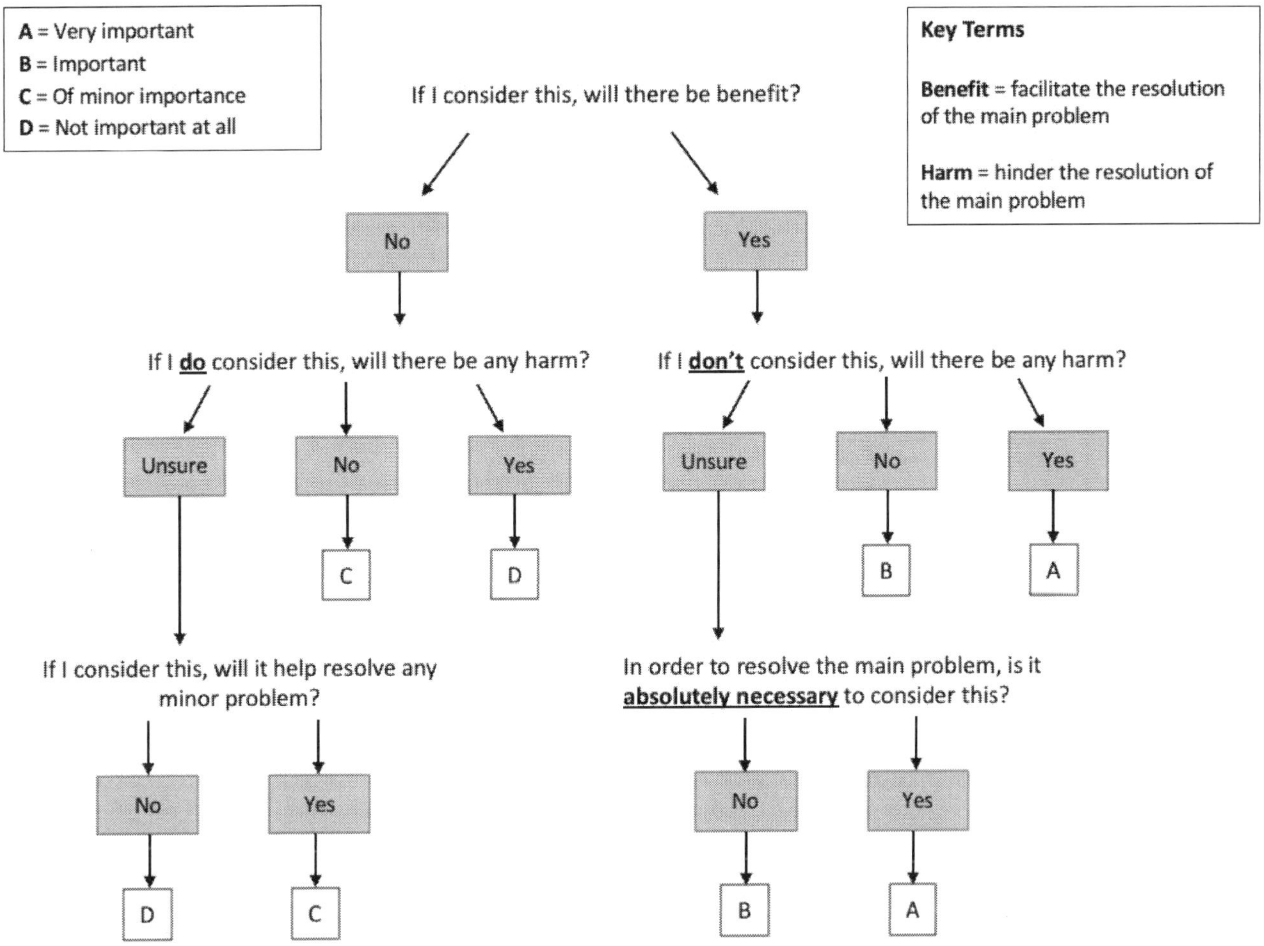

A great deal of research has gone into developing this strategy, and we have found it to be the best method for maximising points in this section. However, like with any other strategy, it is not a be-all and end-all, and thus, should be used attentively.

Try to implement the above strategy to answer the following question.

Example 1

Alisha, a second-year medical student, is pulled aside by a patient during her hospital placement. The patient tells Alisha that he is scared because one of the doctors on the ward is plotting against him. Alisha, unsure of what to do, advises a nurse of what the patient has said. The nurse suggests that the patient is probably making this up for attention, as normally, all patients love that doctor.

How **important** to take into account are the following considerations for **Alisha** when deciding how to respond to the situation?

1. Patients normally love this doctor.
    A. Very important
    B. Important
    C. Of minor importance
    D. Not important at all

2. The doctor might be offended if Alisha brings this up.
    A. Very important
    B. Important
    C. Of minor importance
    D. Not important at all

3. The patient told her he is scared of one of the doctors.
    A. Very important
    B. Important
    C. Of minor importance
    D. Not important at all

Answer 1

The main problem: Patient feels that the doctor is plotting against him.

- Theme: Patient safety

Minor problem(s): None noted in the scenario.
Primary goal: Ensure the safety of this patient.

1. The correct answer is D.
    a. "If I consider this, will there be benefit?" No, considering this will not help resolve the issue of patient safety, as the statement has nothing to do with the fact that *this* patient feels unsafe.
    b. "If I do consider this, will there be any harm?" Yes, there is a possibility of harm. If Alisha chooses to consider that all patients normally love this doctor, she may have a biased approach when dealing with the matter of patient safety and therefore choose to downplay or overlook the concerns of the patient.
    c. Therefore, the answer is D: Not important at all.
2. The correct answer is D.
    a. "If I consider this, will there be benefit?" No, considering this will not help resolve the main issue of **patient safety**, as the statement has nothing to do with the fact that the patient feels unsafe. You must consider the primary goal first and foremost.

b. "If I do consider this, will there be any harm?" This is not very clear cut. However, there is a possibility of harm. Similar to the last question, if this is considered, it may stop Alisha from progressing with her investigation, thus hindering the resolution of the patient safety matter.

c. Therefore, the answer is D: Not important at all.

   Note: Potentially offending a colleague is of minor importance compared to patient safety. Alisha should say this in a polite and non-confrontational manner, but should not shy away from investigating the situation due to fear of offending someone. Because this consideration has a possibility of hindering the resolution, it should not even be considered. Further, it is *not appropriate* of the doctor to be offended when an investigation is ongoing with regards to patient safety, as this should take priority over ones' own ego.

3. The correct answer is A.
   a. "If I consider this, will there be benefit?" Yes, because the main concern is patient safety, and if a patient has declared that they feel unsafe, this is evidence for investigation into the main problem.
   b. "If I don't consider this, will there be any harm?" Yes, because the patient's views are paramount when it comes to patient safety matters. If the patient's views are not considered, it is likely that more harm can occur to the patient, as Alisha may decide not to take action.
   c. Therefore, the answer is A: Very important.

      Note: Doctors have many privileges when it comes to patient care. If a patient says that he is scared of one of the doctors, this should not be taken lightly. Patients can be extremely vulnerable to abuse, and it is essential to prevent this by investigating such complaints. Look into the case of Harold Shipman, a GP who was able to abuse hundreds of patients due to his authority as a doctor.

Hopefully, it makes sense how to implement this strategy to answer importance questions. More of these questions will appear throughout the book, so you can refer back to the flowchart when attempting to answer the questions.

Appropriateness Questions: Format 1

In this type of question, you will be given a scenario alongside actions that can be taken in response to the scenario. This is different to importance questions, where there is no action or response given. You must judge the appropriateness of each action, bearing in mind the role of the person conducting the action. For example, for a medical student to give medication to a patient in need is very inappropriate as they are not qualified to do so, but for a doctor to do this would be very appropriate.

The first format of appropriateness questions consists of the following responses:

A. A very appropriate thing to do
B. Appropriate, but not ideal
C. Inappropriate, but not awful
D. A very inappropriate thing to do

Appropriateness Questions: Format 1 Strategy

When rating the appropriateness, it is essential to consider the main traits required of a medical student or a doctor. Some main points to note are:

- **The worst-case scenario comes first.** For example, if there is a possibility of a patient being in danger, and there is a possibility of you being late to meet your supervisor, the worst thing that could happen here is the violation of patient safety. With regards to professionalism, it is expected of a medical student or doctor to be on time. Further, it is not appropriate to make your supervisor wait, as they may have important things to do, such as seeing patients. However, if there is an immediate threat to patient safety, this triumphs over timeliness with meetings.
- **If an action is based on an assumption, it loses its credibility.** For example, if one patient is in danger, it is still important to consider the safety of other patients. However, it is less important to consider other patients' safety if you have no evidence that their safety is being compromised.
- **Provide a solution**. The most appropriate action will address the main problem in the scenario and *at least* be a step towards finding a solution. If the main problem is not addressed, the answer cannot be "very appropriate".
- **Be careful with suggestions.** Even if you do not directly break the rules, it is inappropriate to even suggest breaking rules. For example, if a friend asks for confidential information about a patient, it is inappropriate to suggest that she instead asks the doctor for these details, as the doctor cannot break confidentiality either. Although it is not awful, as you are not actually breaking the rules, it is not appropriate to make such a suggestion.
- **Act in a timely manner.** If a situation is urgent, an appropriate action will address it as such. For example, if a patient is about to take an overdose, it would be very inappropriate to go to the other end of the hospital to find the consultant in charge, as the patient's safety is in immediate danger.
- **Maintain dignity and respect.** Discussing mistakes of colleagues in front of other colleagues or patients is never ideal. You should maintain privacy and respect their dignity.

Further, consider positive and negative words. Positive words lead towards the response being "appropriate" while negative words lead towards the response being "inappropriate".

Positive Words	Negative Words
Reassure	Threaten
Listen	Intimidate
Explore	Confront
Recommend	Blame
Help	Accuse
Encourage	Warn

You will not always be given clear hints with the use of language. However, you can use all of the strategies above to categorise the response as follows:

Category	Response	What it means
Appropriate (Positive)	A very appropriate thing to do	All positive with no negative terms. The optimal approach. Addresses the key issue and/or suggests a resolution.
	Appropriate, but not ideal	Overall positive but potentially some negativity. Not the best way to respond as it may not address the key issue.
Inappropriate (Negative)	Inappropriate, but not awful	Overall negative but potentially some positivity. Not the worst possible outcome, but will not make the situation worse or cause any harm.
	A very inappropriate thing to do	Only negative terms. Would make the situation worse and/or lead to harm.

If you are unsure of the answer, attempt to place it in an overall category of "appropriate" or "inappropriate". This will likely help you achieve a 50% chance of selecting the correct answer, and a good chance of being awarded partial marks.

Example 2

Leanne is a medical student on placement at a GP practice. She is running clinics with her colleague, who returns after stepping out for a couple of minutes. Her colleague tells her that he has just seen his old friend in the waiting room. He decides to check the system to find out what his friend is there for.

How **appropriate** are each of the following responses by **Leanne** in this situation?

1. "You're not allowed to do that."
   A. A very appropriate thing to do
   B. Appropriate, but not ideal
   C. Inappropriate, but not awful
   D. A very inappropriate thing to do

2. "Maybe he wouldn't want you to check his file."
   A. A very appropriate thing to do
   B. Appropriate, but not ideal
   C. Inappropriate, but not awful
   D. A very inappropriate thing to do

3. "That's breaking his confidentiality. Maybe you can call him later on to see how he's doing."
   A. A very appropriate thing to do
   B. Appropriate, but not ideal
   C. Inappropriate, but not awful
   D. A very inappropriate thing to do

Answer 2

Main concern: Patient confidentiality

1. The correct answer is B. This response vaguely addresses the main concern, but does not do so in an ideal way. It is not absolutely clear what Leanne is referring to by saying her colleague is not allowed to do "that". Further, there is a lack of politeness to the response, thus a hint of negativity here. Patient confidentiality is serious, and thus, her response should be polite and *very clear*, leaving no room for *any doubt* or misinterpretation.
2. The correct answer is B. The answer is mainly positive, as it nicely addresses the concern. However, it is not clear enough and leaves room for doubt. Patient confidentiality is a serious matter, and it is not just the case of the patient "maybe"

not wanting their file to be checked, but actual laws governing and prohibiting anyone from doing so without necessity.

3. The correct answer is A. This response clearly addresses the main concern of patient confidentiality. It also provides a practical solution to the problem. It considers that Leanne's colleague may be concerned about his friend and advises a more suitable option for dealing with this.

Appropriateness Questions: Format 2

The second format of appropriateness questions is the most unique. It is also the one that appears the least often in the Situational Judgement Test. You will be provided with a scenario, followed by 3 options. You are required to select the single "most appropriate" and the single "least appropriate" response. This means that one of the responses is not selected at all. Your answers should be dragged and dropped into their respective boxes, as will be demonstrated below. You must select both the *most* and the *least* appropriate to be awarded any marks.

Appropriateness Questions: Format 2 Strategy

There is often one response that stands out as being the "most appropriate" or the "least appropriate". If you are able to identify it, you can drag it into the box, and have two left to choose from. Consider the following:

1. The "most appropriate action" is not necessarily "a very appropriate thing to do". It is simply more appropriate than the rest. As such, you may have an action that is not ideal, but is better than the rest. E.g. Apologising on behalf of a colleague in order to deescalate a situation is better than doing nothing or making matters worse.
2. Always remember the limitations of the person involved. E.g. Any extensive ethical issues should be relayed directly to a senior, rather than allowing a medical student or someone without experience to attempt to deal with them.
3. Can this response make the situation worse? E.g. It is better to do *nothing* or to ignore the situation than to take a step that might make matters worse.
4. A response that provides a practical solution is always more appropriate than a response that does not. E.g. Asking to hold a group meeting to discuss concerns is better than just expressing to the group that you are unable to complete a task.
5. Responses can be time-sensitive. E.g. If someone is going through depression, it is vital to address this concern and it is less appropriate to "wait and see" or to "give them space". Although, realistically, some people are happier to have time alone in this kind of scenario, in the UCAT, there is not enough room to identity in detail the personal preferences of individuals. Thus, it is never appropriate to leave alone someone who is suffering from mental health problems, and concerns like this should be addressed immediately.

The following example will demonstrate the drag-and-drop format that will appear in the UCAT. Understandably, in this book, you cannot drag and drop. The remainder of this question type throughout the book will appear in plain text format.

Example 3

Maryam, a medical student, is walking home after finishing some shopping, when an elderly man across the road collapses. People start gathering around the man and shouting for a doctor to come help. Although she has learned some basic life support, she cannot fully recall the steps to take.

Choose **both** the **one most appropriate action** and the **one least appropriate action** that **Maryam** should take in response to this situation.

You will not receive any marks for this question unless you select **both** the most and least appropriate actions.

Most Appropriate	
Least Appropriate	

Call her sister who is a doctor and try to get advice from her.

Go to the scene to see what's happening, but not take any action.

Call an ambulance, then rush to the scene to see if she can help in any way.

Answer 3

The most appropriate response here would be to call the ambulance, then rush to the scene to see if she can help in any way. There is an immediate danger, and thus, she must act swiftly within her limits. Even if she is unable to perform any basic life support because she cannot remember how to, she can help by calling an ambulance – an essential and urgent act.

The least appropriate response would be to do nothing. There is an immediate danger, so although she should not act outside of her limits, she should try to help in any way that may be appropriate. However, if there was an option that might make matters worse, doing nothing would be more appropriate.

The option in between would be to call her sister. If Maryam is unsure what to do, it would be good to seek advice from someone who knows better. However, the more urgent and necessary action would be to call an ambulance.

The 4 Pillars of Medical Ethics

Autonomy, justice, beneficence, and non-maleficence: these principles are the foundations of modern medicine. It is essential to understand these pillars their applications in order to succeed in your Situational Judgement Test, interviews, and your medical career.

Autonomy

Autonomy refers to a patient's right to make their own decisions regarding their healthcare. This principle moves us away from the previous paternalistic approach to medicine whereby the doctor was at the centre of making healthcare decisions. It is now mandatory to seek informed and valid consent by patients prior to conducting any investigations, examinations, or providing any treatment. This also gives patients the right to refuse treatments that they do not wish upon themselves, and allows medical care to take a more holistic approach, whereby physical health is not the only domain that is taken into consideration.

Justice

In medical ethics, justice often refers to the fair and equal distribution of resources. This is most easily explained by a scenario whereby there are limited resources, and it would be unjust to provide all of the resources to a single patient at the expense of hundreds of other patients. In real-life scenarios, doctors aim to provide the most cost-effective medications to patients in order to avoid unjustly allocating NHS funds. For example, if an antibiotic costs

£150 for a 7-day course, but a similar and equally effective antibiotic costs £30 for a 7-day course, it is more appropriate to offer the £30 option. Time allocation also comes under the principle of justice. For example, if a standard GP appointment is 10 minutes, it would be unjust to allow a patient to take up 30 minutes, then complete the remaining appointments in 4-5 minutes each in order to finish on time. Often, appointments do run over time as some patients needs more time than others, but it is unjust to then take time away from other patients. Unfortunately, this means for doctors that they are often giving up their own break time for the sake of patients – a reason why *altruism* is an essential quality in the medical profession.

Beneficence

Beneficence refers to the act and intent of always doing good for the patient and acting in their best interests. For example, in an incompetent patient who is unable to make their own decisions, doctors must consider the personal, spiritual and religious values of the patient in order to care for their holistic health. Looking past physical health is an example of beneficence. For example, if a patient refuses to have certain medications made with animal products due to religious or personal beliefs, it would be an act of beneficence to provide alternative medications to the patient. Doing "good" does not just refer to physical health – an important point to note. Beneficence also refers to many of the day-to-day roles of a doctor, such as: listening to patients' concerns, providing valuable insight, prescribing effective medication, performing life support, and performing necessary operations.

Non-maleficence

Non-maleficence means to cause **no harm** to the patient. This is different to beneficence, although students often get confused between the two. Consider a scenario with unnecessary treatments and operations that have their side-effects and potential of harm. If these treatments, such as amputating a fractured leg, are unnecessary, they should not be carried out. Avoiding amputation is not "doing good", but is "doing no harm". Take the example of an elderly patient with a long list of prescribed medications. The GP may recognise that the large number of medications can be harmful for the patient due to some drugs interacting with others, and subsequently advise the patient to stop some medications in order to avoid harm. This is not simply "doing good" but is "avoiding harm".

Common Themes

There are a number of common themes that present in the Situational Judgement Test. These are used to test candidates as it is necessary for medical and dental students to be familiar with these themes and apply them in clinical and non-clinical settings. During your exam, it is essential to identify the main theme of each scenario and answer the subsequent questions accordingly. Some themes take precedence over others. For example, patient safety is paramount in each and every setting. Empathy is necessary, but it would not be appropriate to sacrifice patient safety in order to act empathetically. Therefore, although both are important, patient safety takes precedence over empathy.

The following section will cover each of the main themes and demonstrate them through example questions. The test at the end of this section will have further occurrences of each, so please ensure that you complete the questions and use the answer explanations to further your learning of these themes in practice.

Patient safety

Patient safety is of the utmost importance to every healthcare professional. Examples of patient safety risks can include risk of infection, risk of abuse, and risk of falls. Prior to any action taken, it is vital to consider the wellbeing and safety of all patients involved and avoid any intended or unintended harm. Healthcare professionals should always actively seek to improve patient safety, following the necessary guidelines and standards in their respective trusts. It is crucial that the individual who first identifies a threat to patient safety takes immediate action, and anyone who further identifies this threat also takes action where appropriate. It is inappropriate to pass on this responsibility to someone else, as this act can delay the resolution and put the patient at risk of greater harm.

If there is an investigation into patient safety, all members of staff must cooperate and support the identification of such risks. Further, it is important to create a culture in the workplace that allows all patients and members of staff to openly raise any safety concerns without fear of repercussions. It is inappropriate to take safety concerns lightly or to not act immediately on them.

Example 4

Helen is a medical student on her surgical rotation. She notices that Mr Oligari, the lead surgeon, seems quite distracted today. He made a number of errors in the morning ward round and got extremely flustered each time. He has been calling patients by the wrong name and writing incorrect details in their notes. She has shadowed him for some time and knows that this is extremely out of character for him. Helen will be joining Mr Oligari in the afternoon theatre sessions, where he will be operating on three different patients. After observing his state today, Helen feels uncomfortable about him operating on patients.

Choose **both** the **one most appropriate action** and the **one least appropriate action** that **Helen** should take in response to this situation.

You will not receive any marks for this question unless you select **both** the most and least appropriate actions.

A. Do nothing as Mr Oligari is a fantastic surgeon. He only made minor mistakes and these probably won't affect the surgeries.
B. Talk to Mr Oligari in the staff room during the lunch break to ask if everything is okay.
C. Ask Mr Oligari to talk privately. Explain that he appears stressed and suggest that it may be best to take the rest of the day off.

Answer 4

Most appropriate: C
Least appropriate: A

It is crucial to identify the risk to patient safety here. Doctors should not be treating patients or performing surgery if they are not in the state to do so. It is clear that Mr Oligari has already made numerous errors, and it would be best for him to consider taking the afternoon off to avoid making further, more serious errors. Thus, C is the most appropriate.

B is not the most appropriate answer as sensitive topics should be discussed privately and Mr Oligari may not want everyone in the staff room to hear this conversation. It is empathetic and appropriate in terms of asking if everything is okay, but is less appropriate than option A that does so privately and also suggests a solution to the safety hazard.

A is inappropriate as it puts patient safety at risk. Regardless of how skilled a surgeon is, anyone can have a bad day, and it is important to recognise this.

Confidentiality

Confidentiality means to withhold and protect the security of all private information, including personal identifiable details, medical history, details about a consultation, and anything discussed in confidence by an individual. Healthcare professionals who are not directly involved in the care of a patient have no right to access confidential information about that patient. This concept is crucial to developing trust in doctor-patient relationships, as well as trust from the general public towards the medical profession. This high level of trust prompts patients to be open and honest about their situations, allowing optimal care.

Confidentiality can be breached in some extreme circumstances, where it is of high importance to disclose specific information. These circumstances can be defined as follows:

1. Risk of serious harm to the patient
2. Risk of serious harm to any other individual
3. Risk of a serious crime
4. Risk of harm to the general public

Where confidentiality must be breached, it is important to note that only relevant details can be provided. For example, if a patient has advised a doctor that they plan to cause harm to another individual, this does not give the doctor the right to expose the patient's entire medical history to the public. Rather, the doctor would have the responsibility of firstly trying to convince the patient otherwise. If the patient is insistent that he will implement his plans, the doctor must inform the authorities of the patient's intentions to cause harm. Details that are not necessary in this situation should still remain confidential.

Example 5

Elena is a third-year medical student on her breast surgery rotation. During her placement, she performs a breast examination on Mrs Khan. Elena later meets her friend, Stacey, for lunch. Stacey's next rotation is breast surgery, so she asks Elena to discuss the patients she examined in the morning to give her some insight.

How **important** to take into account is the following consideration for **Elena** when deciding how to respond to the situation?

The chance that revealing too much information might allow Stacey to identify Mrs Khan.

A. Very important
B. Important
C. Of minor importance
D. Not important at all

Answer 5

The correct answer is A. Patient confidentiality must be maintained except in extreme circumstances. There appears to be no reason for Elena to break Mrs Khan's confidentiality. If she considers this, she will remain cautious in her approach and not provide any patient-identifiable details. If she does not consider this, she may accidentally breach patient confidentiality. Thus, it is very important to consider the possibility of revealing any identifiable information about a patient, such as: name, address, date of birth, and NHS number.

Empathy

Empathy is a quality expected of healthcare professionals and is vital to the doctor-patient relationship. It means to fully understand the situation of a patient from their perspective – to *feel* what they are going through. Patients are likely to be more open and honest with a doctor who is empathetic, subsequently improving the care that the doctor is able to provide. If a patient refuses to be honest with their doctor, it is extremely difficult for the doctor to fully appreciate the problem on and be able to provide an effective treatment plan.

Take the example of a patient who continuously attends the GP complaining of various harmless moles and marks on their skin, worrying they might have skin cancer. An empathetic doctor would address this by asking the patient to expand on their concerns. Perhaps the patient had a friend who died from skin cancer, so they are extremely cautious and worry about every mark on their own skin. It is vital to act with empathy, seeing situations from the patient's point of view. The doctor could simply brush this off and sternly advise that the patient has nothing wrong with them. However, if the doctor was in a similar situation and suffered a traumatic bereavement due to skin cancer, they would not appreciate receiving such a response. Further, visiting a doctor who lacks empathy can be an unpleasant experience, and the patient is likely to avoid seeing such a doctor again. Alternatively, if they must visit them, they may not open up about their concerns, knowing that the doctor will not care. Thus, empathy is an essential quality and helps to provide excellent patient care.

Example 6

Karishma is a medical student who was asked by her friend, Amina, to watch her pet bunny for the weekend. Just as Amina enters to pick up her pet, Karishma realises that the bunny has swallowed and appears to be choking on an orange Lego piece that was on the floor.

How **appropriate** is the following response by **Karishma** in this situation?

"It's just Lego, he'll be fine."

A. A very appropriate thing to do
B. Appropriate, but not ideal
C. Inappropriate, but not awful
D. A very inappropriate thing to do

Answer 6

The correct answer is D. This response is extremely inappropriate as it is completely dismissive of Amina's feelings towards her bunny, suggesting that Karishma has a lack of empathy. Further, the animal is just as deserving of her empathy as a human is. There is no solution provided through this response, and it is likely to escalate the situation and make Amina feel worse. It is vital to get help right away, rather than being defensive and suggesting that there is no problem at present.

Knowledge, Skills and Performance

Medicine is an ever-evolving field, with billions of pounds spent every year, in the UK alone, on medical research. Continuous research into every subspecialty of medicine allows for evolvement and progressive improvement of services and patient care. Each healthcare professional is responsible for updating their knowledge base regularly to match the standards of practice, and should not act outside of the limitations of their knowledge. For example, a medical student who has not yet learned how to take bloods should not attempt to take bloods. A surgeon who has not yet been trained on a new procedure should not be performing that procedure until he is competent.

Example 7

Li is a fifth-year medical student on placement in a renal ward. He has been revising all of the renal conditions and drugs lately, so he feels very confident during placement. He visits a patient, Mr Matthews, to conduct an examination. Mr Matthews tells him that he fell asleep during his regular medication time, and was wondering if he should take the medication by his bedside now. Li recognises this medication and is aware that Mr Matthews should probably take it.

How **appropriate** is the following response by **<u>Li</u>** in this situation?

Tell Mr Matthews that he should take the medication.

A. A very appropriate thing to do
B. Appropriate, but not ideal
C. Inappropriate, but not awful
D. A very inappropriate thing to do

Answer 7

The correct answer is D. Li is still a medical student, thus has no right or responsibility to provide or prescribe patients with any medications. It would be very inappropriate for Li to act outside of his limitations and risk causing harm to the patient. In this scenario, Li should ask a more senior member of staff who can better advise the patient.

Communication and Teamwork

These skills are vital in the field of medicine. Communication with patients and with colleagues should be clear, considerate, and professional. Doctors need to be able to work in partnership with other healthcare professionals, including nurses, healthcare assistants, pharmacists, physiotherapists, dieticians, midwives, and the list goes on! Therefore, it is important to have excellent communication and teamwork skills in order to function in a multidisciplinary team. As team leaders, doctors make the overall decisions about patient care, and thus, have the greatest level of responsibility. A good leader is able to recognise the skills and contributions of every member of the team, and allow them to demonstrate their skills accordingly. It is also essential, as a team player, to never undermine other members of the team.

Example 8

Sam, a dental student, has an upcoming deadline for a very important group project. One of his group members, Jill, has stopped being responsive on their group chat, and has not handed in any of her work so far. Sam is starting to worry that Jill will not complete the work on time and that this will impact his grades. He is also aware that Jill has had a recent bereavement.

How **important** to take into account is the following consideration for **Sam** when deciding how to respond to the situation?

The Jill may be undergoing significant life changes and finding it difficult to adjust.

A. Very important
B. Important
C. Of minor important
D. Not important at all

Answer 8

The correct answer is A. The main problem here is that Jill is not contributing to the work. This puts teamwork, professionalism, and communication at stake. However, to be a good team player or a leader, it is vital to consider the individual circumstances of each team member. Knowing his colleague is undergoing difficult personal circumstances, Sam will be able to make a better decision regarding how to respond. If Sam does not consider this, the resolution may be hindered as Sam may assume that Jill is simply being lazy. Therefore, it is important as a team member to show leadership by being accommodating of his team member.

Note: He can accommodate for Jill's circumstances by discussing some adjustments that can be made to the project roles. However, it would not be appropriate to take the entire workload, as each individual has their own responsibilities and roles within a group project. If Jill is unable to complete any work at all, she would have to discuss this with the group supervisor, rather than with the team.

Honesty and Integrity

Integrity means to have a strong moral character that is always present and not shaken under any circumstances. Essentially, it means to be honest and to do the right thing, even when no one is looking.

Any act that dismisses the importance of honesty and integrity is always inappropriate. In a clinical setting, small and large mistakes are made regularly. To have integrity means to accept your errors, apologise for them, and correct them. Take the example of a doctor who happens to prescribe the wrong medication to a patient. Rather than being embarrassed or brushing it off, the doctor needs to explain the situation to the patient and apologise for his mistake. He should further expand on any consequences that this mistake may have on the patient.

Example 9

Elise, a junior doctor, was careless in the morning when she prescribed a medication to a patient. She realises that she wrote the wrong dose, and the patient has probably already taken the medication.

How **appropriate** is the following response by **Elise** in this situation?

Do not do anything as the ward pharmacist will probably check the dose and correct it.

A. A very appropriate thing to do
B. Appropriate, but not ideal
C. Inappropriate, but not awful
D. A very inappropriate thing to do

Answer 9

The correct answer is D. To wilfully ignore a mistake that she has made is dishonest and unethical. This particular mistake also puts patient safety at risk. Further, Elise is hoping that someone else will correct the mistake for her. This does nothing to solve the problem at hand, and instead exacerbates it by leaving it for someone else. Whenever there is an error, the first person to recognise the error should take action immediately. Ideally, the person conducting the error should be the one to correct it. When leaving it for someone, it is possible that no one will notice the mistake, and the patient will continue to take the wrong dose of medication. Bearing all of these factors in mind, it is evident that this is a very inappropriate thing to do.

Responsibility to the Community

Doctors are not just responsible for their individual patients, but for the community and public health. Any decision that undermines the trust and respect from the community towards the medical profession is very inappropriate. Any decision that puts the safety or health of the public at risk is also very inappropriate. Therefore, doctors always need to consider the impact of their decisions on the wider community. Take the example of a doctor who attends work intoxicated. There is a plethora of things wrong with this situation, but we will consider this with regards to responsibility to the wider community. If the patients in the hospital see that this intoxicated doctor has attended work, they are likely to spread this knowledge to their family and friends, who will be just as outraged. This may undermine the public's confidence in the medical profession, and subsequently their trust in their own doctors. If a single doctor attends work intoxicated, who is to say that others do not? How can patients trust that their doctor is providing the correct treatment plan, when they have heard of doctors attending work intoxicated? Therefore, it is vital to consider the impact of individual actions on the wider community.

Example 10

Blessing is junior doctor working on an elderly ward. One of the patients has been diagnosed with COVID-19 and needs to be transferred to a different ward. The patient refuses as he is tired of being in the hospital, and tells Blessing that he will be discharging himself.

How **important** to take into account is the following consideration for **<u>Blessing</u>** when deciding how to respond to the situation?

The patient lives in a care home with many other elderly residents.

A. Very important
B. Important

C. Of minor important
D. Not important at all

Answer 10

The correct answer is A. The main problem here is the contagious nature of COVID-19 and its likelihood to be deadly to an elderly population. This is a public health concern, and so, the wider community needs to be considered. Although the patient has the autonomy to make his own decisions, the doctor has the responsibility to inform the patient of the risks involved. Considering where the patient lives will be of benefit to solving the main problem. If the patient lived on his own, he would be less likely to transmit the disease. Because he lives in a populated care home with other at-risk individuals, their safety should also be a priority. If this is not considered, the resolution of the main problem can be hindered, as Blessing may choose to let him go freely, thus putting his co-residents at risk. By considering this, the healthcare team may be able to devise a practical solution to respect the patient's wishes of discharging himself, but also protect other individuals in the community.

Responding Under Pressure

Healthcare professionals are known to have stressful and high-pressure jobs. This is likely because patients' lives are often at stake, and small mistakes can have major impacts. It is important to be able to rank priorities and respond effectively in a stressful situation. Even a newly qualified doctor can be responsible for covering an entire ward where multiple patients are severely unwell, so the ability to respond appropriately under pressure is critical. It is also important to prioritise personal, family and social life. The inability to handle pressure can lead to the stresses of work accumulating and impacting other aspects of life. This goes to show why admissions tutors for medical school like to see that applicants have methods of coping with stress.

Example 11

Olena, a junior doctor, has many tasks to complete at work today. She also has a deadline for a project proposal in 30 minutes, and is just about to go on her break to submit this. As she is leaving, her supervisor asks her to do urgent bloods for a patient who seems to be deteriorating. Olena is worried about the patient but also wants to submit her project proposal.

How **appropriate** is the following response by **<u>Olena</u>** in this situation?

Rather than going for her break, save time by submitting the project proposal from the ward computer, then proceed to take the patient's bloods.

A. A very appropriate thing to do
B. Appropriate, but not ideal
C. Inappropriate, but not awful
D. A very inappropriate thing to do

Answer 11

The correct answer is D. In this case, the most important action is to take bloods from the deteriorating patient. It is essential that she is able to prioritise the importance of tasks and think calmly under pressure. When struggling, it would be useful to ask a senior for help. Although Olena has a project proposal that is due very soon, her primary duty is to maintain patient safety. As such, doing the bloods of the patient is of the highest priority and is the action that should be taken first. She can then save time on her project proposal by submitting it from the ward computers after she has taken the bloods. If she runs out of time and is unable to submit her project proposal, this will not put anyone's life at risk. However, leaving the care of a patient who is in urgent need can be much riskier.

Negotiating Skills and Conflict Resolution

In any team, conflict is bound to occur. It is vital not to simply ignore conflict, as this can create tension and an uneasy working environment. Problems should be addressed in a professional and appropriate manner. Conflict should be resolved internally within the group, and if there is no resolution, the problem can be escalated to a more senior person.

The key points to keep in mind when dealing with conflict are:

1. Do not over-escalate, as this can lead to further, unnecessary problems. Additionally, it is not necessarily the supervisor's job to deal with trivial arguments. For example, Julie should not run to her supervisor because she does not like how Sal designed the PowerPoint slides. However, if the argument is so great that it cannot be resolved between them, the supervisor can step in and attempt to mediate the resolution. Likewise, there is no use in reporting Sal to the GMC for this.
2. Maintain the respect and dignity owed to team members during conflict resolution. Have the necessary conversations in a private place, rather than public.
3. Formulate an action plan for resolving the conflict. Do not end the conversation without a strategy for moving forward.
4. Do not shift responsibility. Accept your actions and apologise when you are in the wrong. Do not lie to avoid blame.

Example 12

Yahya, a dental student, visits his friend Yusuf's flat after university. When they enter, they find Yusuf's flatmates arguing. Two of them are insistent that the others have been leaving the kitchen messy, while the others are insistent that they always clean up after themselves. Yahya has the opportunity to help resolve this conflict.

How **appropriate** is the following response by **Yahya** in this situation?

Ask them calmly if they would like to discuss their views and allow him to give his impartial opinion.

A. A very appropriate thing to do
B. Appropriate, but not ideal
C. Inappropriate, but not awful
D. A very inappropriate thing to do

Answer 13

The correct answer is A. This response helps to provide a resolution to the conflict. Because it is not Yahya's flat, he is less likely to have any sort of biased opinion regarding the members of the flat. The action is done in a positive way, using words like "calmly" and "discuss". Therefore, this is an appropriate method of conflict resolution.

Important Things to Remember

1. **Do not avoid extreme responses.** Sometimes, students are afraid to select the extreme "very appropriate" or "very inappropriate" responses, and settle for options in between. While it is true that you may still get partial marks, you are unlikely to do well on the test by always avoiding the more extreme responses. Rather, you should familiarise yourself with the format of the Situational Judgement Test as well as the rules that regulate healthcare professionals. Although this test can be subjective, experience will allow you to make a more informed response.
2. **Always remember the character you are playing.** Your response will change depending on who the character is, thus you need to be clear on this before you answer any questions.
3. **Think like an expert.** Often, the correct answer does not represent what a student would normally do. Not everyone would say to their friend "Sorry, I can't sign you in. Maybe you should call up the university and ask them what to do!" However, you need

to think about what would be expected of you as a medical student, and what the experts would want you to do in the situation given.

4. **Read GMC Guidelines!** A good understanding of GMC's Good Medical Practice will help you to fully understand each scenario and formulate a better response.
5. **Learn your ethics.** You can search for ethical dilemmas online and challenge yourself to come up with appropriate responses. This exercise will help you to familiarise yourself with the application of ethical principles and prepare you for your Situational Judgement Test.
6. **Keep practicing.** Some students struggle a lot with this section. The more you practice, the more familiar you will become with the types of scenarios that can come up and the correct responses that will be required. That is not to say that responses will repeat themselves, but some things will become more evident. For example, whenever a question asks how important it is to consider the safety or autonomy of a patient, the answer will always be "very important".

Situational Judgement Mock Test

Scenario 1

Dr Ramanthan, a consultant Paediatrician, has had a very busy shift. A young child has been crying in the waiting room for over 30 minutes. When he steps out to call the child and her parents in for their appointment, he finds the parents speaking very aggressively to the receptionist.

How **appropriate** are the following responses by **Dr Ramanthan** in this situation?

1. Speak to the parents about what has upset them.
    A. A very appropriate thing to do
    B. Appropriate, but not ideal
    C. Inappropriate, but not awful
    D. A very inappropriate thing to do

2. Tell the receptionist to carry on with her work while he deals with the situation.
    A. A very appropriate thing to do
    B. Appropriate, but not ideal
    C. Inappropriate, but not awful
    D. A very inappropriate thing to do

3. Apologise for the long delay.
    A. A very appropriate thing to do
    B. Appropriate, but not ideal
    C. Inappropriate, but not awful
    D. A very inappropriate thing to do

Scenario 2

Jasmine is a junior registrar on a night shift in general surgery. She received a phone call from Eileen who states that she is the daughter of Mr Simpson, one of the patients on the ward. Eileen wants to know how her father is doing, as he does not have a mobile phone that she can contact him with.

How **appropriate** are the following responses by **Jasmine** in this situation?

4. Let Eileen know that her father is doing well and alleviate any concerns she may have.

A. A very appropriate thing to do
B. Appropriate, but not ideal
C. Inappropriate, but not awful
D. A very inappropriate thing to do

5. Check Mr Simpson's records to see whether Eileen is mentioned.
    A. A very appropriate thing to do
    B. Appropriate, but not ideal
    C. Inappropriate, but not awful
    D. A very inappropriate thing to do

6. Ask Mr Simpson whether he is happy for Eileen to know how he is doing.
    A. A very appropriate thing to do
    B. Appropriate, but not ideal
    C. Inappropriate, but not awful
    D. A very inappropriate thing to do

7. Explain to Eileen that she cannot disclose any information over the phone.
    A. A very appropriate thing to do
    B. Appropriate, but not ideal
    C. Inappropriate, but not awful
    D. A very inappropriate thing to do

Scenario 3

Gurleen, a medical student, spent the weekend at home with her family. Her younger siblings miss her a lot when she is at university, and are insistent that she stay with them for a while longer. She has seminars all day tomorrow, and knows that these are important to attend. However, she wishes to spend more time with her siblings, as she hardly gets the chance to come home.

How **appropriate** are the following responses by **Gurleen** in this situation?

8. Call the medical school explaining her situation and ask for advice.
    A. A very appropriate thing to do
    B. Appropriate, but not ideal
    C. Inappropriate, but not awful
    D. A very inappropriate thing to do

9. Report a "sick" absence to the medical school.
   A. A very appropriate thing to do
   B. Appropriate, but not ideal
   C. Inappropriate, but not awful
   D. A very inappropriate thing to do

10. Ask her friends to sign her in to the seminars and send any notes that they have made.
   A. A very appropriate thing to do
   B. Appropriate, but not ideal
   C. Inappropriate, but not awful
   D. A very inappropriate thing to do

11. Tell her siblings that she has no choice, and go back for her seminars.
   A. A very appropriate thing to do
   B. Appropriate, but not ideal
   C. Inappropriate, but not awful
   D. A very inappropriate thing to do

12. Call the medical school and ask if there is any way she can make up for the seminars.
   A. A very appropriate thing to do
   B. Appropriate, but not ideal
   C. Inappropriate, but not awful
   D. A very inappropriate thing to do

Scenario 4

Hamza is a junior doctor who has been seeking the opportunity to practice performing a lumbar puncture. The opportunity finally comes up, as a patient is in need of a lumbar puncture and there is a consultant to supervise and educate him on this. As Hamza is heading to gather his equipment, his alarm goes off reminding him of his meeting with a research supervisor.

How **important** to take into account are the following considerations for **Hamza** when deciding how to respond to the situation?

13. Hamza's supervisor had offered to buy him lunch during the meeting.
   A. Very important
   B. Important

C. Of minor importance
D. Not important at all

14. Hamza's supervisor has taken time out of his schedule to meet with him.
    A. Very important
    B. Important
    C. Of minor importance
    D. Not important at all

15. Someone else will probably end up doing the lumbar puncture while he is at the meeting.
    A. Very important
    B. Important
    C. Of minor importance
    D. Not important at all

Scenario 5

Amit, a medical student, is out doing some shopping, when he sees some students he recognises from his course. As he approaches them, he overhears one of them discussing Daniel, a patient that she examined earlier.

How **appropriate** are the following responses by **Amit** in this situation?

16. Confront her about using patient identifiable details.
    A. A very appropriate thing to do
    B. Appropriate, but not ideal
    C. Inappropriate, but not awful
    D. A very inappropriate thing to do

17. Walk in the other direction so as not to be associated with this breach of confidentiality.
    A. A very appropriate thing to do
    B. Appropriate, but not ideal
    C. Inappropriate, but not awful
    D. A very inappropriate thing to do

18. Report her to the medical school as this is a serious matter.
    A. A very appropriate thing to do

B. Appropriate, but not ideal
C. Inappropriate, but not awful
D. A very inappropriate thing to do

19. Politely remind her that patients' names should not be mentioned, especially in a public place.
    A. A very appropriate thing to do
    B. Appropriate, but not ideal
    C. Inappropriate, but not awful
    D. A very inappropriate thing to do

Scenario 6

Carl is a junior doctor on a surgical rotation. When he enters the doctors' office in the morning, he witnesses one of the surgeons quickly shove a bottle of whiskey in his drawer.

How **appropriate** are the following responses by **Carl** in this situation?

20. Report him immediately as he should not be drinking during work.
    A. A very appropriate thing to do
    B. Appropriate, but not ideal
    C. Inappropriate, but not awful
    D. A very inappropriate thing to do

21. Ask him if everything is okay.
    A. A very appropriate thing to do
    B. Appropriate, but not ideal
    C. Inappropriate, but not awful
    D. A very inappropriate thing to do

22. Confront him about the alcohol and demand that he takes the day off work for the safety of the patients.
    A. A very appropriate thing to do
    B. Appropriate, but not ideal
    C. Inappropriate, but not awful
    D. A very inappropriate thing to do

23. Talk to him to detect whether he appears to have been drinking.
    A. A very appropriate thing to do

B. Appropriate, but not ideal
C. Inappropriate, but not awful
D. A very inappropriate thing to do

24. "Are you okay? It's not like you to be drinking at work."
    A. A very appropriate thing to do
    B. Appropriate, but not ideal
    C. Inappropriate, but not awful
    D. A very inappropriate thing to do

Scenario 7

Emmanuel is a medical student on placement in a hospital. While seeing some patients, he hears a quarrel and immediately runs to find out what is happening. He finds a nurse shouting at one of the healthcare assistants. It appears that the healthcare assistant forgot to complete one of her tasks, potentially jeopardising a patient's safety.

How **important** to take into account are the following considerations for **Emmanuel** when deciding how to respond to the situation?

25. The healthcare assistant is new to the ward and probably did make the mistake.
    A. Very important
    B. Important
    C. Of minor importance
    D. Not important at all

26. The healthcare assistant jeopardised patient safety.
    A. Very important
    B. Important
    C. Of minor importance
    D. Not important at all

27. Emmanuel is only a medical student and it may not be his place to step in.
    A. Very important
    B. Important
    C. Of minor importance
    D. Not important at all

28. Patients are listening to the quarrel.
    A. Very important

B. Important
C. Of minor importance
D. Not important at all

29. The doctor had told the nurse to reprimand the healthcare assistant.
    A. Very important
    B. Important
    C. Of minor importance
    D. Not important at all

Scenario 8

Sonia, a GP, is visited by Mr Atkinson. He is a long-time alcoholic and has been advised many times to quit drinking. He feels no desire to stop, so he has refused the advice each time. He previously had some tests done and has come in today for the results. It turns out that Mr Atkinson has liver failure, likely as a result of his excessive drinking. Sonia needs to refer him to be put on the waiting list for a liver transplant.

How **important** to take into account are the following considerations for **Sonia** when deciding how to respond to the situation?

30. Mr Atkinson's liver failure is his own fault, as he refused to quit drinking.
    A. Very important
    B. Important
    C. Of minor importance
    D. Not important at all

31. Mr Atkinson drinks as a coping mechanism for problems in his personal life.
    A. Very important
    B. Important
    C. Of minor importance
    D. Not important at all

Scenario 9

Josephine, a dental student, has just arrived at her morning tutorial. She gets a text message from one of her friends, Cameron, asking her to sign him in to the session. She had seen his pictures on social media and knows he was out all night.

How **appropriate** are the following responses by **Josephine** in this situation?

32. Sign him in as he is probably hung over and it would not be appropriate for him to come to class in such a state.
    A. A very appropriate thing to do
    B. Appropriate, but not ideal
    C. Inappropriate, but not awful
    D. A very inappropriate thing to do

33. Ignore his text message.
    A. A very appropriate thing to do
    B. Appropriate, but not ideal
    C. Inappropriate, but not awful
    D. A very inappropriate thing to do

34. Advise him that she cannot sign him in, but can take some notes and share them with him later.
    A. A very appropriate thing to do
    B. Appropriate, but not ideal
    C. Inappropriate, but not awful
    D. A very inappropriate thing to do

35. Show the text message to the class tutor, as it is an unethical thing to do and someone more senior should be made aware of it.
    A. A very appropriate thing to do
    B. Appropriate, but not ideal
    C. Inappropriate, but not awful
    D. A very inappropriate thing to do

Scenario 10

Coleen is a dental student who has just moved in with her friend, Charlotte, who is also a dental student. They will soon be starting clinics with patients, and Coleen is concerned about Charlotte. She has been expressing inappropriate ideas about the position of a dentist in relation to the patients that they treat. Coleen thinks that Charlotte has been negatively influenced by a television series that she has been watching.

How **important** to take into account are the following considerations for **Coleen** when deciding how to respond to the situation?

36. The impact that Charlotte's behaviour might have on patients that she sees in her clinics.
    A. Very important
    B. Important
    C. Of minor importance
    D. Not important at all

Scenario 11

Adam is a third-year medical student on placement in a respiratory department. It is his first day, so his supervisor has asked him to have a quick 15-minute meeting after his morning session. As he is leaving the ward to attend his meeting, he sees a large pool of blood on the floor.

How **important** to take into account are the following considerations for **Adam** when deciding how to respond to the situation?

37. His supervisor is likely to find him very unprofessional for being late.
    A. Very important
    B. Important
    C. Of minor importance
    D. Not important at all

38. The blood may be infectious.
    A. Very important
    B. Important
    C. Of minor importance
    D. Not important at all

39. A patient may be actively bleeding.
    A. Very important
    B. Important
    C. Of minor importance
    D. Not important at all

40. He is unaware of the protocol for safely disposing of potentially infectious fluids.
    A. Very important
    B. Important
    C. Of minor importance

D. Not important at all

41. Someone else has probably already seen the blood and is planning to deal with it.
    A. Very important
    B. Important
    C. Of minor importance
    D. Not important at all

Scenario 12

Henry, a medical student, is on placement in a cardiology ward. He is going through patient notes and prescription charts to learn of different medications that are prescribed on the ward. He notices that Mr Xiu's notes declare that he is allergic to a specific medication. Upon checking his prescription chart, Henry notices that Mr Xiu had been prescribed the medication he is allergic to earlier this morning. The doctor who wrote the prescription is nowhere in sight.

How **appropriate** are the following responses by **Henry** in this situation?

42. Spend time trying to locate the doctor responsible for writing the prescription.
    A. A very appropriate thing to do
    B. Appropriate, but not ideal
    C. Inappropriate, but not awful
    D. A very inappropriate thing to do

43. Cross out the prescription so no one uses it.
    A. A very appropriate thing to do
    B. Appropriate, but not ideal
    C. Inappropriate, but not awful
    D. A very inappropriate thing to do

44. Urgently inform the first doctor or nurse in sight.
    A. A very appropriate thing to do
    B. Appropriate, but not ideal
    C. Inappropriate, but not awful
    D. A very inappropriate thing to do

Scenario 13

Ellie is a second-year medical student on placement in a GP surgery. The GP is conducting a questionnaire on lifestyle factors of each patient. He asks one of the patients, Mrs Corfield, how many bottles of wine she drinks in a week. She advises that she drinks seven bottles a week, but Ellie notices that the GP accidentally presses "8" on his keyboard as he enters this in Mrs Corfield's file.

How **appropriate** is the following response by **Ellie** in this situation?

45. Immediately inform the GP of his error so that he can correct it.
    A. A very appropriate thing to do
    B. Appropriate, but not ideal
    C. Inappropriate, but not awful
    D. A very inappropriate thing to do

Scenario 14

Lola is a first-year medical student and is about to go into the operating theatre for the first time. She is extremely excited, and tells her partner, Daniel, that she can't wait. Daniel appears a bit nervous. During the surgery, there is a lot of blood, and Lola notices Daniel becoming very pale.

Choose **both** the **one most appropriate action** and the **one least appropriate action** that **Lola** should take in response to this situation.

You will not receive any marks for this question unless you select **both** the most and least appropriate actions.

46.
    A. Immediately inform the surgeon conducting the operation so he can help Lola to deal with this.
    B. Immediately take Daniel out of the operating room without telling anyone, as it may disrupt the operation.
    C. Take Daniel to the side and sit him down, informing one of the other staff members what has happened.

Scenario 15

Natalia, a dental student, is enjoying some lunch with her colleagues in a busy canteen. Some of them start to make jokes about "the role of a woman" and "feminists". She starts to feel extremely uncomfortable as she finds their comments very offensive.

How **important** to take into account are the following considerations for **<u>Natalia</u>** when deciding how to respond to the situation?

47. Others may also be feeling uncomfortable.
    A. Very important
    B. Important
    C. Of minor importance
    D. Not important at all

48. The people making the remarks are her colleagues.
    A. Very important
    B. Important
    C. Of minor importance
    D. Not important at all

49. People in the canteen may overhear the jokes.
    A. Very important
    B. Important
    C. Of minor importance
    D. Not important at all

50. She is a dental student.
    A. Very important
    B. Important
    C. Of minor importance
    D. Not important at all

Scenario 16

Dr Jerome, a dentist, is at the cinema with her children. A patient of hers, Mrs Phillips, finds her in the queue for tickets. Mrs Phillips asks how Hannah, her friend's daughter, is doing after her wisdom teeth removal. Mrs Phillips is close with Hannah's family who are also patients at Dr Jerome's practice.

How **important** to take into account are the following considerations for **Dr Jerome** when deciding how to respond to the situation?

51. That Hannah is doing well.
    A. Very important
    B. Important
    C. Of minor importance
    D. Not important at all

52. She knows that Mrs Phillips is very close with Hannah's family.
    A. Very important
    B. Important
    C. Of minor importance
    D. Not important at all

53. Hannah is not present during this encounter.
    A. Very important
    B. Important
    C. Of minor importance
    D. Not important at all

Scenario 17

Sally, a dental student, is working on a group project. Aiman is visibly frustrated at one of the other group members, Linda. Aiman begins to use harsh language and insults the quality of Linda's work. Sally notices that this seems to have upset Linda, who remains quiet.

How **appropriate** are the following responses by **Sally** in this situation?

54. Immediately demand that Aiman apologises for insulting Linda.
    A. A very appropriate thing to do
    B. Appropriate, but not ideal
    C. Inappropriate, but not awful
    D. A very inappropriate thing to do

55. Talk to Aiman privately afterwards to discuss what had happened.
    A. A very appropriate thing to do
    B. Appropriate, but not ideal
    C. Inappropriate, but not awful

D. A very inappropriate thing to do

56. Report Aiman's behaviour to the group supervisor as he is likely to help resolve the issue.
    A. A very appropriate thing to do
    B. Appropriate, but not ideal
    C. Inappropriate, but not awful
    D. A very inappropriate thing to do

Scenario 18

Candice is a medical student on placement in a busy GP surgery. A patient comes in with a long list of problems and wants to discuss each of them in-depth with Dr Sheffield. There are many other patients waiting, so Candice is concerned that he is allowing too much time for this patient.

How **appropriate** are the following responses by **Candice** in this situation?

57. Interrupt the consultation to remind Dr Sheffield that other patients are waiting.
    A. A very appropriate thing to do
    B. Appropriate, but not ideal
    C. Inappropriate, but not awful
    D. A very inappropriate thing to do

58. Do nothing as there are other doctors in the surgery that can see the other patients.
    A. A very appropriate thing to do
    B. Appropriate, but not ideal
    C. Inappropriate, but not awful
    D. A very inappropriate thing to do

59. Interrupt the consultation and ask the patient to leave, as there are other patients who need to be seen.
    A. A very appropriate thing to do
    B. Appropriate, but not ideal
    C. Inappropriate, but not awful
    D. A very inappropriate thing to do

Scenario 19

Alex is a medical student on his clinical placement. While he is taking a history from one of the patients on a bay, he hears another patient start to choke. A nurse immediately rushes to the patient and starts to perform the necessary manoeuvres. Alex has been trained on dealing with choking, and feels that the nurse is performing the manoeuvres inadequately.

How **important** to take into account are the following considerations for **Alex** when deciding how to respond to the situation?

60. Choking is very dangerous.
    A. Very important
    B. Important
    C. Of minor importance
    D. Not important at all

61. She is just a nurse and might not know what she is doing.
    A. Very important
    B. Important
    C. Of minor importance
    D. Not important at all

62. The nurse is more qualified than Alex and probably knows what she is doing.
    A. Very important
    B. Important
    C. Of minor importance
    D. Not important at all

63. Alex feels very confident in his ability to deal with a choking patient.
    A. Very important
    B. Important
    C. Of minor importance
    D. Not important at all

Scenario 20

Peter and Beth are both junior doctors working in the emergency department. Peter mistakenly uses the incorrect pronoun for a patient after the patient had advised him of their preferences.

Choose **both** the **one most appropriate action** and the **one least appropriate action** that **Beth** should take in response to this situation.

You will not receive any marks for this question unless you select **both** the most and least appropriate actions.

64.

A. Quickly apologise on Peter's behalf to deescalate the situation.
B. Do nothing as Peter should deal with his own mistakes.
C. Explain to the patient that Peter is not required to call patients by their preferred pronouns.

Scenario 21

Sidney, a dental student, notices that her friend, Rhiannon, has been very quiet lately. She decides to check on her, and Rhiannon confesses that she has been having very negative and depressed thoughts.

How **appropriate** are the following responses by **Sidney** in this situation?

65. Remind her that her exams are coming up, so it would be best to try to resolve any issues she is having immediately.
    A. A very appropriate thing to do
    B. Appropriate, but not ideal
    C. Inappropriate, but not awful
    D. A very inappropriate thing to do

66. Ask her if she wants to talk about what has been going on.
    A. A very appropriate thing to do
    B. Appropriate, but not ideal
    C. Inappropriate, but not awful
    D. A very inappropriate thing to do

67. Advise her to visit her GP, as they can be helpful in dealing with depression.
    A. A very appropriate thing to do
    B. Appropriate, but not ideal
    C. Inappropriate, but not awful
    D. A very inappropriate thing to do

68. Inform the university of this, as they should be aware of the mental health of their students.
    A. A very appropriate thing to do
    B. Appropriate, but not ideal
    C. Inappropriate, but not awful
    D. A very inappropriate thing to do

69. Advise Rhiannon to inform the university, as they can help her if they are aware of her situation.
    A. A very appropriate thing to do
    B. Appropriate, but not ideal
    C. Inappropriate, but not awful
    D. A very inappropriate thing to do

Situational Judgement Test Answers

Scenario 1

1. The correct answer is A. It is essential for Dr Ramanthan to address the obvious fact that they are upset. Without addressing this, it will be difficult to solve the problem. This is a positive response and demonstrates empathy. Although he is having a busy shift, he is taking the time to speak to the patient's parents about their concerns.
2. The correct answer is C. It is not appropriate to dismiss another staff member in the middle of a conflict, as this may indicate that they have done something wrong. It may also be offensive to the staff member, who is not sure why they are being sent away. Although it may seem that he is doing nothing wrong, and is simply trying to help, the receptionist was involved in the conflict and thus it is important for her to be present while he attempts to deal with it. However, this does demonstrate an attempt to resolve the main issue of the parents' frustration, so it is not entirely bad.
3. The correct answer is A. Remember, this does not have to be the only action that is taken. Beginning by apologising for the delay is likely to deescalate the situation. This will allow the parents to speak in a calmer manner, and hopefully discuss what the issue is.

Scenario 2

4. The correct answer is D. Without any confirmation of who the person on the phone is, and whether Mr Simpson has given explicit consent for that person to be given information about him, Jasmine cannot make any comments. It is highly inappropriate to even confirm that Mr Simpson is on this ward. Patient confidentiality is crucial. If he does not want her to know he is there, it is not Jasmine's right to inform her. Further, from a patient safety point of view, it may even be someone pretending to be his daughter. Therefore, Jasmine must exercise caution and avoid giving away any information.
5. The correct answer is A. If there are identifiable details about Eileen on Mr Simpson's record, and it has been stated that she has permission to obtain information about him, then Jasmine can pass on information. Therefore, it would be very appropriate to check his record for such information.
6. The correct answer is A. If Jasmine has any doubt, and the patient is available and able to make an informed decision, it is best to ask him directly. If he gives his explicit consent, Jasmine can answer Eileen's questions over the telephone.

7. The correct answer is A. Patient confidentiality and patient safety are at risk. It is appropriate to explain to Eileen that she is unable to confirm or deny any information about any of the patients on the ward without explicit consent.

Scenario 3

8. The correct answer is A. As a medical student, it is essential to maintain professionalism at all times. However, it is also important to maintain a good personal life and family ties. The medical school should be understanding of her situation, and it would be best to seek advice on what she can do. This is a positive step towards resolving the issue, and she is doing nothing wrong here.
9. The correct answer is D. Lying is always unacceptable and should always be "very inappropriate".
10. The correct answer is D. This is also lying, which is unethical and unacceptable. It is good to ask friends for support and any notes from something that she has missed, but this must be "very inappropriate" due to the unethical act of requesting to be signed in.
11. The correct answer is C. This maintains her professionalism as a medical student, but does not deal with her own personal problem. It is important to have a good work-life balance and maintain good mental health, and although she should not miss any important seminars, Gurleen should try to find a solution to spend more time with her siblings. This response shows no effort towards finding a solution, but is not entirely bad as she is not doing anything wrong.
12. The correct answer is A. This is appropriate, although would not be a solo action. It is always good to reach out to the medical school and to be honest. If any important sessions might be missed, it is vital to catch up on them. Therefore, this is a good step to take. She may even find out that the seminars are not mandatory or that she can view the recordings online.

Scenario 4

13. The correct answer is C. Considering this will not impact the main problem in a positive or a negative way. The main problem is the time commitment and professionalism, not the promise of lunch. However, it would be beneficial to consider this in order to solve a minor problem. Because the doctor had offered lunch, he may take some offence if Hamza does not accept this invitation, thus it is of minor importance to consider.
14. The correct answer is A. The main problem here is the professionalism associated with keeping time commitments. It is very important for Hamza to ensure that he respects his commitments to others, and considers commitments that others have made for

him. A doctor who does not uphold their professional commitments is likely to struggle upholding commitments to patients.

15. The correct answer is C. This does not address the main problem. Nowhere does it say that it is necessary for Hamza to perform this procedure. It is clear that Hamza wants this for his own education and learning, which is important, but it is more essential to uphold the commitments that others have made for him. However, it does help to solve a minor problem, which is Hamza's desire to perform a lumbar puncture. By considering this, he may be able to find a solution to this minor problem, such as asking the consultant to wait until he is back. If the procedure is not urgent, this may be possible.

Scenario 5

16. The correct answer is C. This response is quite negative, as outlined by the term "confront". It is important to maintain politeness, as this kind of mannerism can lead to a defensive response and problems between colleagues. However, Amit is clearly attempting to solve the problem by reminding her that she should not be breaking confidentiality. Therefore, although he has not used the correct tone for resolving the problem, it is not entirely inappropriate.
17. The correct answer is D. Patient confidentiality is a serious issue, and anyone breaching it should be advised not to do so. By walking away, Amit is ignoring this problem, which can make matters worse. This is very inappropriate.
18. The correct answer is D. This is a severe escalation which is inappropriate as the individual involved has not been consulted prior to escalation. Further, it does not address the issue at hand, which is the current and ongoing breach of confidentiality. Therefore, there is nothing immediately positive about this response.
19. The correct answer is A. This response is well-mannered and will help maintain the relationship with his colleague. Further, it addresses the issue immediately in order to resolve it.

Scenario 6

20. The correct answer is D. It is vital to solve the danger to patient safety, but the consultant must first be approached before any escalation. It is unclear whether or not he has been drinking, thus no assumption should be made.
21. The correct answer is A. This is an appropriate and empathetic response which aims to resolve any misinterpretation of the circumstances. It is non-confrontational, non-judgemental and non-accusatory. This open question is an ideal response to the circumstances. If the consultant had been drinking, he is less likely to be defensive with such a response.

22. The correct answer is D. There is no evidence that the consultant has been drinking, thus harsh and negative terms such as "confront" and "demand" are very inappropriate.
23. The correct answer is A. Carl has just walked into the room and seen the consultant with a bottle of whiskey. He has not seen him drink anything, and has not yet observed his actions. Therefore, it is very appropriate to try to assess the situation further and respond accordingly. This action will help Carl to resolve the problem and clarify any misunderstanding he may have.
24. The correct answer is C. It is inappropriate to make any assumptions, as Carl has not seen him drink, therefore he should not accuse him of doing so. However, the response has an empathetic tone and attempts to deal with the situation. Therefore, it is not awful.

Scenario 7

25. The correct answer is D. It is not right for any member of the team to shout at anyone. Poor leadership and teamwork skills are being demonstrated by the nurse, and this matter should be resolved. If Emmanuel considers that the healthcare assistant probably made the mistake, it may stop him from doing anything to resolve the issue at hand, as he may feel that the nurse's actions are necessary.
26. The correct answer is D. If Emmanuel considers this, it may stop him from doing anything to resolve the issue at hand. Shouting is never an appropriate way to deal with anything, regardless of what the issue is. If he considers that patient safety was at risk, he may justify the shouting and do nothing about it. It is important to identify the main issue here, which is *not* patient safety.
27. The correct answer is D. When something wrong is happening, anyone who is there to witness it should do something about it. There should not be a culture in a healthcare environment whereby, due to a hierarchy of roles, people stay quiet and let abusive situations progress. Therefore, considering that he is "only" a medical student may stop him from resolving this issue. As such, it is not important at all to consider.
28. The correct answer is A. The main issues at hand are the poor leadership and teamwork skills displayed. However, another major issue has presented in this question – responsibility towards patients and the wider community. Such incidences should never occur in front of patients, as they can lead to patients losing confidence and trust in the healthcare profession. If someone makes a mistake, they should be advised privately, rather than in front of patients. Thus, if Emmanuel considers that patients are listening, it will urge him to act promptly to resolve the situation.
29. The correct answer is D. The doctor has no right to make such a request. It is appropriate to explain the errors made, but is not appropriate to shout. So, if Emmanuel considers that the doctor requested this, he may think that the nurse is allowed to shout at the healthcare assistant and therefore not take any action. Thus,

this is not important at all to consider. The situation is wrong in and of itself, so the reason for the shouting is not relevant.

Scenario 8

30. The correct answer is D. Mr Atkinson, like any other patient, has the right to make his own decisions. Lifestyle choices are his own, and it is not the doctor's right to be biased against patients who choose to make seemingly unwise choices. Therefore, it is not appropriate to blame a patient for diseases that they may be suffering from. If she considers the fact that his drinking has caused this, she may not wish to refer him for any further treatment, which can be detrimental to his health and his life.
31. The correct answer is B. It is important to understand the reason why someone with an addiction or an unhealthy lifestyle choice makes specific decisions. Understanding a patient's holistic problems can help the doctor to be more empathetic, and therefore to offer more effective treatment. However, regardless of the reason why he drinks, she should treat him with the same level of respect and dignity that is given to all patients.

Scenario 9

32. The correct answer is D. It is not appropriate of him to attend class hungover, but it is complete unethical of Josephine to sign him in, regardless of his situation.
33. The correct answer is C. By ignoring the situation, Josephine is not technically doing anything wrong. However, she is doing nothing to resolve the problem, so this is not an appropriate response. Further, if she simply ignores him, he may just ask someone else to sign him in. Therefore, it would be best to advise him of a solution to the problem.
34. The correct answer is A. This is an honest and dignified approach, thus it is appropriate. It also includes a helpful solution for Cameron, so it is an ideal response.
35. The correct answer is D. It is unnecessary to escalate the situation without first speaking to Cameron. This level of escalation can severely impact her relationship with her colleague, and it is always recommended to deal with matters internally before escalating.

Scenario 10

36. The correct answer is A. It is always essential to consider patient safety. Patients are always a top priority, and to *not* consider patients is wrong. If Coleen considers this, it will help her to take necessary actions to prevent any harm from occurring to patients.

Scenario 11

37. The correct answer is C. The main concern here is patient safety. This pool of blood can be contaminated and pose a risk to himself, to patients, and to other staff members. This is the primary issue that needs to be dealt with, so considering the impact of his unpunctuality will not help solve this. However, considering this can help him to deal with the minor problem of professionalism. As such, if he considers this, he can try to contact his supervisor to explain the situation.
38. The correct answer is A. Patient safety is the main priority. Considering the possibility of contamination or infection will help Adam to respond urgently and effectively. Anything that is infectious needs to be dealt with in an appropriate manner in order to remove all traces of contaminants, thus, this is vital to consider.
39. The correct answer is A. Again, patient safety is the main priority. If there is a patient who may be in danger, this needs to be dealt with immediately. As such, it is very important to consider this in order to locate the patient or the source of the blood. If this is not considered, the main concern of patient safety may not be dealt with appropriately.
40. The correct answer is A. Infectious material poses a risk of harm to anyone in contact. Therefore, it is vital that it is disposed of properly. Adam must consider this in order to make an appropriate decision about what to do. He can help clean the blood, but he needs to be aware of his limitations in order to seek guidance from someone who is more aware of the protocol. If he does not consider the limitations to his knowledge, he may clean it in an inappropriate manner, thus maintaining the risk to patients.
41. The correct answer is D. Workplace safety is everybody's responsibility. He cannot make the assumption that someone is already dealing with it, nor can he base his actions on this assumption. There does not appear to be anyone there dealing with it, thus, he should not consider this when deciding how to act. If he happens to consider this, it may prevent him from taking urgent action, thus increasing the risk to patients and other staff members.

Scenario 12

42. The correct answer is D. The threat to patient safety should be urgent and immediate. Therefore, after knowing that the doctor is nowhere in sight, it would be very inappropriate to spend time looking for the doctor. In this time, someone may give Mr Xiu the medication, resulting in him having an allergic reaction. This action would increase the risk to the patient, thus is very inappropriate.
43. The correct answer is D. As a medical student, Henry is not qualified to change a prescription. Although patient safety is at risk, he must not do anything outside the scope of his limitations. Rules and limitations are set to ensure patient safety, so it is not appropriate to break them in an attempt to maintain patient safety.

44. The correct answer is A. This is the appropriate measure in this scenario as Henry will deal with the problem in a time-sensitive manner and successfully resolve his concerns. Nurses are responsible for administering medications, so informing a nurse will be useful to ensure that the medication is not administered. If a doctor is found, they will communicate this to the nurse in charge of the patient, and if a nurse is found, they will communicate this to the doctor in charge of the patient. Healthcare is a team effort, and in this scenario regarding patient safety, informing either a doctor or nurse would be useful in beginning to resolve the problem. Although it would be ideal for the doctor who wrote the prescription to check it, the scenario has made it clear that he is not available.

Scenario 13

45. The correct answer is C. It is important to correct this error, but it is not urgent or life-threatening, as there will be no immediate harm from this mistake. Correcting the doctor in front of the patient can undermine the patient's trust in the doctor and in the healthcare profession. Therefore, it is best to wait until the patient has left and then correct the doctor privately. If there is any doubt, the doctor can contact the patient to clarify what the response to his question was.

Scenario 14

46. Most appropriate: C

    Least appropriate: A

    A is the least appropriate, as Lola should not disrupt the surgeon conducting the operation. This may cause him to make a mistake and potentially risk patient safety. B is slightly appropriate, but it is unprofessional to leave the room without telling anyone. Therefore, C is the best option, as it deals with the issue at hand, and maintains professionalism. It is important to inform one of the staff members who is not currently conducting the operation so they can help deal with the matter. They likely have a lot of experience with students feeling faint in operations, so they can offer their help and advice.

Scenario 15

47. The correct answer is A. It is important to consider that others may also find this offensive and may be feeling uncomfortable. If she considers this, it will help her resolve the matter in a way that is suitable for everybody. If she does not consider this, she may only take into account her own feelings and therefore not resolve the

matter in the most appropriate way. The feelings of others are paramount and should always hold importance.

48. The correct answer is C. The main problem is the fact that they are making offensive remarks. Their positions do not give them any special privileges to be offensive. Therefore, considering this will not help solve the main problem. However, it is of minor importance as it is important to maintain good relationships with colleagues, thus she should deal with it in an appropriate and professional way.
49. The correct answer is A. If she finds the jokes offensive, anyone overhearing them may also find them offensive. Moreover, this can shed negative light on dental students and on the profession. If she considers this, she may take more urgent action to resolve the issue.
50. The correct answer is A. It is essential to maintain professionalism at all times, regardless of whether Natalia is on the job, at university, or in a completely different environment. Therefore, when associating with a group making offensive jokes, she should remember her position as a dental student and her responsibility of professionalism. This will help her to solve the matter at hand, and to act in the most professional way possible.

Scenario 16

51. The correct answer is D. The outcomes of the surgery have no impact on whether her private information should be released to a third party or not. Considering this may actually cause harm, as it could lead Dr Jerome to making a passive remark such as "She's doing well!" which may seem harmless but is still a breach of confidentiality.
52. The correct answer is D. Hannah's confidentiality is not any less important in the presence of a family friend. It is vital to maintain patient confidentiality at all times. Considering this may lead to a more relaxed approach, and Dr Jerome may happen to casually mention details that she should not. Therefore, this should not even be considered.
53. The correct answer is C. The main problem is patient confidentiality. Regardless of whether or not Hannah is present, Dr Jerome must maintain patient confidentiality. Considering her presence will not help her resolve this problem, nor will it hinder the resolution. If Hannah was present, she may be able to give consent to discuss her, but her absence has no impact on confidentiality. Therefore, this is of minor importance.

Scenario 17

54. The correct answer is D. The language used is harsh. By "demanding" that she apologise, Sally would appear unreasonable and would be making the situation worse.
55. The correct answer is A. This is an ideal approach as it is empathetic rather than blaming Aiman for her actions. It allows a calm environment to discuss the situation,

and is a better form of conflict resolution than confronting or teaming up against a certain individual who appears to be in the wrong.

56. The correct answer is D. It is not appropriate to escalate the situation prior to dealing with it internally. There are steps to escalation that should be followed.

Scenario 18

57. The correct answer is C. It is not appropriate to interrupt the consultation, or to give the doctor such advice in front of the patient. Both parties may find this disrespectful, and it may undermine the patient's trust in the doctor. However, nothing directly offensive is said about the patient, and this action is attempting to deal with the issue, so it is not entirely inappropriate.
58. The correct answer is C. It is not appropriate to relay responsibilities to others, as each individual should take responsibility for patients. However, it is true that there are other doctors, and sometimes it is important to give extra time to specific patients. Therefore, this is inappropriate, but not awful.
59. The correct answer is D. Candice is a medical student and should not interrupt the consultation, nor should she be the one to determine that the consultation is over and the patient should leave. It is inappropriate to step outside of her limits. Each patient should be prioritised, and oftentimes, doctors need to give slightly more time to specific patients. Sometimes, patients need to wait a bit longer for their appointments in busy clinics. They should still get their full appointment time in an unrushed manner. There is no indication to suggest that Dr Sheffield is giving this patient time at the expense of other patients' time.

Scenario 19

60. The correct answer is A. Patient safety is a primary concern at all times, and therefore is very important. He must consider this and act urgently.
61. The correct answer is D. The problem at hand is patient safety. Regardless of her qualifications, Alex needs to act urgently for the sake of the patient. Perhaps she has made a mistake, or is newly qualified and has not had much practice. Regardless, it is inappropriate to undermine other healthcare professionals. Nurses are trained in life support, and should be very well-versed in dealing with choking. Thus, this is not something to consider.
62. The correct answer is D. Alex needs to respond immediately to the threat to patient safety. If he suspects there is danger, he should not let the idea that the nurse is more qualified than him get in the way of acting. Therefore, this should not be considered.
63. The correct answer is A. If he considers his confidence, he may be able to step in and help out. Most importantly, he will be able to identify that the manoeuvres are not being performed correctly, and act urgently to address the patient safety concern. If

he does not recognise his own knowledge of choking, he may lack confidence and not act promptly.

Scenario 20

64. Most appropriate: A
Least appropriate: C
Although it is not ideal to apologise on behalf of someone else, this is the best option out of the three as it can help to deescalate the situation. Doing nothing can cause the patient to proceed with further complaints. The last option is completely inappropriate, as patients' wishes should be respected.

Scenario 21

65. The correct answer is C. The main priority is Rhiannon's mental wellbeing. Sidney should act with empathy. Exams are of minor concern in this situation, however, they are not entirely inappropriate to mention as this shows some level of concern that Sidney has for her friend.
66. The correct answer is A. Rhiannon has confided in Sidney, and it appears that she would like her help. Sidney has already noticed that Rhiannon has been reserved, so it would be appropriate to help her where possible. Talking about things can be helpful for a lot of people, especially with a trustworthy friend. This is an empathetic response that Rhiannon was likely hoping for.
67. The correct answer is A. Although this does not show immediate empathy and help from Sidney, it provides a practical and longer-term solution, so is highly appropriate. If someone is depressed, they should seek help, and oftentimes just talking to a friend is not enough. Remember, this does not have to be the only response in order to be "very appropriate". Sidney can advise her to visit the GP *and* also do everything she can to help out.
68. The correct answer is D. There is no evidence of immediate threat to Rhiannon, such as mention of suicidal thoughts. Therefore, there is no justification for breaking her confidentiality and informing the school of her situation.
69. The correct answer is A. It is important for students to contact their supervisor or university to inform them of personal circumstances that may be impacting their ability to attend classes, placement, or to see patients. Informing the university gives them the opportunity to provide support to the student. Therefore, this is very appropriate as it provides a practical solution.

Congratulations!

Congratulations on getting through the book! By now, you should have learned a lot about the UCAT and had a fair number of opportunities to practice your skills. If you haven't already, now is a great time to get in touch with us about booking an expert UCAT tutor to help you perfect your techniques and skills in order to excel in each section. You can book a tutor or book a consultation to discuss your learning needs on https://www.medichut.com/ucat.

UCAT Mock Test

Put your knowledge to the test with the end-of-book mock starting on the next page. Please complete this test within 2 hours, and each section within its allocated time:

- Verbal Reasoning: 21 minutes
- Decision Making: 31 minutes
- Quantitative Reasoning: 24 minutes
- Abstract Reasoning: 13 minutes
- Situational Judgement Test: 26 minutes

Note down your answers, and mark against the correct answers at the end. All the best!

Verbal Reasoning Questions

Passage 1

The Battle of Gallipoli occurred on 29 May 1416 between a squadron of the Venetian navy and the fleet of the Ottoman Empire off the Ottoman naval base of Gallipoli. The battle was the main episode of a brief conflict between the two powers, resulting from Ottoman attacks against Venetian possessions and shipping in the Aegean Sea in late 1415. The Venetian fleet, under Pietro Loredan, was charged with transporting Venetian envoys to the Sultan, but was authorized to attack if the Ottomans refused to negotiate. The subsequent events are known chiefly from a letter written by Loredan after the battle. The Ottomans exchanged fire with the Venetian ships as soon as the Venetian fleet approached Gallipoli, forcing the Venetians to withdraw.

On the next day, the two fleets manoeuvred and fought off Gallipoli, but during the evening, Loredan managed to contact the Ottoman authorities and inform them of his diplomatic mission. Despite assurances that the Ottomans would welcome the envoys, when the Venetian fleet approached the city on the next day, the Ottoman fleet sailed to meet the Venetians and the two sides quickly became embroiled in battle. The Venetians scored a crushing victory, killing the Ottoman admiral, capturing a large part of the Ottoman fleet, and taking large numbers prisoner, of whom many—particularly the Christians serving voluntarily in the Ottoman fleet—were executed. The Venetians then retired to Tenedos to replenish their supplies and rest. Although a crushing Venetian victory, which confirmed Venetian naval superiority in the Aegean Sea for the next few decades, the settlement of the conflict was delayed until a peace treaty was signed in 1419.

Source: https://en.wikipedia.org/wiki/Battle_of_Gallipoli_(1416)

1. Why did the Venetians step back from the battle?
   - A. Due to the Ottomans exchanging fire.
   - B. Due to the command of Pietro Loredan.
   - C. Due to transport issues in the Aegean Sea.
   - D. Due to the death of the Ottoman admiral.

2. Where did the Venetians head to after the battle?
   - A. Gallipoli
   - B. Tenedos
   - C. Aegean Sea
   - D. Loredan

3. What did the Ottomans promise the Venetians?

A. That they would defeat them in the battle.
B. That they would welcome them.
C. That they would not enslave any of the captives.
D. That they would help them to travel back home.

4. Which of the following can best be inferred from the passage?
   A. The Ottomans and Venetians were long-time enemies.
   B. The Ottomans and Venetians set aside their differences during the Battle of Gallipoli.
   C. Pietro Loredan was present during the Battle of Gallipoli.
   D. The Venetians were known for always executing their captives of war.

Passage 2

Coal is a black or brownish-black sedimentary rock that can be burned for fuel and used to generate electricity. It is composed mostly of carbon and hydrocarbons, which contain energy that can be released through combustion (burning). Coal is the largest source of energy for generating electricity in the world, and the most abundant fossil fuel in the United States. Fossil fuels are formed from the remains of ancient organisms. Because coal takes millions of years to develop and there is a limited amount of it, it is a nonrenewable resource.

The conditions that would eventually create coal began to develop about 300 million years ago, during the Carboniferous period. During this time, the Earth was covered in wide, shallow seas and dense forests. The seas occasionally flooded the forested areas, trapping plants and algae at the bottom of a swampy wetland. Over time, the plants (mostly mosses) and algae were buried and compressed under the weight of overlying mud and vegetation. As the plant debris sifted deeper under Earth's surface, it encountered increased temperatures and higher pressure. Mud and acidic water prevented the plant matter from coming into contact with oxygen. Due to this, the plant matter decomposed at a very slow rate and retained most of its carbon (source of energy).

These areas of buried plant matter are called peat bogs. Peat bogs store massive amounts of carbon many meters underground. Peat itself can be burned for fuel, and is a major source of heat energy in countries such as Scotland, Ireland, and Russia. Under the right conditions, peat transforms into coal through a process called carbonization. Carbonization takes place under incredible heat and pressure. About 3 meters (10 feet) of layered vegetation eventually compresses into a third of a meter (1 foot) of coal!

Coal exists in underground formations called "coal seams" or "coal beds." A coal seam can be as thick as 30 meters (90 feet) and stretch 1,500 kilometers (920 miles). Coal seams exist on every continent. The largest coal reserves are in the United States, Russia, China, Australia, and India. In the United States, coal is mined in 25 states and three major regions. In the Western Coal Region, Wyoming is the top producer—about 40% of the coal mined in the country is extracted in the state. More than one-third of the nation's coal comes from the Appalachian Coal Region, which includes West Virginia, Virginia, Tennessee, and Kentucky. Coal extracted from Texas in the Interior Coal Region supplies mostly local markets.

Source: https://www.nationalgeographic.org/encyclopedia/coal/

5. Which of the following statements is best supported by the passage?
   A. 40% of the coal mined in the United States is in Wyoming.
   B. There is not enough coal in the world.
   C. Coal can be renewed.
   D. Peat bogs are made from coal.

6. Which of the following can be inferred from the passage?
   A. Peat bogs are made from coal.
   B. Coal is made from plants.
   C. Coal from Texas cannot be transported to other parts of the country.
   D. Carbonization can take millions of years.

7. What best describes the condition of Earth around 300 million years ago?
   A. Deep seas and wide forests
   B. Lots of vegetation
   C. Large amounts of algae
   D. Wide seas and deep forests

8. Which of the following statements is correct regarding the formation of coal?
   A. It begins as plant matter, then forms peat, which forms coal.
   B. It begins as plant matter, which forms coal seams which are carbonised to form coal.
   C. It begins as peat bogs which then break down into plant matter to form coal.
   D. It begins as mud, which is carbonised to form coal.

Passage 3

History in Bahrain is nowhere more intriguing than among the 85,000 burial mounds that now lump, curdle and honeycomb 5% of the island's landmass. Archaeologists have recently confirmed Bahrain as the seat of the lost and illustrious empire of Dilmun (3200–330 BC), whose influence spread as far north as modern Kuwait and as far inland as Al Hasa Oasis in eastern Saudi Arabia. According to Sumerian, Babylonian and Assyrian inscriptions, the island's residents were not only commercially active but also attentive to matters at home. The proper burial of the sick, disabled and young in elaborate chambers, together with their chattels of ceramics, glass and beads (carefully displayed at the Bahrain National Museum),

suggest an enlightened civilisation of considerable social and economic development, assisted by the perpetual abundance of 'sweet', or potable, water on the island.
Little wonder, then, that Dilmun (which means 'noble') was often referred to as the fabled Garden of Eden and described as 'paradise' in the Epic of Gilgamesh, the world's oldest poetic saga. Dilmun's economic success was due in no small part to the trading of Omani copper, which was measured using the internationally recognised 'Dilmun Standard' (the weights can be seen in the Bahrain National Museum). When the copper trade declined around 1800 BC, Dilmun's strength fell with it, leaving the island vulnerable to the predatory interests of the surrounding big powers. By 600 BC Dilmun was absorbed entirely by Babylon and was subsequently ceded to Greece. The Greeks called the island Tylos, a name it kept for nearly a thousand years (from 330 BC to AD 622), despite Greek rule enduring for less than 100 years. Little distinguishes the history of Bahrain from that of the rest of the Gulf thereafter until the 16th century.

Source: https://www.lonelyplanet.com/bahrain/a/nar/ff4cd0f8-9a6f-4a9c-8b10-2d871bcbe572/361009

9. Which of the following statements can best be inferred from the passage?
   A. Oman is a different country to Bahrain.
   B. It took 1200 years from the beginning of Dilmun's decline to its end.
   C. The language of ancient Bahrain was Assyrian.
   D. Bahrain is north of Kuwait.

10. What was Dilmun described as in old poetry?
   A. Successful
   B. Noble
   C. Paradise
   D. Dilmun Standard

11. Which of the following statements best describes why Dilmun lost its power?
   A. Due to surrounding countries having power.
   B. Due to the decrease in copper trading.
   C. Due to the conquest by Greece.
   D. Due to the Bahrain International Museum.

12. Which of the following statements is best supported by the passage?
   A. The water in Dilmun was portable.
   B. Bahrain was formed in the 16th century.
   C. The residents of Saudi Arabia were commercially active.
   D. The behaviours of the people of Dilmun suggested that the empire was well-developed.

Passage 4

The American effort to send astronauts to the moon had its origins in an appeal President Kennedy made to a special joint session of Congress on May 25, 1961: "I believe this nation should commit itself to achieving the goal, before this decade is out, of landing a man on the moon and returning him safely to Earth." At the time, the United States was still trailing the Soviet Union in space developments, and Cold War-era America welcomed Kennedy's bold proposal. In 1966, after five years of work by an international team of scientists and engineers, the National Aeronautics and Space Administration (NASA) conducted the first unmanned Apollo mission, testing the structural integrity of the proposed launch vehicle and spacecraft combination.

Then, on January 27, 1967, tragedy struck at Kennedy Space Center in Cape Canaveral, Florida, when a fire broke out during a manned launch-pad test of the Apollo spacecraft and Saturn rocket. Three astronauts were killed in the fire. Despite the setback, NASA and its thousands of employees forged ahead, and in October 1968, Apollo 7, the first manned Apollo mission, orbited Earth and successfully tested many of the sophisticated systems needed to conduct a moon journey and landing. In December of the same year, Apollo 8 took three astronauts to the dark side of the moon and back, and in March 1969 Apollo 9 tested the lunar module for the first time while in Earth orbit. That May, the three astronauts of Apollo 10 took the first complete Apollo spacecraft around the moon in a dry run for the scheduled July landing mission.

Source: https://www.history.com/topics/space-exploration/moon-landing-1969

13. What was the adversity that took place before the successful orbit around Earth?
    A. Difficulty landing on the moon.
    B. Death of astronauts.
    C. Thousands of employees were killed in a fire.
    D. Problems with the structural integrity of the launch.

14. According to the passage, which Apollo mission landed on the moon?
    A. Apollo 11
    B. Apollo 9
    C. Apollo 10
    D. Can't tell.

15. Which of the following can be inferred from the passage?
    A. The Soviet Union was ahead of the United States in space development.
    B. The first unmanned Apollo mission was in 1971.
    C. President Kennedy led the Apollo missions to ensure that man would step foot on the moon.
    D. President Kennedy's appeal was granted in 1967.

16. When was the first unmanned Apollo mission?
    A. 1971
    B. 1968
    C. 1966
    D. 1969

Passage 5

Italian Renaissance artists became anatomists by necessity, as they attempted to refine a more lifelike, sculptural portrayal of the human figure. Indeed, until about 1500–1510, their investigations surpassed much of the knowledge of anatomy that was taught at the universities. Opportunities for direct anatomical dissection were very restricted during the Renaissance. Giorgio Vasari's Lives of the Artists states that the great Florentine sculptor, painter, and printmaker Antonio Pollaiuolo (ca. 1432–1498) was the "first master to skin many human bodies in order to investigate the muscles and understand the nude in a more modern way." Giving credence to Vasari's claim, Pollaiuolo's highly influential engraving of the Battle of Naked Men displays the figures of the nude warriors with nearly flayed musculature, seen in fierce action poses and from various angles. The later innovators in the field, Leonardo da Vinci (1452–1519) and Michelangelo (1475–1564), who are known to have undertaken detailed anatomical dissections at various points in their long careers, set a new standard in their portrayals of the human figure. The patrons commissioning art in this period also came to expect such anatomical mastery. In the words of the Florentine sculptor Baccio Bandinelli (1493–1560), who was trying to impress a duke to hire him, and who also appears to have run an academy for the teaching of young artists, "I will show you that I know how to dissect the brain, and also living men, as I have dissected dead ones to learn my art". Circumstantial evidence suggests that a number of other artists also attempted direct dissections. Some later great masters produced écorchés, studies of the peeled away or ripped apart forms of muscles, to explore their potential for purely artistic expression. The majority of artists, however, limited their investigations to the surface of the body—the appearance of its musculature, tendons, and bones as observed through the skin—and recorded such findings in exquisitely detailed studies after the live nude model.
Source: https://www.metmuseum.org/toah/hd/anat/hd_anat.htm

17. Most of the artists of the time conducted thorough full body dissections.
    A. True
    B. False
    C. Can't tell

18. Giorgio Vasari was a great Florentine sculptor.
    A. True
    B. False

C. Can't tell

19. All Italian Renaissance artists had greater knowledge of anatomy than was taught at universities.
    A. True
    B. False
    C. Can't tell

20. Pollaiuolo conducted his own research to learn about the human body.
    A. True
    B. False
    C. Can't tell

Passage 6

Many thousands of years ago, late in the Ice Age, humans journeyed across the Bering land bridge, from Asia into Alaska. Their descendants explored along the west coast of North America. As early as 1000 BC, they had covered nearly the entire continent. It is not known when the first people arrived in the Americas. Some archaeologists (scientists who study the remains of past human lives) believe it might have been about 12000 BC.

Over thousands of years, as they migrated across the continents, American Indians have developed a wide range of languages, customs, and civilizations. There are as many different tribal nations in the Americas as there are nations in Europe, Asia, or Africa, and there is as much variety among them.

Ten thousand years ago, when the Ice Age ended, changes in climate and increasing populations inspired some Native American tribes to experiment with growing different crops. Some became highly skilled farmers. As early as about 5500 BC, tribes in Mexico cultivated corn and squash. They raised turkeys, llamas, and guinea pigs for food and they hunted deer and bison. They regularly burned off patches of land to keep it in pasture, so the animals would come to graze. Many tribes on the coasts hunted sea mammals from boats and caught fish, using a variety of efficient methods.

After 2000 BC, some Native Americans developed states, each governing thousands of people. They established extensive trade routes across the continents. And they used cargo rafts and other boats to ship their goods from one trading point to another. In South America, llamas provided transportation on land.

From the present-day region of the mid-western United States to southern Peru in South America, centers of government were marked by enormous mounds of earth. Most of these mounds were flat on top, with palaces and temples built on them. Some were burial sites of honored leaders. American Indian cities were as big as the cities in Europe and Asia at that time. Their fine architecture is still greatly admired.

Source: https://www.scholastic.com/teachers/articles/teaching-content/history-native-americans/

21. Around 1000 BC, the first people arrived in the Americas.
    A. True
    B. False
    C. Can't tell

22. Tribes in Mexico fed on deer and bison.
    A. True
    B. False
    C. Can't tell

23. There was a climate change around 10,000 years ago.
    A. True
    B. False
    C. Can't tell

24. Boats were exclusively used for travel by the Native Americans.
    A. True
    B. False
    C. Can't tell

Passage 7

The 16th-century Spanish explorer and conquistador Hernando de Soto (c. 1496-1542) arrived in the West Indies as a young man and went on to make a fortune in the Central American slave trade. He supplied ships for Francisco Pizarro's southward expedition and ended up accompanying Pizarro in his conquest of Peru in 1532. Seeking greater glory and riches, de Soto embarked on a major expedition in 1538 to conquer Florida for the Spanish crown. He and his men traveled nearly 4,000 miles throughout the region that would become the southeastern United States in search of riches, fighting off Native American attacks along the way. In 1541, de Soto and his men became the first Europeans to encounter the great Mississippi River and cross it; de Soto died early the next year. Hernando de Soto's Early Life and Career. Like many of the era's conquistadors, Hernando de Soto was a native of the impoverished Extremadura region of southwestern Spain. He was born in 1496 in Jerez de los Caballeros, Bajadoz province. De Soto's family was of minor nobility and modest means, and at a very young age he developed dreams of making his fortune in the New World. Around the age of 14, de Soto left for Seville, where he got himself included on an expedition to the West Indies led by Pedro Arias Dávila in 1514. De Soto earned a fortune from Dávila's conquest of Panama and Nicaragua, and by 1530 he was the leading slave trader and one of the richest men in Nicaragua. In 1531, he joined

Francisco Pizarro on an expedition in pursuit of rumors of gold located in the region that is now northwestern Colombia, on the Pacific coast. In 1532, De Soto acted as Pizarro's chief lieutenant in the former's conquest of Peru. Before Spanish forces defeated the Incas at Cajamarca that November, de Soto became the first European to make contact with the Inca emperor Atahualpa.

Source: https://www.history.com/topics/exploration/hernando-de-soto

25. What was the main reason for Hernando's major expedition mentioned in the passage?
    A. Conquering land
    B. Glory and riches
    C. To gain the Spanish crown
    D. To gain power as the leader of his army

26. Which year did Hernando de Soto pass away?
    A. 1532
    B. 1541
    C. 1538
    D. 1542

27. Who was the leader of the expedition that Hernando went on at the age of fourteen?
    A. Jerez de los Caballeros
    B. Francisco Pizarro
    C. Bajadoz
    D. Pedro Arias Dávila

28. Which statement best describes de Soto's family?
    A. They were not that wealthy.
    B. They were very wealthy.
    C. They were slaves.
    D. They were explorers.

Passage 8

Mediterranean Sea, an intercontinental sea that stretches from the Atlantic Ocean on the west to Asia on the east and separates Europe from Africa. It has often been called the incubator of Western civilization. This ancient "sea between the lands" occupies a deep, elongated, and almost landlocked irregular depression lying between latitudes 30° and 46° N and longitudes 5°50′ W and 36° E. Its west-east extent—from the Strait of Gibraltar between Spain and Morocco to the shores of the Gulf of Iskenderun on the southwestern coast of Turkey—is approximately 2,500 miles (4,000 km), and its average north-south extent, between Croatia's southernmost shores and Libya, is about 500 miles (800 km). The Mediterranean Sea, including the Sea of Marmara, occupies an area of approximately 970,000 square miles (2,510,000 square km).

The western extremity of the Mediterranean Sea connects with the Atlantic Ocean by the narrow and shallow channel of the Strait of Gibraltar, which is roughly 8 miles (13 km) wide at its narrowest point; and the depth of the sill, or submarine ridge separating the Atlantic from the Alborán Sea, is about 1,050 feet (320 metres). To the northeast the Mediterranean is connected with the Black Sea through the Dardanelles (with a sill depth of 230 feet [70 metres]), the Sea of Marmara, and the strait of the Bosporus (sill depth of about 300 feet [90 metres]). To the southeast it is connected with the Red Sea by the Suez Canal.

A submarine ridge between the island of Sicily and the African coast with a sill depth of about 1,200 feet (365 metres) divides the Mediterranean Sea into western and eastern parts. The western part in turn is subdivided into three principal submarine basins. The Alborán Basin is east of Gibraltar, between the coasts of Spain and Morocco. The Algerian (sometimes called the Algero-Provençal or Balearic) Basin, east of the Alborán Basin, is west of Sardinia and Corsica, extending from off the coast of Algeria to off the coast of France. These two basins together constitute the western basin. The Tyrrhenian Basin, that part of the Mediterranean known as the Tyrrhenian Sea, lies between Italy and the islands of Sardinia and Corsica.

Source: https://www.britannica.com/place/Mediterranean-Sea

29. Which of the following countries does the Algerian Basin touch?
    A. Croatia
    B. Libya
    C. Sardinia
    D. France

30. Which side of the Mediterranean connects with the Atlantic Ocean?
    A. Southeast
    B. West
    C. Southwest
    D. Northeast

31. Which of the following is not connected to the northeast of the Mediterranean Sea?
    A. Black Sea
    B. The Strait of Gibraltar
    C. Sea of Marmara
    D. The strait of the Bosporus

32. Which of the following statements is true, based on the passage?
    A. Libya is on the southern end of the Mediterranean Sea.
    B. The Sea of Marmara is on the northwest of the Mediterranean Sea.
    C. The Gulf of Iskenderun is on the northern end of the Mediterranean Sea.
    D. The Alborán Basin is east of the Algerian Basin.

Passage 9

Most modern roses sold today bloom somewhat regularly throughout the growing season. In contrast, some old garden roses and climbing roses bloom once a year or bloom only in the spring and fall. Roses that bloom on a regular basis are called "repeat" bloomers.
The speed with which a rose forms a new bloom-producing cane (stem), develops a bud, and the bud opens to a flower varies. When we cut off a dead spent bloom (deadheading) we signal to that stem to grow a new flower-producing stem. In repeat-blooming roses, the timing of the blooming process begins with the removal of an aged flower.
Generally it takes 4 to 10 weeks (28 to 70 days) for reblooming to occur. Roses having a lot of petals take longer to re-bloom than roses with only a few petals. Miniature roses, single roses (those with 5 to 12 petals) and some old garden roses (especially Chinas, noisettes and polyanthas) tend to re-bloom the fastest (28 – 32 days). Roses with a lot of petals (45 – 50) take longer to re-bloom, usually 6 weeks. While densely-petaled roses like Belinda's Dream and Quietness (100+ petals) take the longest to rebloom, these roses hold their blooms on the bush a lot longer than their lesser-petaled counterparts. It is common for 100-petaled roses to last on the bush 10 to 14 days, making it worth the wait from a landscape impact perspective. A good rule of thumb is "more petals = more time."
Source: https://arborgate.com/blog/garden/how-often-do-roses-bloom/

33. Which of the following statements can be inferred from the passage?
    A. Repeat-blooming roses will only grow once a year.
    B. A new rose will not grow in a repeat-blooming rose until the old rose has been removed.
    C. A rose with 60 petals would rebloom in under 30 days.
    D. Roses with less petals are more likely to live longer.

34. Which of the following statements is true based on the passage?
    A. Reblooming generally occurs in under 28 days.
    B. The less petals a rose has, the longer it will take to rebloom.
    C. The bud of the rose is formed before the stem.
    D. New stems are formed due to deadheading.

35. Which of the following conclusions can be drawn from the passage?
    A. Quietness will most likely take over 42 days to bloom.
    B. A miniature rose will definitely bloom within 32 days.
    C. A noisette will take more than 28 days to bloom.
    D. Belinda's Dream will most likely take over 100 days to bloom.

36. The majority of roses sold in stores are:
    A. Have between 5 and 12 petals.
    B. Last for 10-14 days.
    C. Are repeat bloomers.
    D. Will rebloom in 28-32 days.

Passage 10

Candles have been used as a source of light and to illuminate celebrations for more than 5,000 years, yet little is known about their origin. The earliest use of candles is often attributed to the Ancient Egyptians, who made rushlights or torches by soaking the pithy core of reeds in melted animal fat. However, the rushlights had no wick like a true candle. While the Egyptians were using wicked candles in 3,000 B.C., the ancient Romans are generally credited with developing the wicked candle before that time by dipping rolled papyrus repeatedly in melted tallow or beeswax. The resulting candles were used to light their homes, to aid travelers at night, and in religious ceremonies. Historians have found evidence that many other early civilizations developed wicked candles using waxes made from available plants and insects. Early Chinese candles are said to have been molded in paper tubes, using rolled rice paper for the wick, and wax from an indigenous insect that was combined with seeds. In Japan, candles were made of wax extracted from tree nuts, while in India, candle wax was made by boiling the fruit of the cinnamon tree. It is also known that candles played an important role in early religious ceremonies. Hanukkah, the Jewish Festival of Lights which centers on the lighting of candles, dates back to 165 B.C. There are several Biblical references to candles, and the Emperor Constantine is reported to have called for the use of candles during an Easter service in the 4th century.
Source: https://candles.org/history/

37. Which of the following can be inferred from the passage?
    A. From the first noted use of candles, to the first noted use of wicked candles by the same population, there is a gap of 2000 years.
    B. The Ancient Egyptians were the first civilisation to use wicked candles.
    C. Many different populations of people around the world have been using candles for thousands of years.
    D. Constantine was the first emperor to use candles in his ceremonies.

38. Which of the following statements is correct?
   A. Candles were made from cinnamon trees in Japan.
   B. Candles were made from insect wax in China.
   C. Candle wicks were made from reeds in Ancient Egypt.
   D. Candle wicks were made from tree nuts in India.

39. What best describes the usage of candles mentioned by the passage between the years 300 and 399?
   A. Easter
   B. Hannukah
   C. Illuminating celebrations
   D. Religious ceremonies

40. Which of the following is not mentioned by the passage as a use of wicked candles by the ancient Romans?
   A. To celebrate Easter
   B. Providing light inside their houses
   C. For use by travellers on their night journeys
   D. To celebrate certain religious ceremonies

Passage 11

Malaysia does not have a good record in traffic law enforcement. According to the WHO, the enforcement of laws in Malaysia related to speed limits, drink-driving, motorcycle helmets and seat belts was ranked between 4 to 5 in a range of 0 to 10. Singapore's enforcement was ranked between 7 to 9. Strict traffic law enforcement is partly responsible for the low traffic fatalities in Singapore where there are only 4 deaths per 100,000 population. Malaysia has about 24 deaths per 100,000 population.
In 2013 Singapore saw an annual 10.6 percent decrease in the number of fatal and injury accidents on their roads. Meanwhile in 2012 Malaysia had an annual 2.98 percent increase in the number of road accidents. The Perception of Being Caught (POBC) rate among Malaysian road users is low, at a 25 percent rate on regular days and a 50 percent rate during the festive seasons. In developed countries, the POBC rate is between 80-90 percent. We have to raise the POBC rate to a high level to instil discipline among Malaysian drivers and to do this we have to drastically improve our culture of enforcement among our authorities and reduce the culture of lawlessness among our drivers. Our enforcement of traffic laws has been lackadaisical, inefficient, corrupt and seasonal, leading to motorists not fearing the laws and breaking them at will.

Motorists simply do not fear being caught as traffic summonses are often not paid, can be negotiated or cancelled through corruption and even discounts can be officially given.
Source: https://www.malaysiakini.com/letters/269749

41. Which of the following can be inferred from the passage?
    A. Lenient traffic law enforcement can contribute to higher rates of traffic fatalities.
    B. Vehicle-related deaths are caused by poor enforcement of traffic laws.
    C. Malaysia may have more deaths due to a larger population than Singapore.
    D. There is poor law enforcement in Malaysia.

42. Which of the following would best confirm POBC as being a cause of breaking traffic laws?
    A. There are more car accidents as the drivers do not fear being caught breaking traffic laws.
    B. Drivers that abide by traffic laws in a different country choose not to abide by traffic laws in Malaysia due to its reputation of lenient law enforcement.
    C. When motorists are caught speeding, they will carry on speeding in the future as they do not think they will get caught again.
    D. Drivers from Malaysia do not follow the traffic laws in other countries either.

43. Which of the following can be inferred as a reason for the greater POBC during festive seasons?
    A. There is greater law enforcement.
    B. People are less likely to be on the roads.
    C. People are more willing to follow the laws.
    D. There is a greater influence from Singapore's law enforcement forces.

44. Which of the following would best reduce the number of road traffic accidents in Malaysia?
    A. Improved vehicle safety
    B. Enforced hefty fines
    C. Increased police force
    D. Prohibition of healthcare to those responsible for collisions

Decision Making Questions

Question 1

Figure 1: The number of cancer registrations by the 24 major sites, Persons, England, 2015

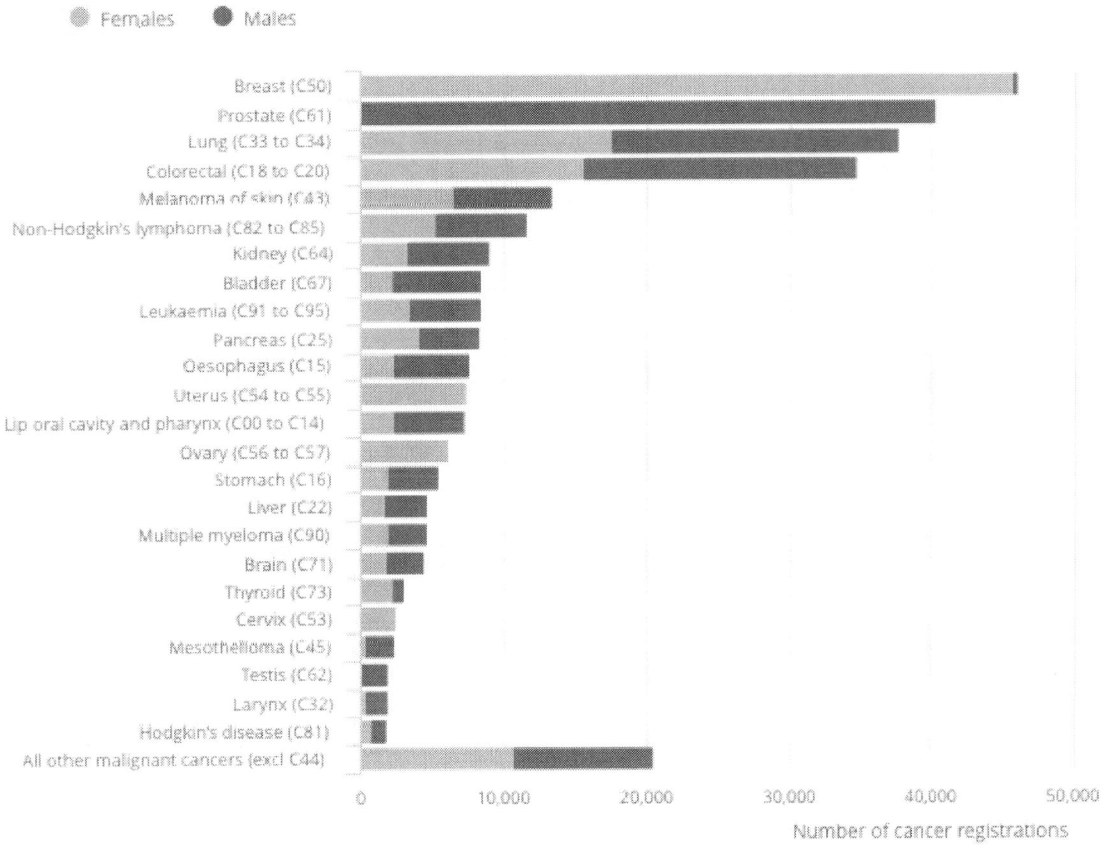

Source: Office for National Statistics

Place "Yes" if the conclusion does follow. Place "No" if the conclusion does not follow.

1. From all cancers, breast cancer is the biggest killer in the UK for females. YES/NO
2. Any of the above types of cancer are non-contagious. YES/NO
3. At least 10,000 people were diagnosed with melanoma of the skin. YES/NO
4. Prostate cancer was the most commonly diagnosed cancer in males. YES/NO
5. Amongst men and women, colorectal cancer was the 3rd most commonly diagnosed cancer. YES/NO

Question 2

Consider the following statements to be true: “Some smart people are athletic”, “All artistic people are smart”, “No athletic people are artistic”, “All musicians are athletic”, “Some musicians are smart”.

Which of the following diagrams represents the information given?

A.

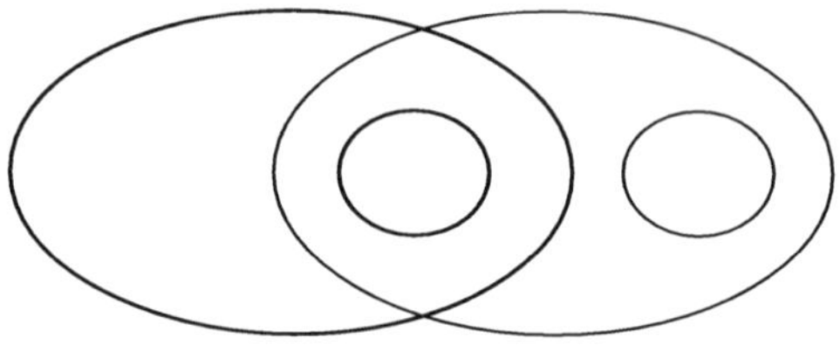

B.

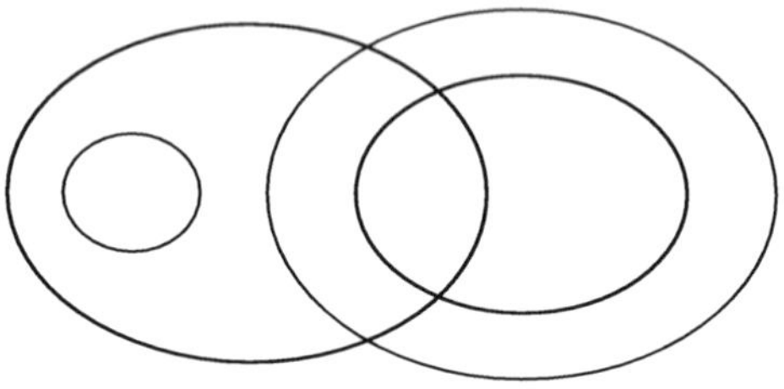

C.

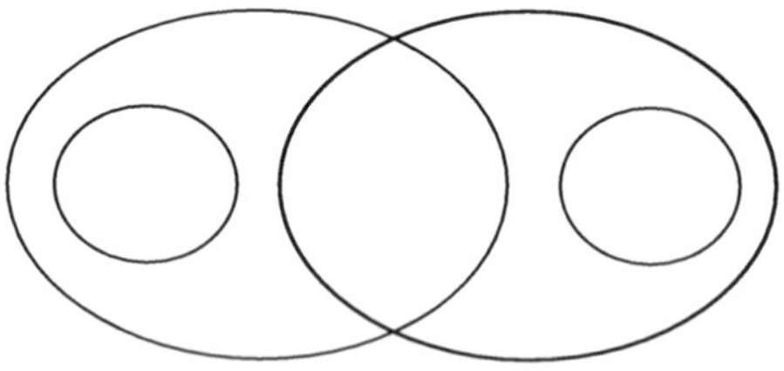

D.

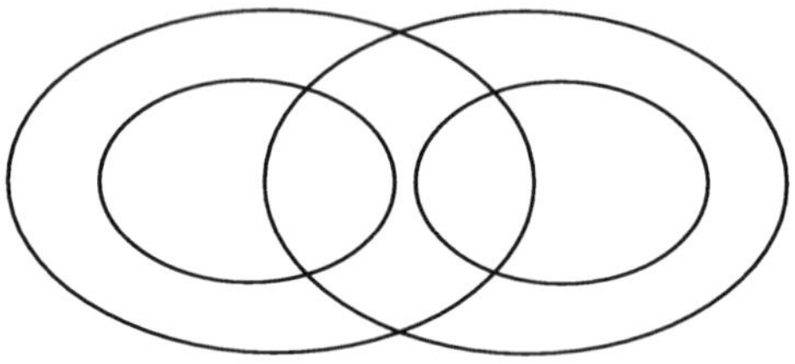

Question 3

David has recently moved apartments and needs a new TV for his living room. There are 3 sizes available in store; pequena, mediana and grande. Each size differs only in length. When 3 pesquena, 6 mediana & 4 grande are lined up together, the total length is 231 inches.

Pequena are 2 inches shorter than mediana TVs. When 2 pequena and 1 grande are lined up, the length is 51 inches. The difference between pequena and mediana TV sizes is half the difference between mediana and grande.

What is the length of grande in inches?

A. 15
B. 17
C. 21
D. 29

Question 4

All bees are insects. No insects crawl. If an insect has wings it must be a bee.

Place "Yes" if the conclusion does follow. Place "No" if the conclusion does not follow.

1. If a bee has yellow and black stripes, it is an insect. YES/NO
2. No insects without wings are bees. YES/NO
3. Some winged insects crawl. YES/NO
4. Bees crawl or do not have wings. YES/NO
5. An insect is a bee or it does not have wings YES/NO

Question 5

Should all children be given tablets in schools in order to maintain interactivity and interest?

Select the strongest argument from the statements below.

A. Yes, because children are more likely to achieve higher grades if they are given ipads for learning.
B. Yes, because studies show that tablet devices increase a child's attention span and keep them engaged.
C. No, because a lack of tablets is not the reason why children are uninterested in schools.
D. No, because tablets should only be given tablets if they attain a high grade.

Question 6

The average height of a male in the United Kingdom is 170cm.
The average height of a female in the United Kingdom is 140cm.

The average height of a male and female in Canada is 10% more than the UK averages. Jaspreet and Harvin are from Canada and have a combined height of 336cm. Harvin's height is double that of Jaspreets.

Which of the following statements must be true?

A. Jaspreet has a height above average for Canada.
B. Harvin is 170cm tall.
C. Jaspreet and Harvin are both above the average height values for the UK.
D. Harvin is above the Canadian average.

Question 7

A shopkeeper in the Isle of Man sells mangoes, strawberries, baskets & apples in his grocery store. Some mangoes are yellow. Some strawberries are also yellow. All baskets are strawberries. All the other items are red.

Place "Yes" if the conclusion does follow. Place "No" if the conclusion does not follow.

A.	Some apples are red.	YES/NO
B.	Strawberries are either red or yellow.	YES/NO
C.	Some baskets are mangoes.	YES/NO
D.	No mangoes are baskets.	YES/NO
E.	All baskets are yellow.	YES/NO

Question 8

Should voting in the general election be made compulsory for citizens of France in order to increase the number of voters?

Select the strongest argument from the statements below.

A. Yes, because research suggests people who should vote do not due to lack of public transport.
B. Yes, because we have the choice to do what we want and the government should not force things on us.
C. No, because research shows that there was no increase in voters from 2014 to 2015 when Pakistan made it compulsory to vote.
D. No, because the whole point of a democracy is to give a choice to people and here you are going against that.

Question 9

There are 6 people standing in a queue to buy their lunch; Huzefa, Demetrius, Billy, Jared, Fabrice & Sky. There is only 1 person ahead of Demetrius. Only Billy is standing behind Jared. Fabrice is 3 places ahead of Billy. Sky is 2 places behind Demetrius.

Which of the following statements is true?

A. Sky is last in line behind Fabrice.
B. Huzefa is 2 places ahead of Fabrice.
C. Jared is 4th in line.
D. Demetrius is 3 places ahead of Billy.

Question 10

Consider the following statements to be true: "All apples are fruits", "All fruit is food", "No apples taste good", "Some fruits taste good", "Something must be food to taste good".

Which of the following diagrams represents the information given?

A)

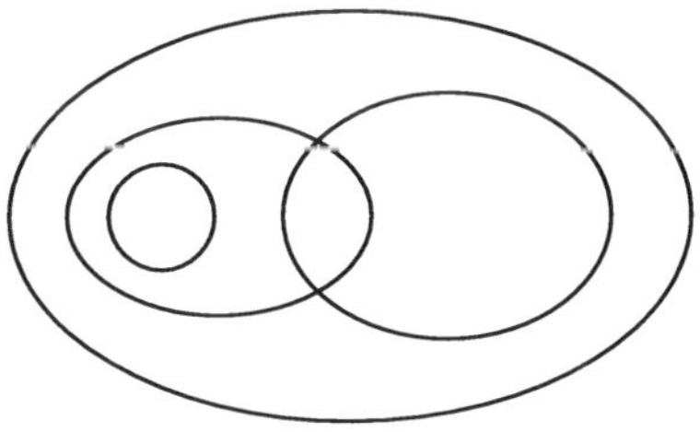

B)

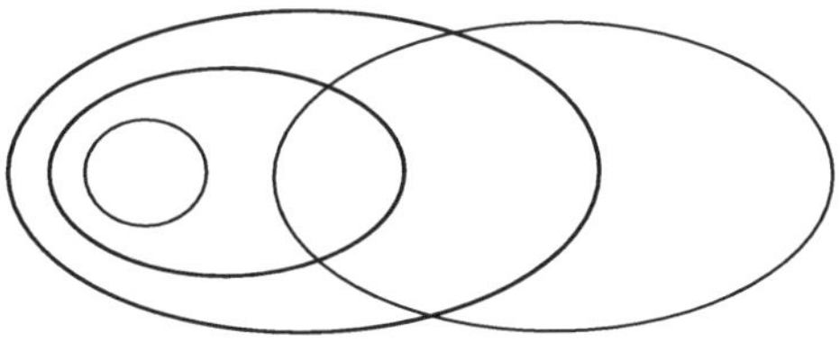

C)

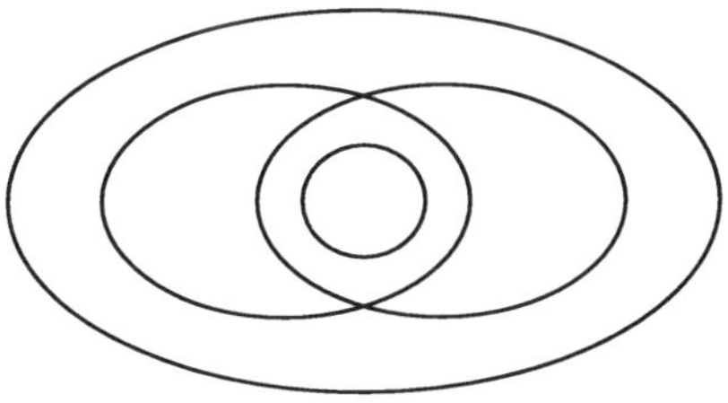

D)

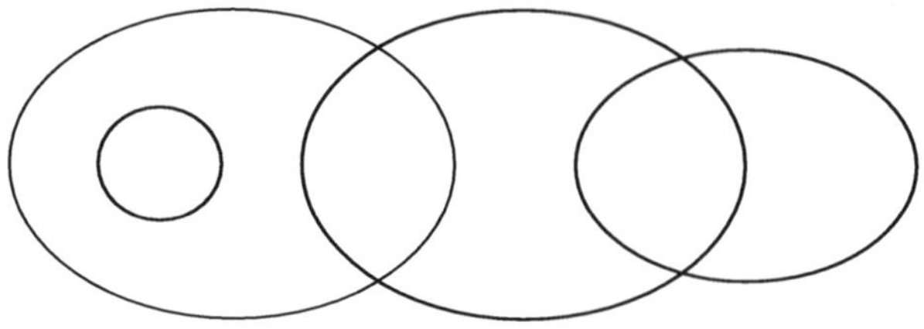

Question 11

Should the U.K government help tackle obesity by giving bicycle grants to citizens with a body mass index (BMI) of 28+?

Select the strongest argument from the statements below.

A. Yes, because this will help people purchase bicycles who otherwise could not afford to pay for them.
B. Yes, because this was done in Italy in 2015 and an analysis of the changes showed that more people with obesity were able to exercise.
C. No, because people with a BMI of 28+ are unlikely to exercise.
D. No, because there has been no correlation found between weight and cycling.

Question 12

Armani and Dora both have playing cards. None of Armani's playing cards are black. Some of Dora's playing cards are blue but none of them are shiny.

Place "Yes" if the conclusion does follow. Place "No" if the conclusion does not follow.

A. All of Dora's playing cards are blue.	YES/NO
B. Neither Armani nor Dora has black playing cards.	YES/NO
C. Neither Armani nor Dora has black playing cards which are shiny.	YES/NO
D. Armani and Dora both have some blue playing cards.	YES/NO
E. Blue playing cards can never be shiny.	YES/NO

Question 13

22 boys and 7 girls are asked to select what sports they play during a survey. 7 people said they play tennis and 5 people said they play football. Hockey is played by 11 people and only 4 people play cricket. 2 people did not play any sports. We also are told that, 2 people play tennis and football, 1 person plays hockey and football, and 3 people play tennis and cricket.

Select the most accurate representation from the choices below.

A.

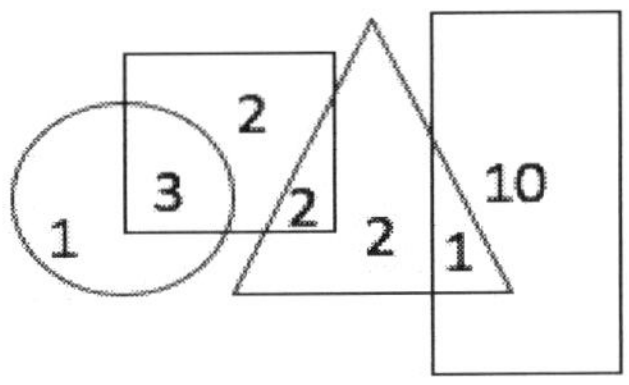

C.

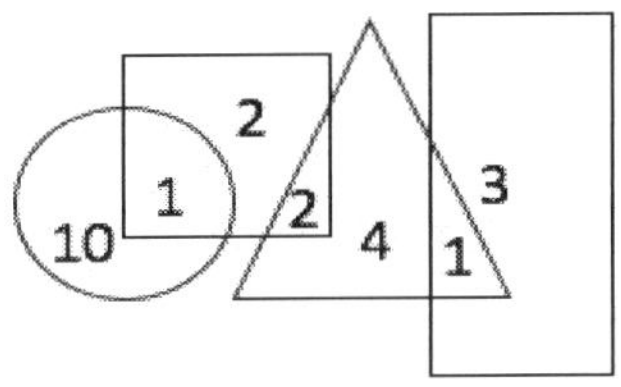

B.

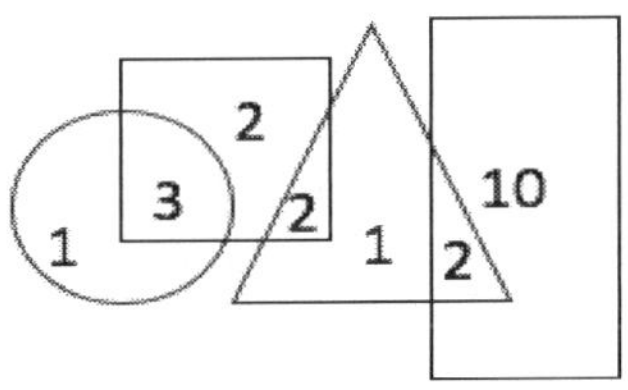

D.

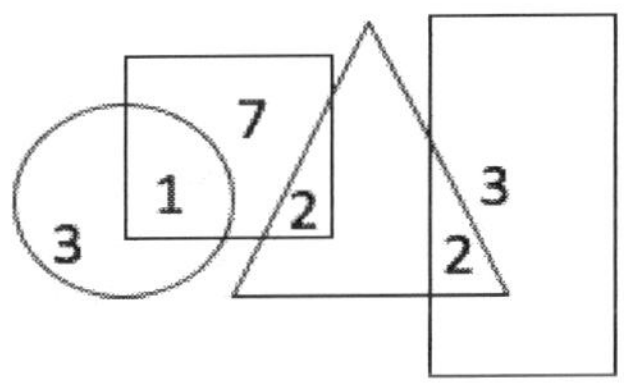

Question 14

The diagram below represents the number of students taking various modules during their 2nd year in university:

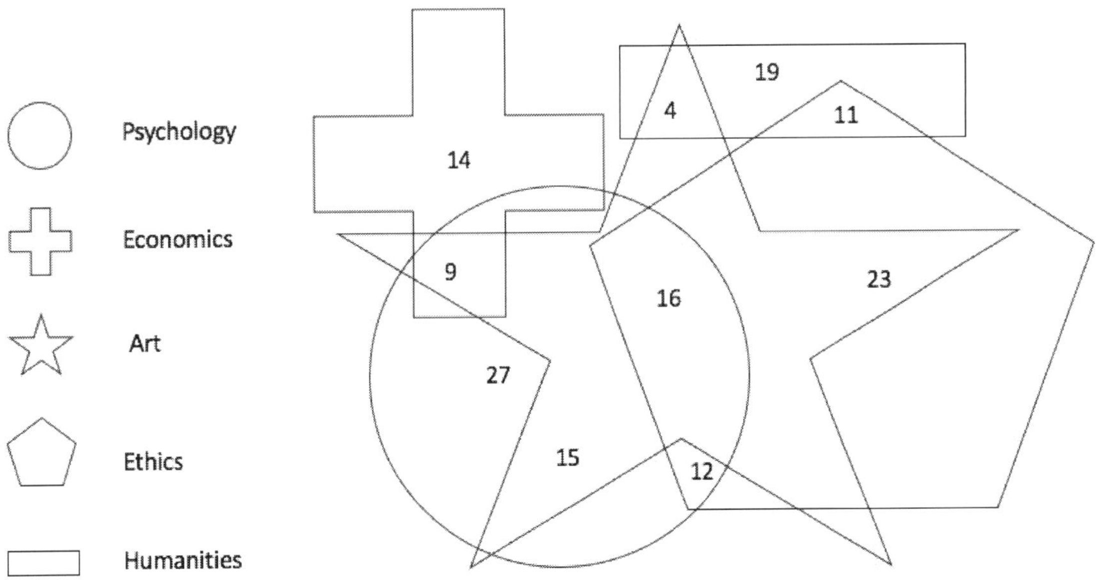

In a particular year, the university announces that all students who study 3 or more modules in year 2 will receive an additional grant. How many students will receive this grant?

A. 25
B. 60
C. 9
D. 37

Question 15

The graph shows information about COVID-19 testing during some months in 2020.

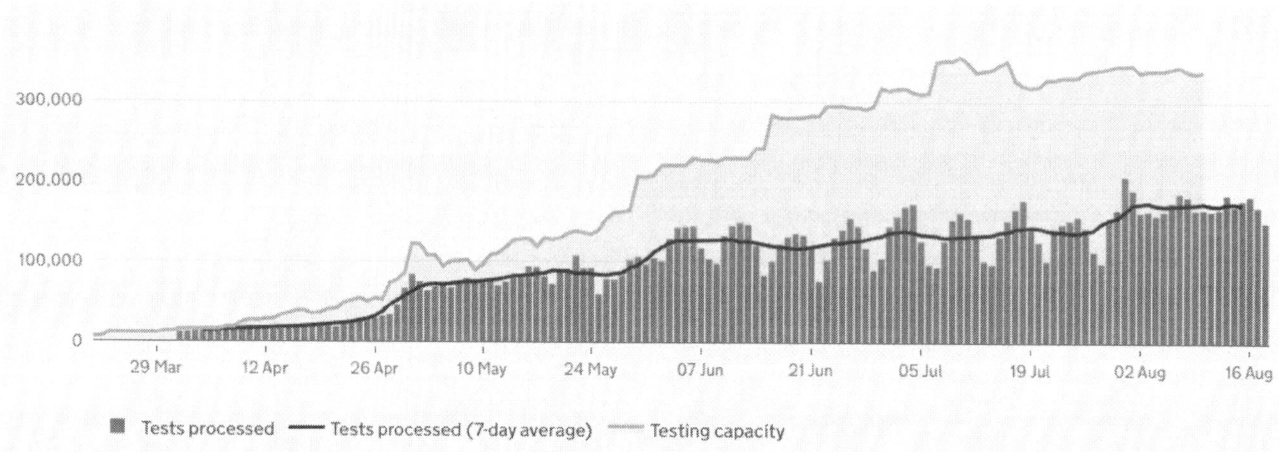

Source: https://coronavirus.data.gov.uk/testing

Place "Yes" if the conclusion does follow. Place "No" if the conclusion does not follow.

A. There were cases of COVID-19 prior to 29th March 2020. YES/NO
B. In April, May, June and July of 2020, there was always a larger testing capacity than tests processed. YES/NO
C. In the data above, the final day of July had the most tests processed. YES/NO
D. The number of tests is directly proportionate to the number of infections. YES/NO
E. The first COVID-19 case diagnosed in the UK was on 29th March 2020. YES/NO

Question 16

There are 85 boys in year 7 at Pep's school. 5 do not participate in any after school sports club. 27 go to badminton club, while 12 play rugby. 8 go to running club, while 42 play soccer. 4 play soccer and tennis. 22 play tennis in total, and 5 play both badminton and tennis.

A.

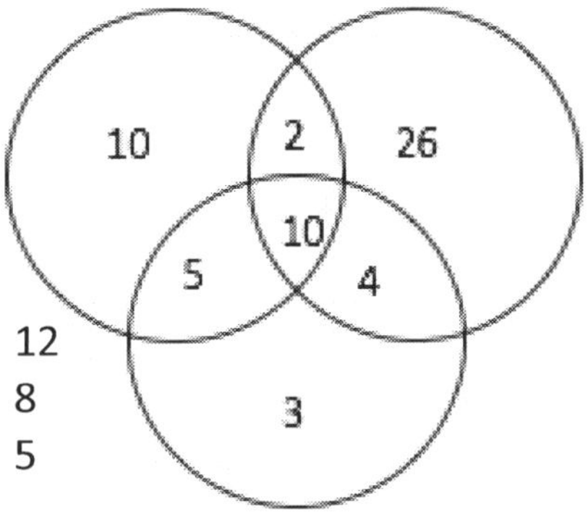

B.

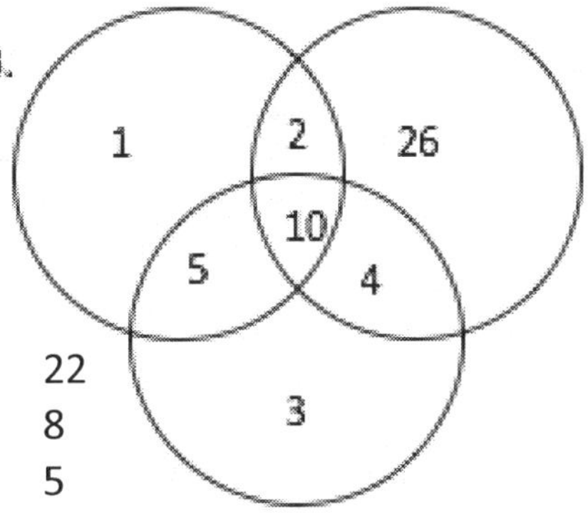

C.

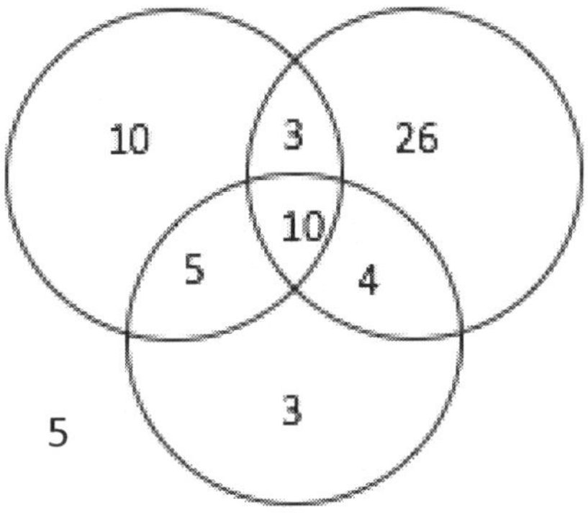

D.

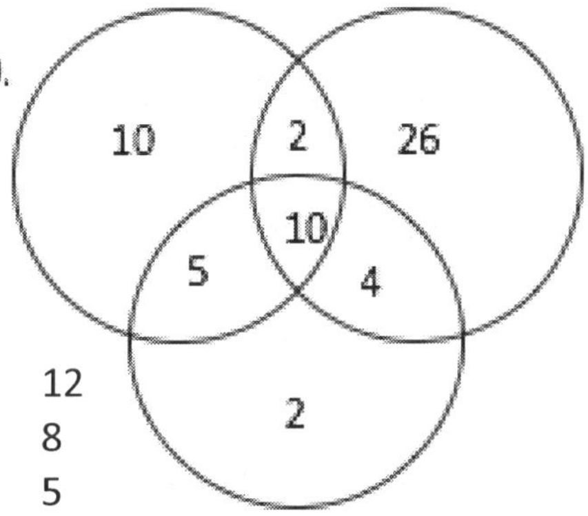

Question 17

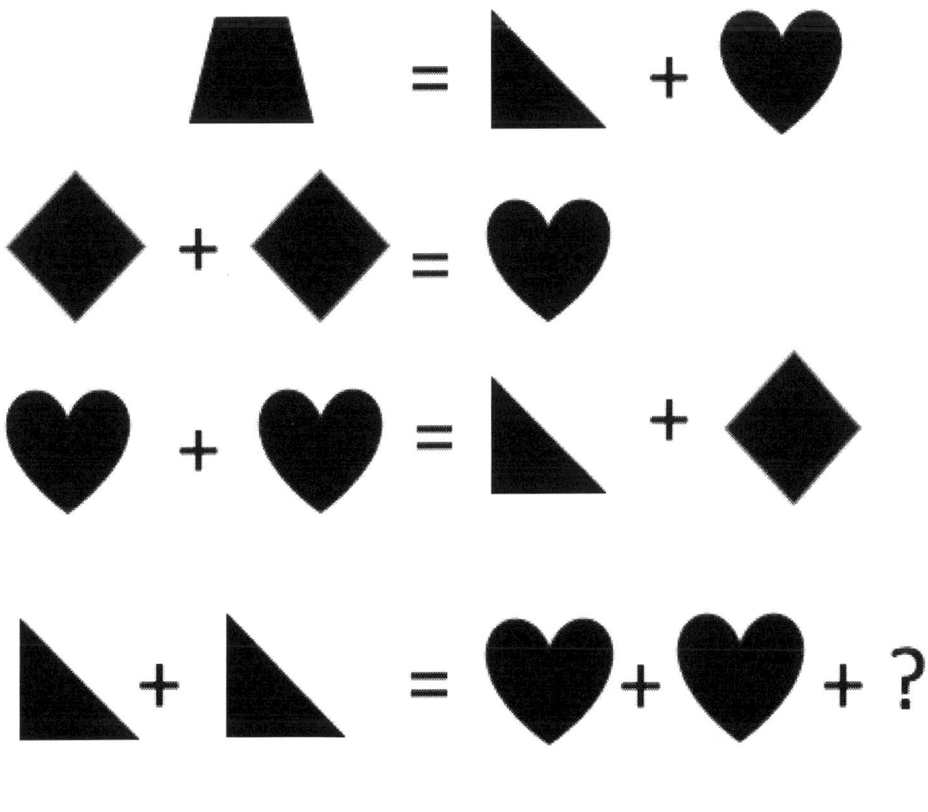

Which of the following makes the last equation true?

A. Heart
B. Diamond
C. Trapezium
D. Triangle

Question 18

Should the government make it compulsory for all students to study History at A-level to ensure they are aware of Britain's colonial past?

Select the strongest argument from the statements below.

A. Yes, as this will boost their chances of progressing to university.
B. Yes, because its important that students realise the importance of History.
C. No, because studying History at A-level does not necessarily mean the students will be exposed to the correct narrative of Britain's history.
D. No, as everyone should have be able to make their own decisions of what they want to study.

Question 19

Should certain drugs like marijuana be legalised to reduce drug crime in the United Kingdom?

Select the strongest argument from the statements below.

A. Yes, because this may reduce the number of citizens arrested for crime every year.
B. Yes, because the greatest marijuana-related crime is for possession, so legalising marijuana will reduce crime rates.
C. No, because marijuana-related crime is scarce, so this will likely not have a large impact on crime rates.
D. No, because studies have shown that marijuana is not as addictive as other drugs, so there should be a bigger emphasis placed on reducing crime related to other drugs.

Question 20

COVID infection rates are recorded for various cities in Yorkshire. Results show a 27% rise in infection rates during September in Leeds. Leeds has 3 universities all of which open during September and 10% of students returning from overseas have tested positive for COVID.

Which of the following statements can be concluded from the passage?

A. The increased infection rates are mainly due to the return of students to universities.
B. Leeds should go on a local lockdown immediately to prevent further spread.
C. Students returning to university in Leeds are a contributory factor in the increased infection rates.
D. Students poor hygiene is to blame for the increased infection rates.

Question 21

Costi, Stari, Nervo & Boti visit the park during their lunch time break. They all decide to purchase some ice cream from the park shop. They buy 1 ice cream each costing; £1.15, £1.43, £1.12, £1.55 in no particular order. The names of the ice creams are; Melon on ice, Rosewater, Blue freeze and Rockstar in no particular order.

Stari purchased a Blue Freeze

The prices of Blue Freeze and Melon on Ice have the same first and last digits

Nervo purchased a Rosewater or Rockstar

The Rockstar was the cheapest

Costi purchased the more expensive of the the following; Blue Freeze and Melon on ice.

What was the cost of Boti's ice cream?

A. £1.21
B. £1.43
C. £1.15
D. £1.55

Question 22

A survey is performed to identify how many patients use a blue inhaler, brown inhaler & pink inhaler. 45 patients used the pink inhaler, 19 used the brown inhaler and only 8 used a blue inhaler. 8 use a pink and brown inhaler while 2 use a blue and brown inhaler. No patients used a pink and blue inhaler. There were 110 participants in the survey.

What is the probability that a patient picked at random from the survey used a brown inhaler only?

A. 37/110
B. 8/110
C. 6/110
D. 9/110

Question 23

A businesswoman is selling some new furniture products in her store: chairs, tables, cupboards & rugs. She has a total of 25 new furniture products.

Some of the new furniture products are made from wood. None of the rugs are made from wood. There are 2 more chairs than cupboards & there are an equal number of tables and chairs. Only chairs and tables are made from wood. There are 3 rugs.

Place "Yes" if the conclusion does follow. Place "No" if the conclusion does not follow

A.	There are more rugs than cupboards.	YES/NO
B.	There are 4 wooden chairs.	YES/NO
C.	The total number of tables is 8.	YES/NO
D.	Some of the cupboards are wooden.	YES/NO
E.	All of the rugs are cotton.	YES/NO

Question 24

Ilyas has a biased coin. There is a 2 in 3 chance of it landing on heads. Ilyas tosses the coin 14 times and lands on heads each time.

"If Ilyas tosses the coin 1 more time, he will have the same chance of landing on tails as he did previously."

A. Yes, because there is no conditional probability.
B. Yes, because 2 in 3 is greater than 1 in 3.
C. No, because he hasn't yet once landed on tails.
D. No, because his coin is biased.

Question 25

Some phones have black cases and all black cases are shiny. Many grey cases are clear but none are shiny.

Place "Yes" if the conclusion does follow. Place "No" if the conclusion does not follow.

A. All shiny cases are black	YES/NO
B. No clear cases are black	YES/NO
C. Grey cases must not be shiny	YES/NO
D. Blue cases could be shiny.	YES/NO
E. Non-grey cases cannot be clear.	YES/NO

Question 26

Should university fees be reduced in order to attract more students from disadvantaged backgrounds?

Select the strongest argument from the statements below.

A. Yes, because fees may be the biggest factor in students not taking up places in universities.
B. Yes, because disadvantaged students cannot afford to study at the moment due to the tuition fee hike and are only able to study If successful in scholarship programmes.
C. No, because education does have a cost to it and people should work hard to have this privilege.
D. No, because disadvantaged students are better suited to non-university based courses.

Question 27

Aaqib, Mahdi, Habib, Mustafa, Amin and Sadiq visit a theme park together just before closing time. They only had enough time to go on one ride. The rides are either water, roller-coaster or skyscrapers in type and either small, medium or large in size.

Only one of them went on a large rollercoaster
Sadiq went on a large water ride
Habib did not go on a skyscraper
3 people in total went on a water ride
All skyscrapers are small

2 people had small sized rides only
Aaqib went on the exact same ride as Sadiq
Mahdi did not go on a rollercoaster or a skyscraper
Only Mustafa went on a medium sized ride
Only 1 person went on a skyscraper

Who went on a skyscraper?

A. Habib
B. Sadiq
C. Mahdi
D. Amin

Question 28

There are 12 fruits, 8 frozen foods and a number of drinks in a shopping trolley. ¼ of the fruits are apples, ½ of the fruits are bananas and the rest are strawberries. Some of the frozen foods are pizzas and half of the frozen foods are garlic bread. There are the same number of drinks as bananas and all the drinks are not fizzy.

Place "Yes" if the conclusion does follow. Place "No" if the conclusion does not follow.

A. There are more non fizzy drinks than fruits.	YES/NO
B. There are twice as many fruits as drinks.	YES/NO
C. There are 4 pizzas	YES/NO
D. There are more strawberries than fizzy drinks.	YES/NO
E. The shopping trolley can hold a maximum of 26 items.	YES/NO

Question 29

The diagram below shows the number of shoppers that purchased particular items from their local supermarket:

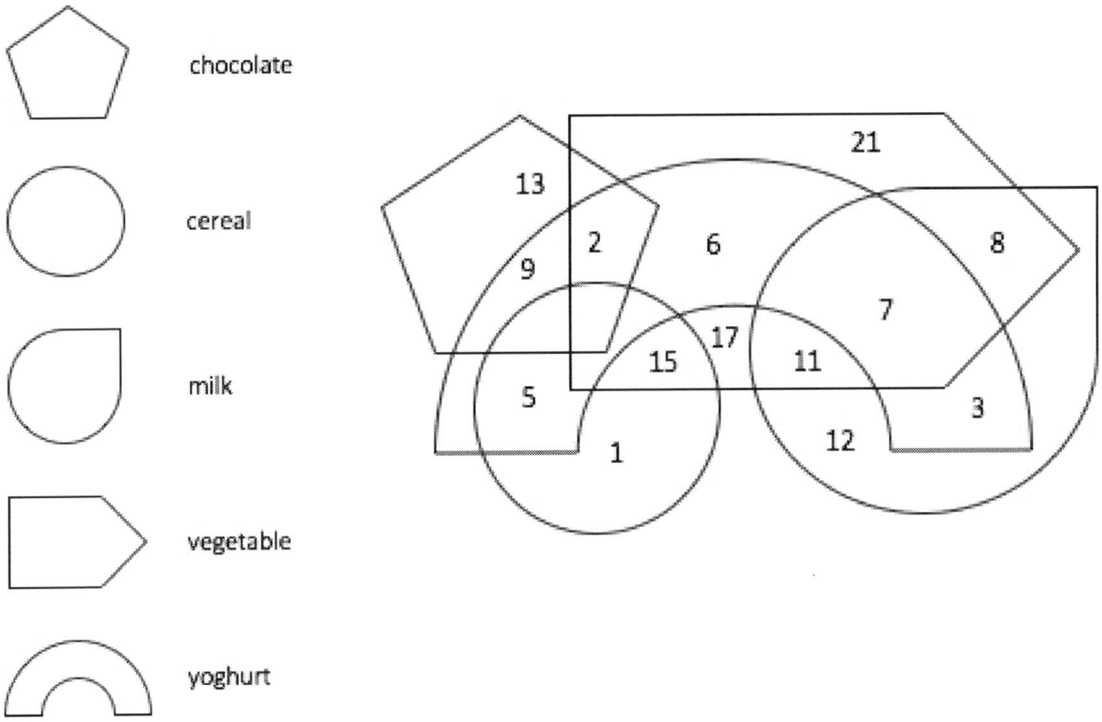

How many shoppers purchased exactly 2 items?

A. 29
B. 32
C. 48
D. 57
E. 10

Quantitative Reasoning Questions

Scenario 1

The following table shows the exchange rate for £1 (GBP) to Euro (EUR), Canadian dollar (CAD), American dollar (USD), Kuwait Dinar (KWD), Pakistan Rupee (PKR) and Hong Kong dollar (HKD).

GBP	Exchange
1.00	1.11 EUR
1.00	1.75 CAD
1.00	1.31 USD
1.00	0.40 KWD
1.00	217.98 PKR
1.00	10.12 HKD

1. Tyson wants to book a surprise holiday to Kuwait for his wife Judith's 60th birthday. The cost of the plane ticket is £436 per person unless it is a child ticket which costs £212. Tyson and Judith have 3 children; Andy 16, Ian 14 & Martin 6. Anyone under the age of 12 is considered a child.

   If Tyson decides to book the plane tickets for his full family, how much will he pay to the nearest Kuwaiti Dinar (KWD)?

   A. 603 KWD
   B. 782 KWD
   C. 1945 KWD
   D. 4100 KWD
   E. 842 KWD

2. Jamal is booking a flight to Canada using his 50% discount coupon for all flights with Qatar Airways. He is also eligible for a further 15% NHS discount. If the total cost of the ticket is 1,650 CAD, how much will he save to the nearest GBP after the discounts are applied?

   A. 401 GBP
   B. 542 GBP
   C. 701 GBP
   D. 948 GBP
   E. 445 GBP

3. 15 friends decide to travel to Hong Kong to watch the Asia Cup Final. Their hotel costs 42 HKD plus a 2.5% service fee each per night. They purchase 15 Cup final tickets which cost 2900 HKD in total. They paid 455 EUR each for their flights and spent an additional 100HKD per day each. If they stayed for 6 days and 6 nights, how much did they pay each in pounds?
   A. £464.41
   B. £513.82
   C. £482.93
   D. £384.55
   E. £762.95

4. Lola has 1,310 USD in her account. She spends all of this during her holiday in New York. How much did she spend in Euros (EUR)?
   A. 1000 EUR
   B. 1400 EUR
   C. 1110 EUR
   D. 1220 EUR
   E. 1320 EUR

Scenario 2

	Hair	Beard	Wax	Facial	Scalp Massage
2016	5,645	2,981	1,022	3,657	0
2017	4,316	1,054	2,792	1,790	0
2018	5,750	5,634	1,313	3,778	1,294
2019	5,249	2,088	3,182	3,118	0
2020	5,309	5,713	1,899	2,626	544

The table shows the number of different services a barbershop was booked for over a 5-year period.

5. What was the most popular service in 2020?
   A. Hair
   B. Beard
   C. Wax
   D. Facial
   E. Scalp massage

6. By what percentage did hair bookings fall between 2016 and 2017?

A. 23.5%
B. 76.5%
C. 28.6%
D. 30.8%
E. 63.2%

7. In 2019, what percentage of bookings were for beard?
   A. 15%
   B. 38%
   C. 23%
   D. 42%
   E. 18%

8. The barbershop opened in 2015 and the total number of bookings in its first year was 6,763. What was the percentage increase in bookings between 2015 and 2016?
   A. 92.4%
   B. 96.7%
   C. 196.7%
   D. 192.4%
   E. 78.6%

Scenario 3

The diagram below shows a floor plan of the first floor of Yaqoob's new house. Both the living room and front room are square-shaped and identical in dimension.

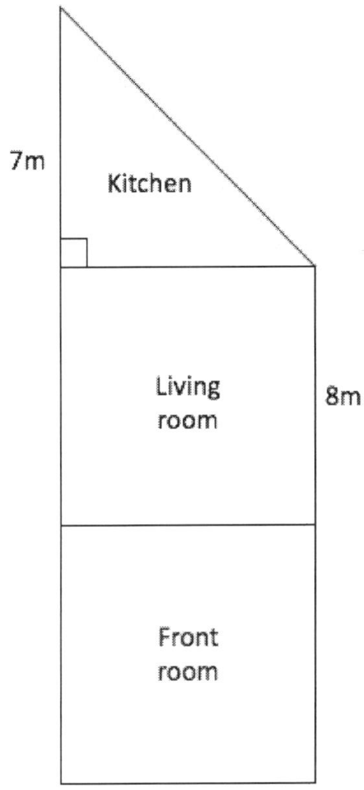

9. Yaqoob's wife Noor wants to put tiles in the living room and kitchen. The living room is square-shaped. Each tile is $0.5m^2$ and costs £2.30. How much will it cost to put tiles in the kitchen and living room.
   A. £184.00
   B. £211.60
   C. £386.40
   D. £423.20
   E. £288.70

10. Yaqoob now wants to extend his front room by 3m in length. By what percent will the front room be bigger than the living room?
    A. 28.4%
    B. 25%
    C. 37.5%
    D. 45%
    E. 27%

11. Noor would like to put new carpet in the extended front room. If the carpet comes in pieces that are 0.8m in length and 1.2m in width, how many pieces will she need to cover the extended front room's floor?
    A. 92
    B. 48

C. 88
D. 91
E. 102

12. Yaqoob's son Yusuf would like to store his boxes in the living room, which is a cube. The boxes have dimensions of 0.2m in height x 0.3m in length x 0.5m in width. How many boxes can he store if he covers half the space of the living room with boxes?
    A. 8534
    B. 8533
    C. 9042
    D. 17066
    E. 17067

Scenario 4

Annual Income	Tax percentage
£0 - £22,000	12%
£22,001 - £50,000	20%
£50,001 - £75,000	32%
£75,001 +	40%

13. Alfonso has recently started working in his local Post Office. He earns £12.50 per hour and works 8-hour shifts. If Alfonso works 5 days a week during each week of the year, how much tax will he pay per month?
    A. £286.67
    B. £433.33
    C. £788.90
    D. £5200.00
    E. £4639.80

14. The Post Office made £276,000 in 2019. Sergio is the owner of the Post Office and has two employees whose salaries he pays. Alfonso works during the week and Bella works over the weekend. If Bella works for 16 hours over the weekend and is paid 50p more than Alfonso per hour, how much tax will Sergio pay annually after removing his staff salary costs?
    A. £82,000.00
    B. £78,420.10

C. £92,257.60
D. £142,886.40
E. £81,913.60

15. Mr Kante owns the meat shop next door to the Post Office. Mr.Kante pays £1,250 tax every month. How much taxable income does he make every year?
    A. £6760
    B. £21125
    C. £15000
    D. £50000
    E. £71125

16. If Mr Kante's monthly income is increased by 7%, how much more tax must he pay every month?
    A. £165.96
    B. £140.13
    C. £1103.75
    D. £441.50
    E. £1390.13

Scenario 5

Karam, Nav & Abraham are 3 friends who have recently started their studies at different universities in Canada. Karam studies in Calgary which is 299km from Edmonton, where Nav studies. Abraham studies in Saskatoon which is 521km from Edmonton.

1mile= 1.6km

17. Nav decides to travel to Saskatoon over the winter holidays. He drives for 3 hours before taking a 30-minute rest to get some food. He then continues his journey and drives for a further 180 minutes before he reaches his destination. What was his average speed during this trip in miles per hour?
    A. 54.3 miles/hour
    B. 80.2 miles/hour
    C. 86.8 miles/hour
    D. 50.1 miles/hour
    E. 75.4 miles/hour

18. Karam travels from Calgary to Saskatoon via train at a speed of 120 miles per hour. If he had travelled on car, it would have taken him 6 hours and 20 minutes. By

travelling on train he saves 32 minutes of travel time. What is the distance between Calgary and Saskatoon?

A. 696 miles
B. 488 miles
C. 600 miles
D. 658 miles
E. 566 miles

19. Lucinda lives in Toronto and wants to catch a flight to Calgary. The time zone in Toronto is 3 hours ahead of Calgary. If Lucinda's flight is scheduled to take off at 2.30 PM Toronto time and lasts for 5 hours, what will the local time be when she arrives in Calgary?

A. 10:30 PM
B. 7:30 PM
C. 3:30 PM
D. 8:30 PM
E. 4:30 PM

20. After arriving in Calgary, Lucinda travels to Edmonton. She then travels to Saskatoon to visit Abraham. She catches a return flight from Saskatoon to Toronto. If the distance travelled by air on the return flight is 6,442 miles, how many kilometres did she travel after landing in Calgary, to the nearest whole number?

A. 6442
B. 4846
C. 11127
D. 7824
E. 5250

Scenario 6

Olive works for a bakery in the town centre. She is contracted to bake chocolate cakes and strawberry tarts. She works 10 hour shifts on Mondays, Wednesdays & on the weekends. She is paid £7.65 an hour on weekdays and £8.65 an hour on the weekends. Her pay is doubled if she works on bank holidays.

21. Olive worked her usual shifts over 4 weeks, including 2 bank holiday Monday shifts. How much did she earn in total?

A. £1304
B. £1111
C. £1457
D. £1532

E. £1409

22. Olive has recently passed her driving test and is looking to purchase her dream car. The car will cost her £99,999 but she is eligible for a 10% discount. Not considering any bank holiday shifts, what is the minimum amount Olive must save every month from her salary in order to have enough money to purchase her dream car within 10 years?
    A. £833.33
    B. £676.70
    C. £412.52
    D. £748.40
    E. £749.99

23. During a normal hour of her work shift, Olive bakes 4 chocolate cakes and 8 strawberry tarts. How many chocolate cakes and strawberry tarts does she make every year during her contracted working hours?
    A. 24,000
    B. 12,480
    C. 24,960
    D. 13,960
    E. 25,000

24. There has been a change in management at the bakery and the new manager demands that staff produce 7% more bakery items each shift. How many more chocolate cakes is Olive now expected to bake every week, to the nearest whole number?
    A. 170
    B. 171
    C. 10
    D. 168
    E. 11

Scenario 7

The table shows the number of students studying particular healthcare courses at five different universities in the UK. Each course is at its maximum capacity this year.

	Medicine	Pharmacy	Dentistry	Radiography	Physiotherapy
University of Liverpool	72	16	27	44	9

University of Plymouth	59	43	37	19	5
University of Luton	125	56	89	21	40
University of Sutton	16	19	60	12	17
University of Newcastle	80	20	40	30	10

25. What is the mean number of students studying Medicine in the above universities, to the nearest whole number?
    A. 70
    B. 34
    C. 80
    D. 42
    E. 31

26. Which university has the highest total number of students studying the above healthcare courses?
    A. University of Liverpool
    B. University of Plymouth
    C. University of Luton
    D. University of Sutton
    E. University of Newcastle

27. The University of Sutton will increase all its course cohorts by 25% next year. How many fewer students will study radiography at Sutton than Luton next year?
    A. 11
    B. 9
    C. 6
    D. 7
    E. 3

28. Which university has the median number of students studying Dentistry from the list table above?
    A. University of Liverpool
    B. University of Plymouth
    C. University of Luton
    D. University of Sutton
    E. University of Newcastle

Scenario 8

The following table shows the local times of some cities around the world when it is 9 AM in London.

Medina	11 AM
Buenos Aires	5 AM
Tokyo	5 PM
Dakar	8 AM
Istanbul	11 AM
Montreal	4 AM
Wellington	8 PM
Islamabad	1 PM

29. The Champions League final is set to kick off at 7.30 PM on Saturday in London and will last 3 hours. What time will it finish in Wellington?
    A. 11:30 PM on Saturday
    B. 9:30 AM on Saturday
    C. 9:30 PM on Sunday
    D. 9:30 AM on Sunday
    E. 11:30 AM on Sunday

30. Cameron begins writing a text message at 10 PM on Friday in Dakar to send to his friend Abigail. If Cameron takes 30 minutes to write the email before sending, and Abigail opens it 1 hour after it reaches her inbox, when will Abigail read the email if she is living in Tokyo?
    A. 8:30 AM on Saturday
    B. 11:30 PM on Friday
    C. 2:30 PM on Saturday
    D. 10:30 PM on Saturday
    E. 8:00 AM on Saturday

31. Zaid who lives in Islamabad enjoys speaking to his family over video call every evening. His sister lives in Medina while his brother Talha is in Buenos Aires. On Friday the call lasted 1.5 hours and Zaid ended the call at 12 PM local time. If everyone joined the call together, when did Talha join the call?
    A. 8:30 AM
    B. 2:30 AM
    C. 6:30 PM
    D. 7:30 AM
    E. 4:30 AM

32. 3 friends decided to travel from Tokyo to Montreal. They had a layover in Islamabad which lasted 3 hours. If the plane set off on Monday at 6 PM from Tokyo and the journey took 8 hours to Islamabad and 14 hours to Montreal, what time did they land in Montreal on the following day?
   A. 5:00 PM
   B. 5:00 AM
   C. 7:00 PM
   D. 6:00 PM
   E. 6:00 AM

Scenario 9

Westbrook is a small town in the south of England and it has 4 main gyms. Some gyms have a one-off joining fee. The table shows the price plans for all 4 gyms. Only Runners and Gymnastics have swimming pools.

	Muscle House	Gymnastics	All-time Fitness	Runners
Joining fee	-	£14.99	£7.99	-
Daily pass	£3	£5	£4.75	£10
Weekly pass	£20	£25	£25	£40
Monthly pass	£24.99	£29.99	£25.99	£59.99
3-month pass	£40	£35	£39.99	£99.99
1-year pass	£100	£95	£100	£200
2-year pass	£150	£180	£190	£350

33. Kieta would like to join a gym which has a swimming pool. What percent would he save if he chose to sign up for a 1-year pass at Gymnastics compared to Runners?
   A. 33%
   B. 25%
   C. 12.5%
   D. 40%
   E. 45%

34. If the gym passes for Runners and Gymnastics have 25% off any of their memberships, while Muscle House and All-time fitness have 20% off, which gym is the cheapest for Jonas to join for a 3-month membership?
   A. Muscle House

B. Gymnastics
C. All-time Fitness
D. Muscle House and All-time Fitness would be the same
E. Runners

35. Muscle House made £150,000 more than Gymnastics in 2020. Gymnastics made a loss of 18% compared to its 2019 income. If Gymnastics earned £89,000 in 2019, how much did Muscle House make in 2020?
    A. £72,980
    B. £222,980
    C. £166,020
    D. £172,980
    E. £264,120

36. All of the gyms decide to start a lifetime membership deal. Muscle House decides it will give lifetime membership to anyone who signs up for at least 10 years. Gymnastics will give lifetime membership to anyone who purchases 7 yearly passes. At All-time Fitness, a lifetime membership is given to anyone that purchases 20 3-month passes. Finally, Runners will give a lifetime membership to anyone who purchases 5 yearly passes. What is the cheapest lifestyle membership?
    A. Muscle House and All-time Fitness
    B. All-time Fitness
    C. Runners
    D. Gymnastics and Muscle House
    E. Gymnastics

Abstract Reasoning Questions

Question 1

Set A

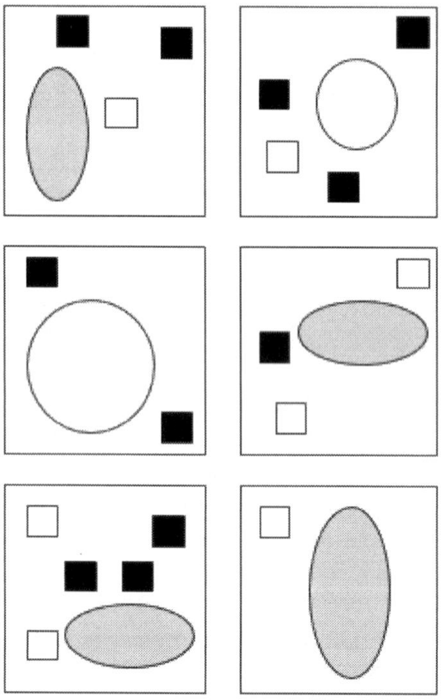

Set B

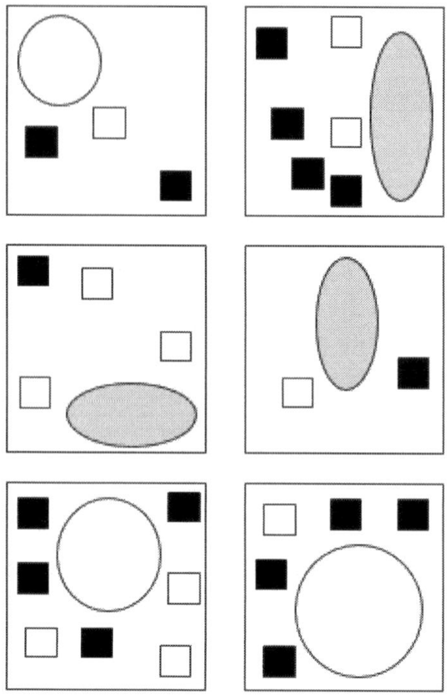

Determine whether the test shapes belong to Set A, Set B or neither.

Test shape 1	Test shape 2	Test shape 3	Test shape 4	Test shape 5

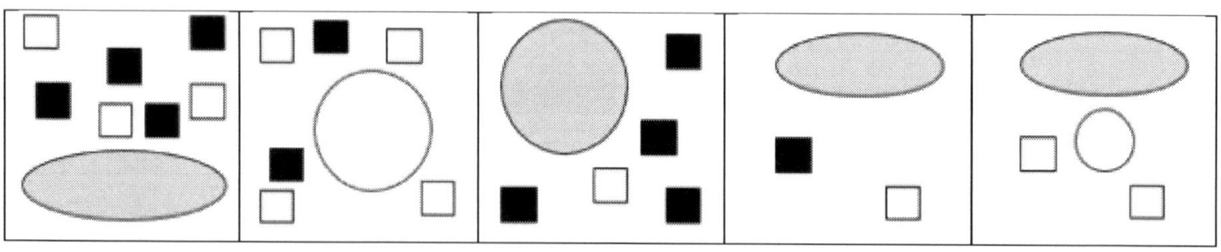

Test shape 1	Test shape 2	Test shape 3	Test shape 4	Test shape 5
A. Set A	A. Set A	A. Set A	A. Set A	A. Set A
B. Set B	B. Set B	B. Set B	B. Set B	B. Set B
C. Neither	C. Neither	C. Neither	C. Neither	C. Neither

Question 2

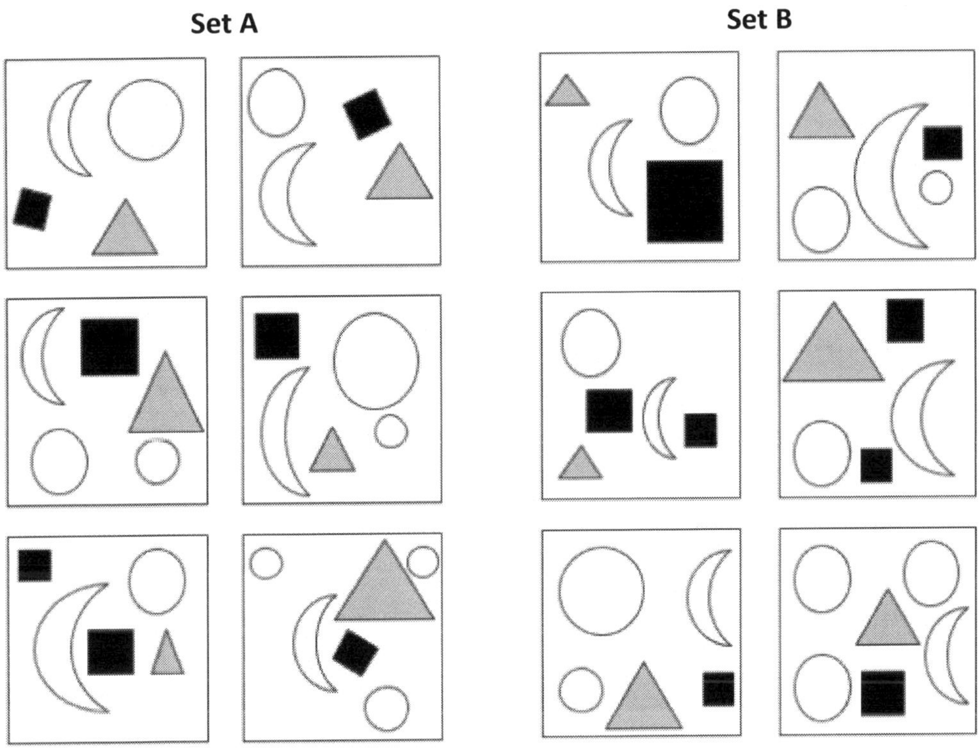

Determine whether the test shapes belong to Set A, Set B or neither.

Test shape 6	Test shape 7	Test shape 8	Test shape 9	Test shape 10

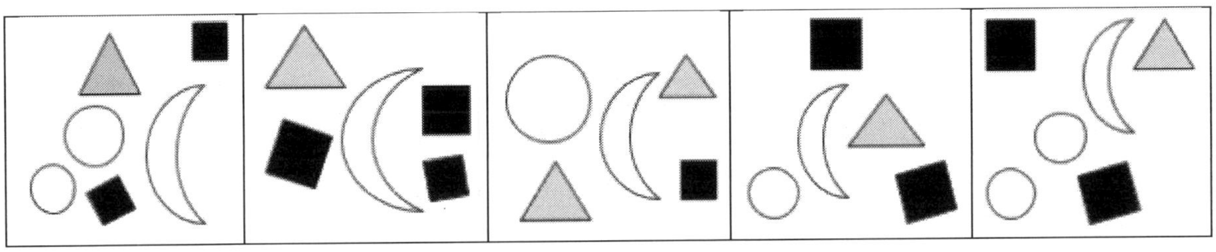

A. Set A	A. Set A	A. Set A	A. Set A	A. Set A
B. Set B	B. Set B	B. Set B	B. Set B	B. Set B
C. Neither	C. Neither	C. Neither	C. Neither	C. Neither

Question 3

Set A | Set B

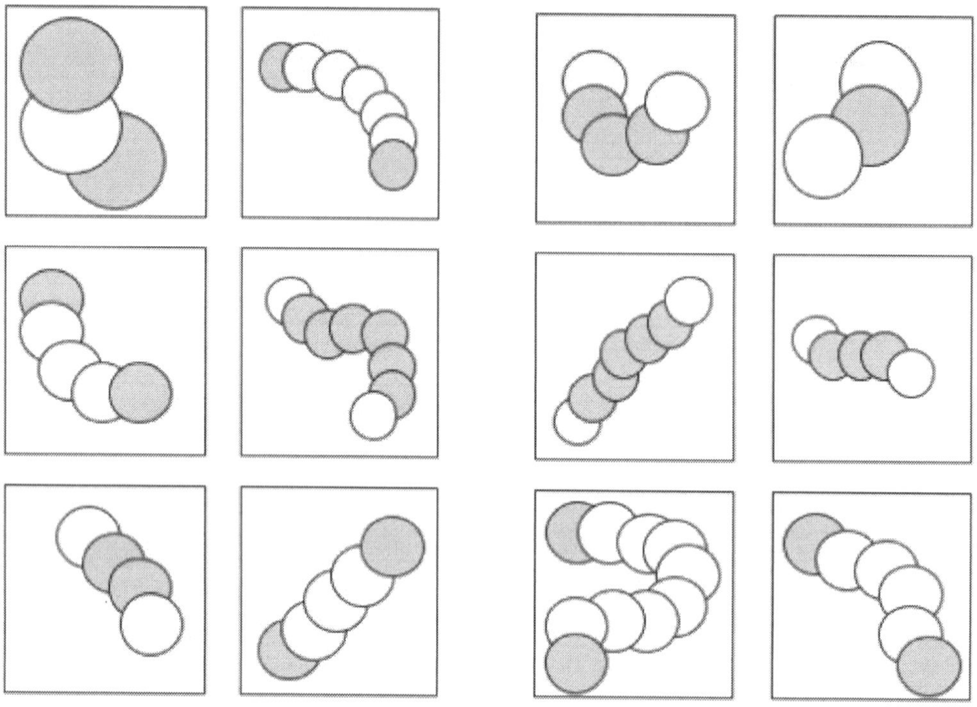

Determine whether the test shapes belong to Set A, Set B or neither.

Test shape 1	Test shape 12	Test shape 13	Test shape 14	Test shape 15

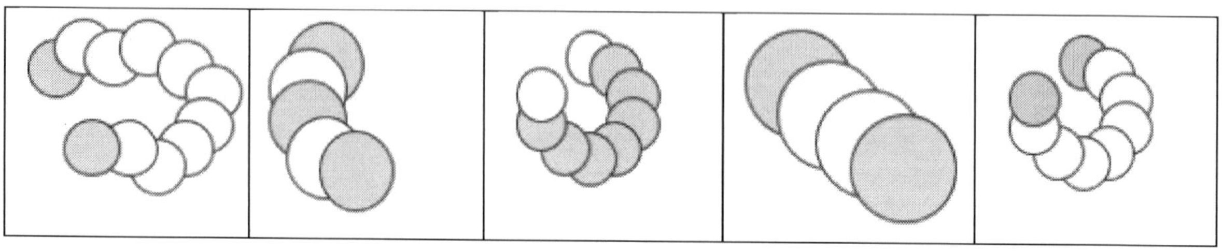

Test shape 1	Test shape 12	Test shape 13	Test shape 14	Test shape 15
A. Set A B. Set B C. Neither	A. Set A B. Set B C. Neither	A. Set A B. Set B C. Neither	A. Set A B. Set B C. Neither	A. Set A B. Set B C. Neither

Question 4

Set A **Set B**

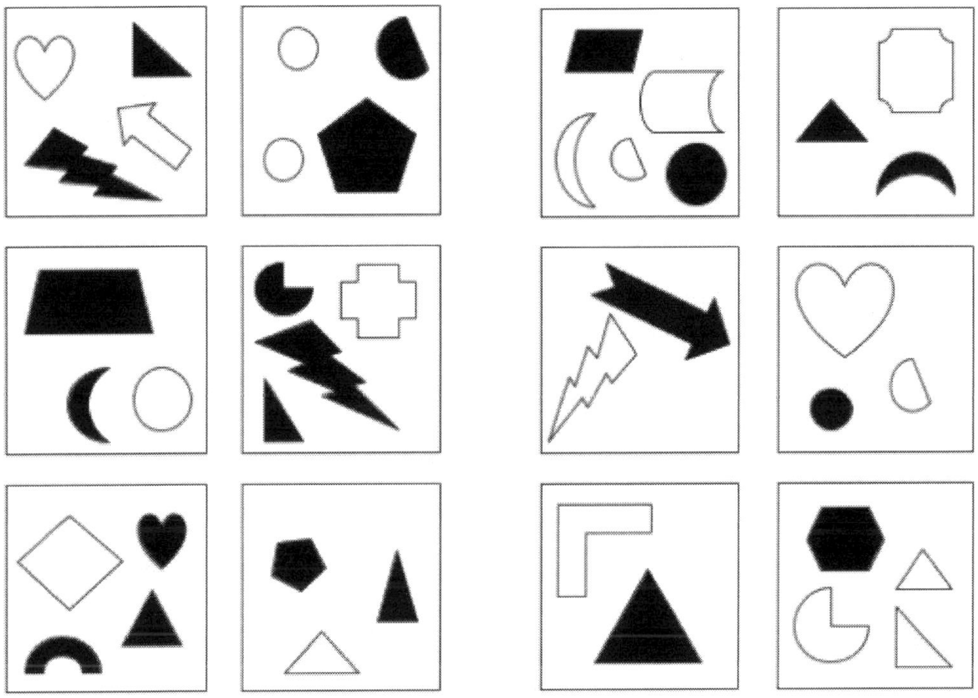

Determine whether the test shapes belong to Set A, Set B or neither.

Test shape 16 | Test shape 17 | Test shape 18 | Test shape 19 | Test shape 20

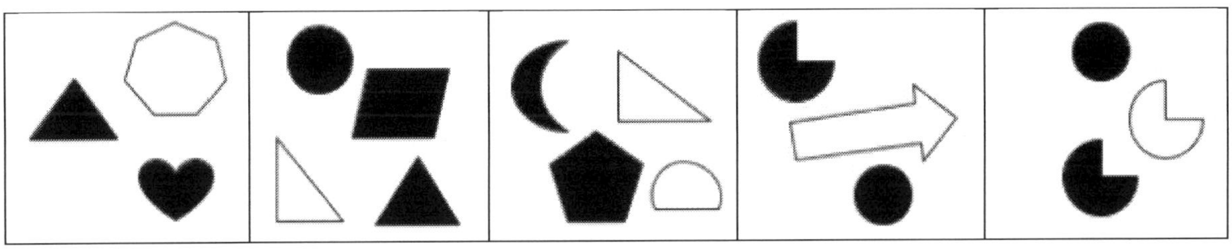

Test shape 16	Test shape 17	Test shape 18	Test shape 19	Test shape 20
A. Set A	A. Set A	A. Set A	A. Set A	A. Set A
B. Set B	B. Set B	B. Set B	B. Set B	B. Set B
C. Neither	C. Neither	C. Neither	C. Neither	C. Neither

Question 5

Set A **Set B**

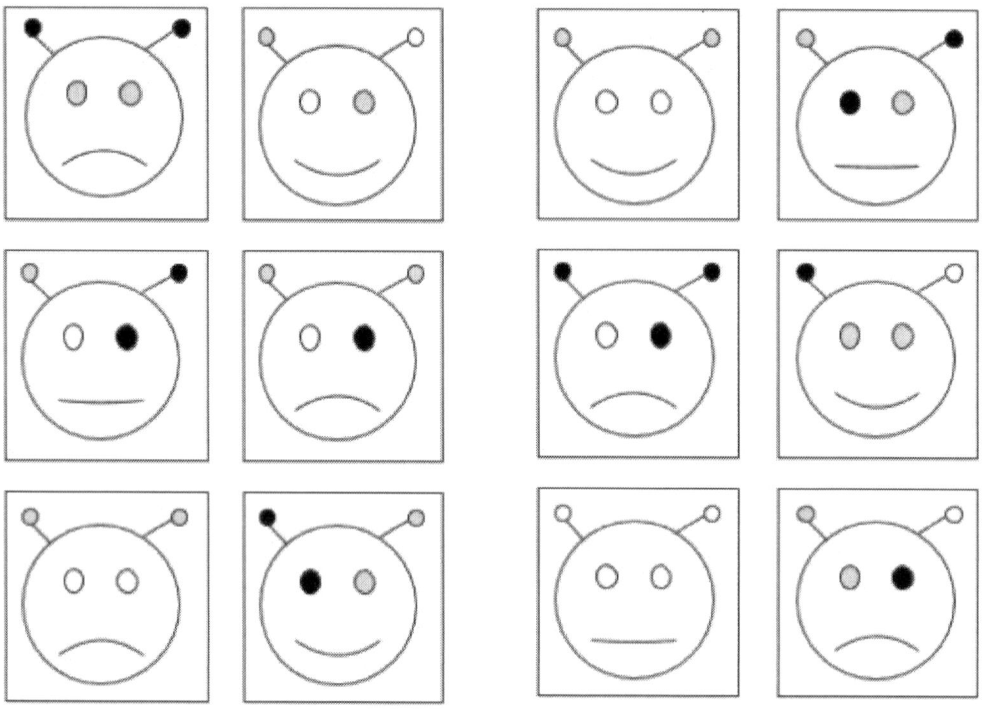

Determine whether the test shapes belong to Set A, Set B or neither.

Test shape 21	Test shape 22	Test shape 23	Test shape 24	Test shape 25

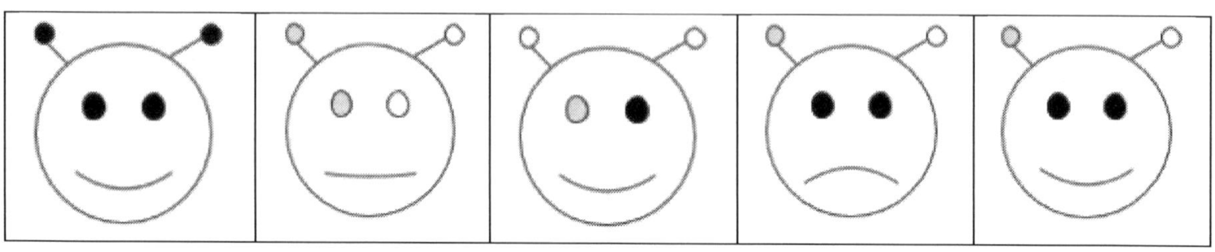

A. Set A	A. Set A	A. Set A	A. Set A	A. Set A
B. Set B	B. Set B	B. Set B	B. Set B	B. Set B
C. Neither	C. Neither	C. Neither	C. Neither	C. Neither

Question 6

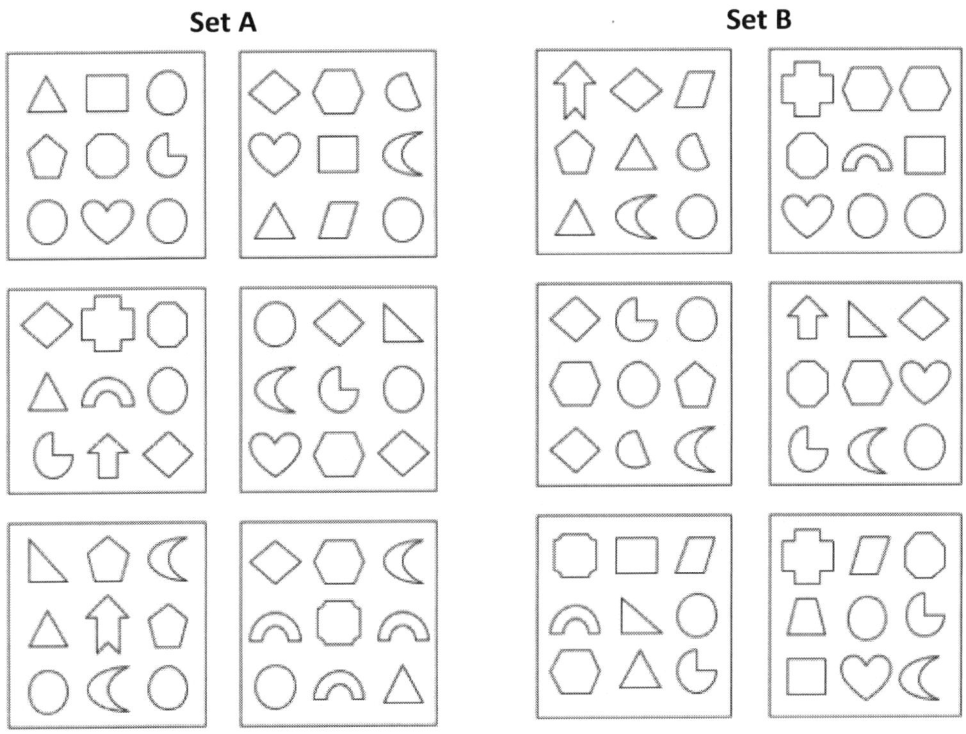

Determine whether the test shapes belong to Set A, Set B or neither.

Test shape 26 | Test shape 27 | Test shape 28 | Test shape 29 | Test shape 30

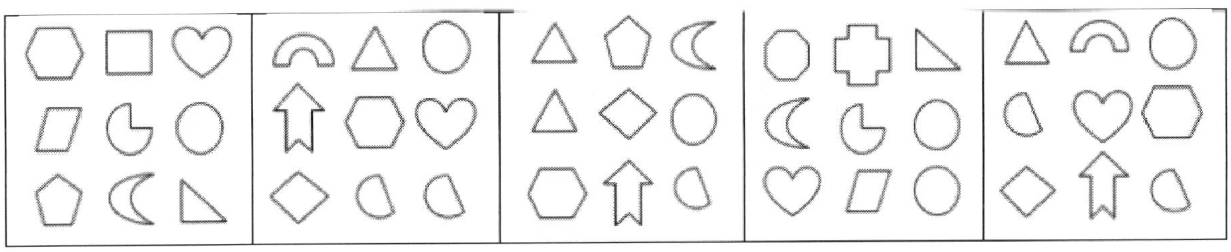

Test shape 26	Test shape 27	Test shape 28	Test shape 29	Test shape 30
A. Set A	A. Set A	A. Set A	A. Set A	A. Set A
B. Set B	B. Set B	B. Set B	B. Set B	B. Set B
C. Neither	C. Neither	C. Neither	C. Neither	C. Neither

Question 7

Set A **Set B**

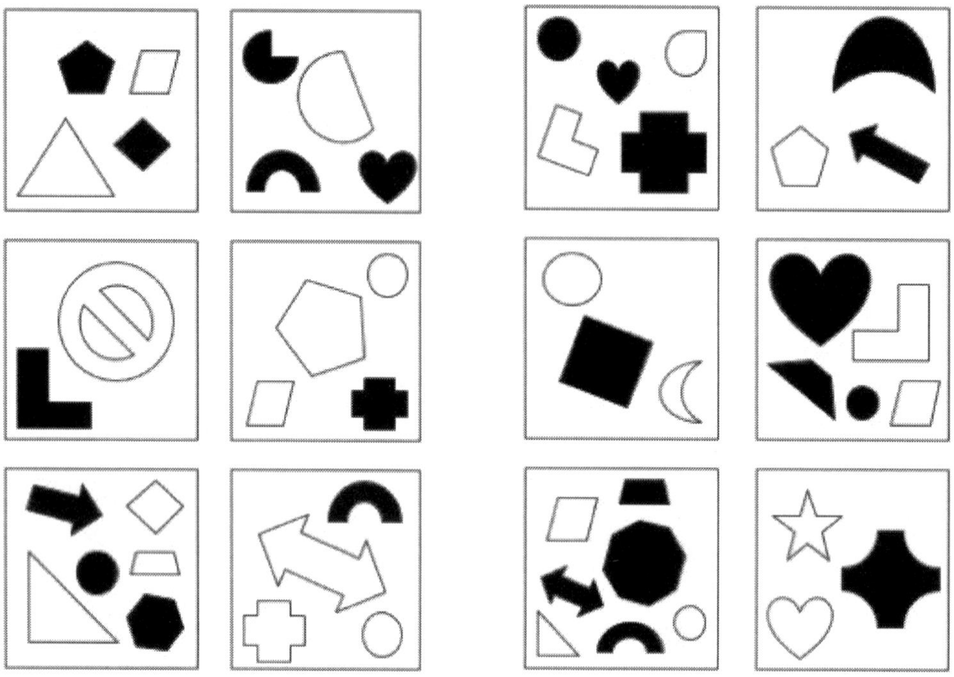

Determine whether the test shapes belong to Set A, Set B or neither.

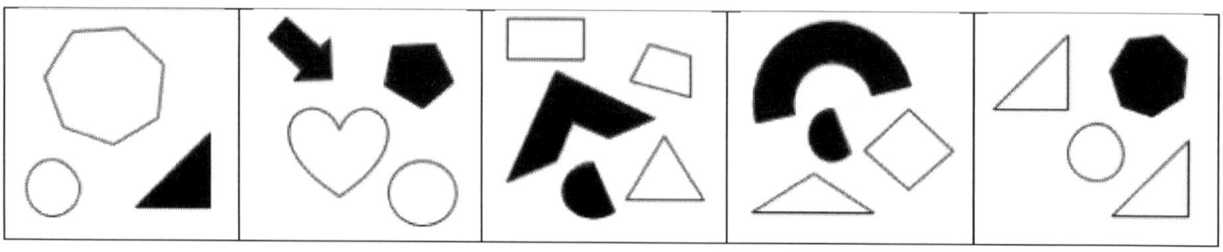

Test shape 31	Test shape 32	Test shape 33	Test shape 34	Test shape 35
A. Set A	A. Set A	A. Set A	A. Set A	A. Set A
B. Set B	B. Set B	B. Set B	B. Set B	B. Set B
C. Neither	C. Neither	C. Neither	C. Neither	C. Neither

Question 8

Set A

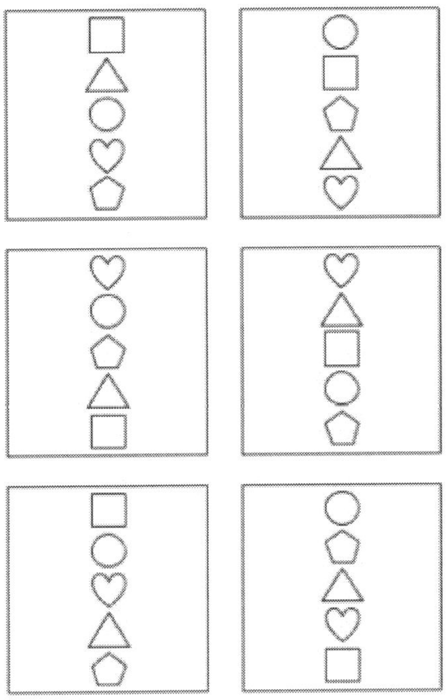

Set B

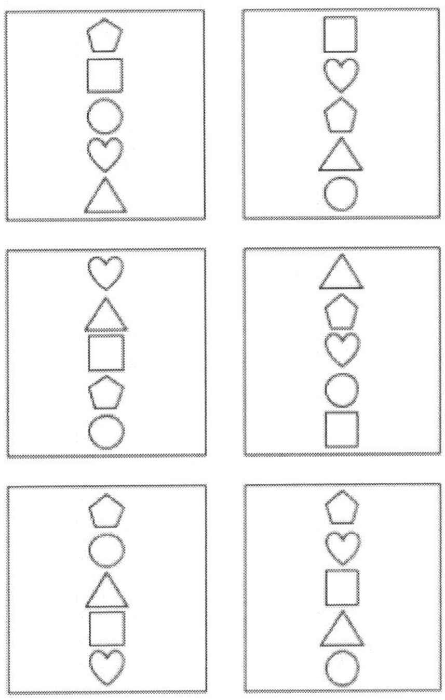

Determine whether the test shapes belong to Set A, Set B or neither.

Test shape 36 | Test shape 37 | Test shape 38 | Test shape 39 | Test shape 40

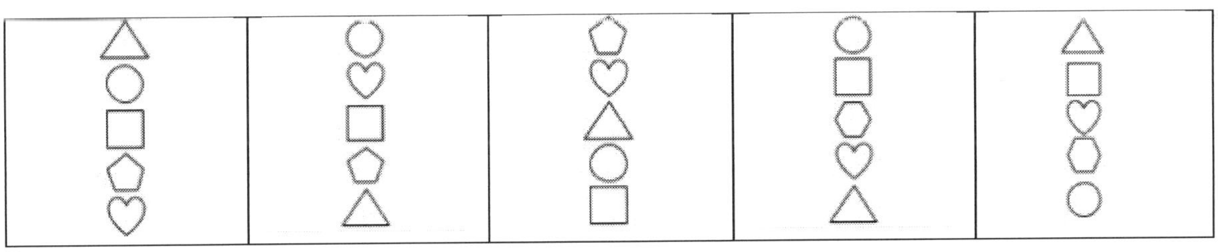

Test shape 36

A. Set A
B. Set B
C. Neither

Test shape 37

A. Set A
B. Set B
C. Neither

Test shape 38

A. Set A
B. Set B
C. Neither

Test shape 39

A. Set A
B. Set B
C. Neither

Test shape 40

A. Set A
B. Set B
C. Neither

Question 9

Set A

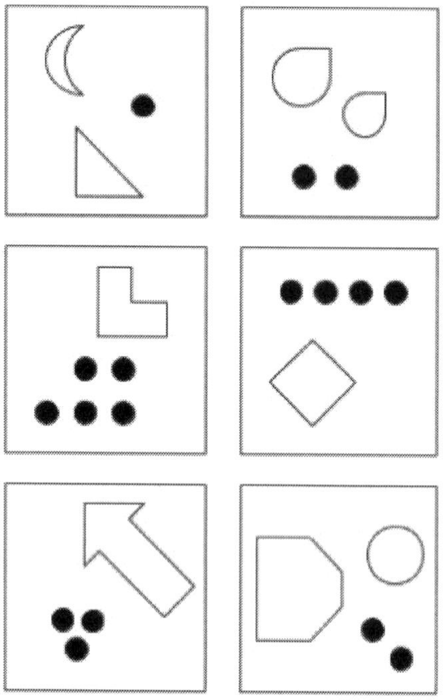

Set B

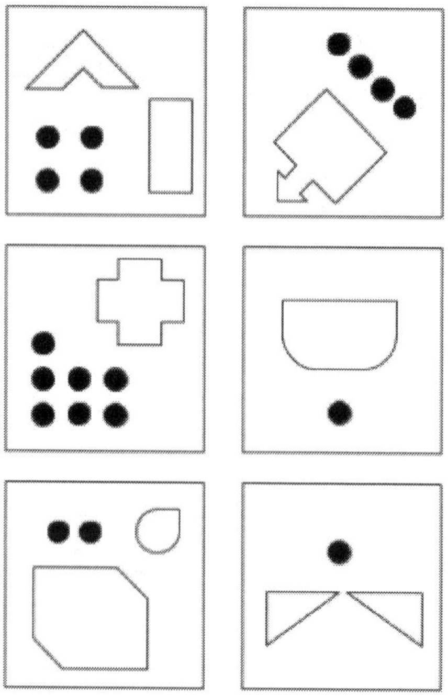

Determine whether the test shapes belong to Set A, Set B or neither.

Test shape 41 | Test shape 42 | Test shape 43 | Test shape 44 | Test shape 45

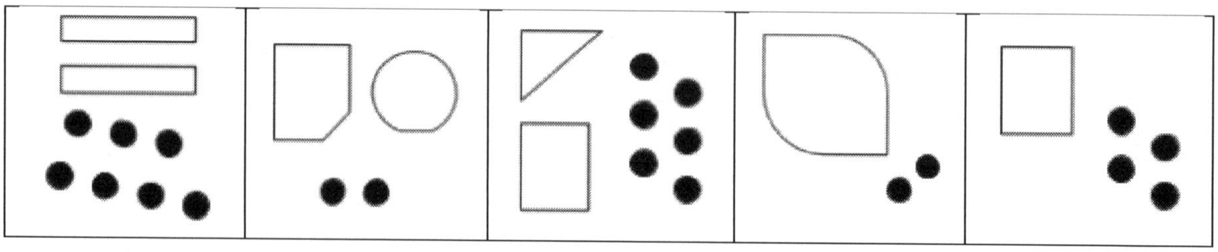

Test shape 41:
A. Set A
B. Set B
C. Neither

Test shape 42:
A. Set A
B. Set B
C. Neither

Test shape 43:
A. Set A
B. Set B
C. Neither

Test shape 44:
A. Set A
B. Set B
C. Neither

Test shape 45:
A. Set A
B. Set B
C. Neither

46.

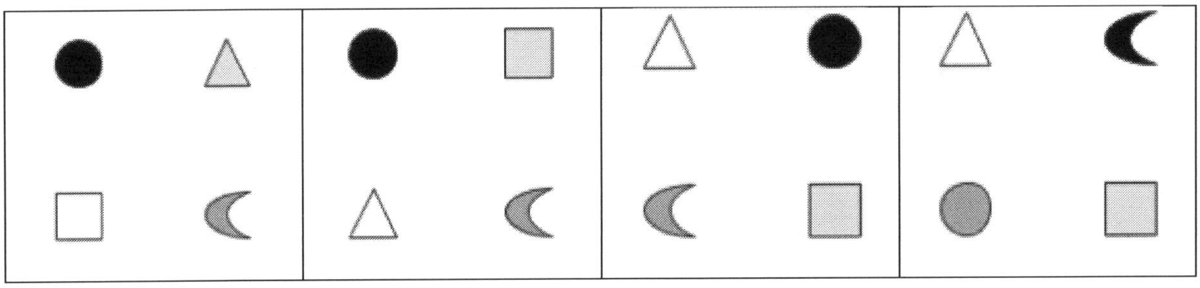

Which figure completes the series?

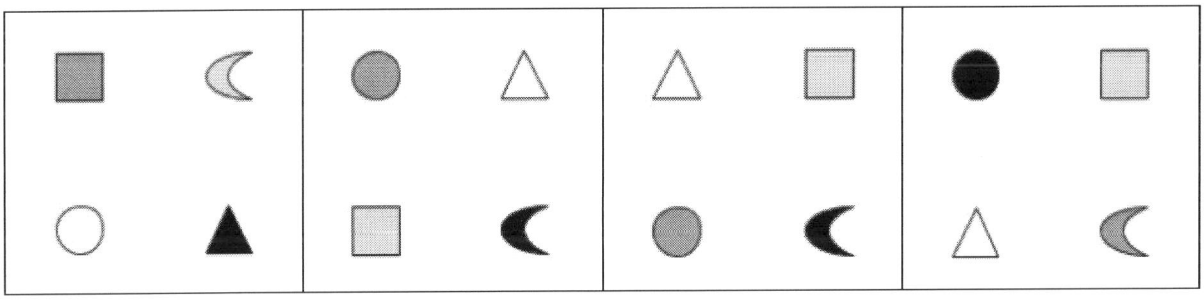

A. **B.** **C.** **D.**

47.

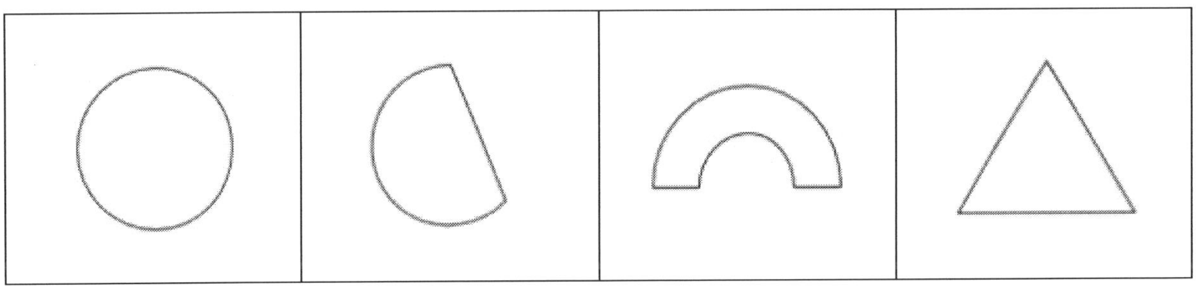

Which figure completes the series?

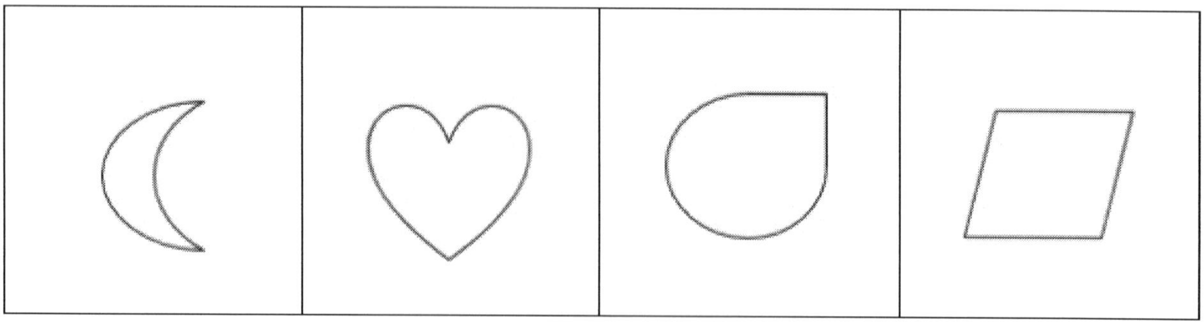

A. B. C. D.

48.

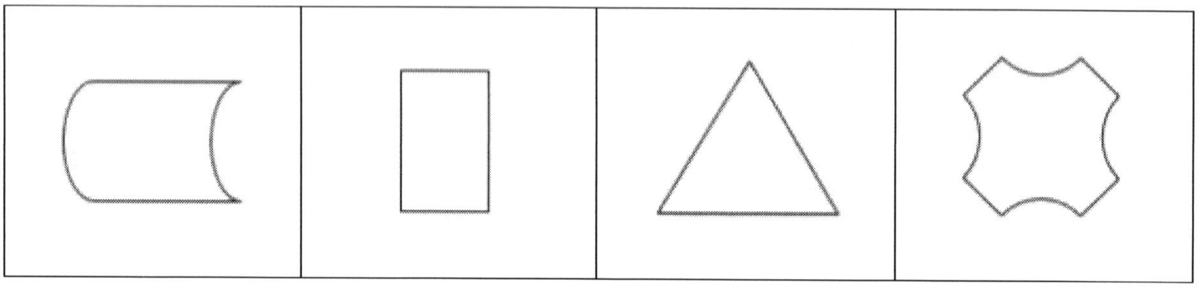

Which figure completes the series?

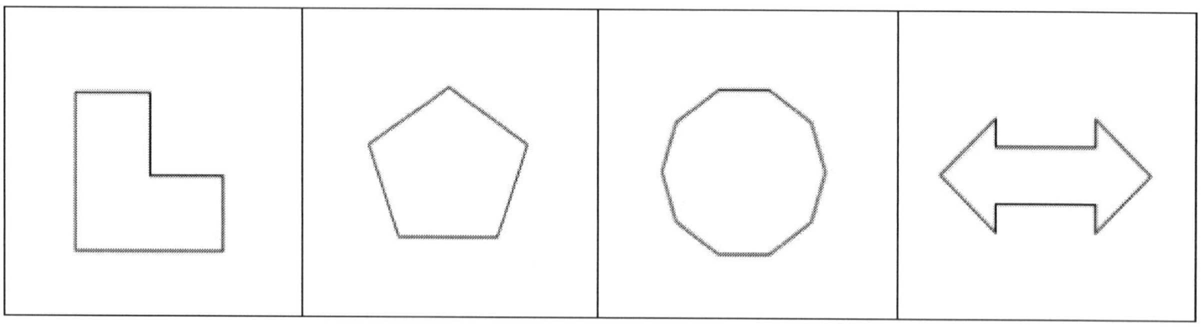

A. B. C. D.

49.

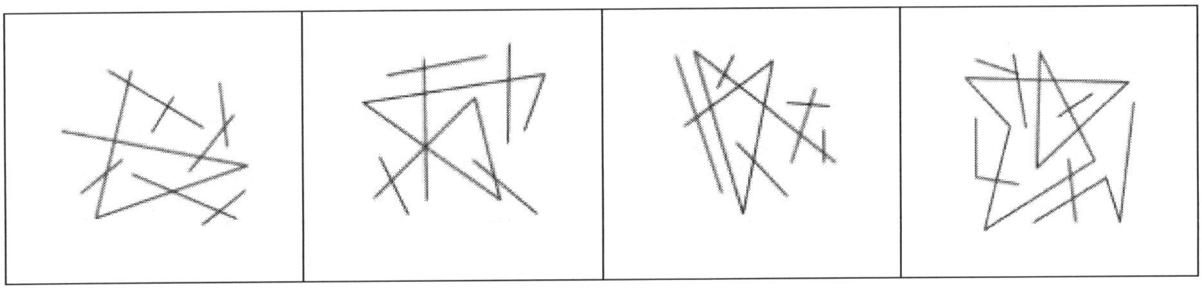

Which figure completes the series?

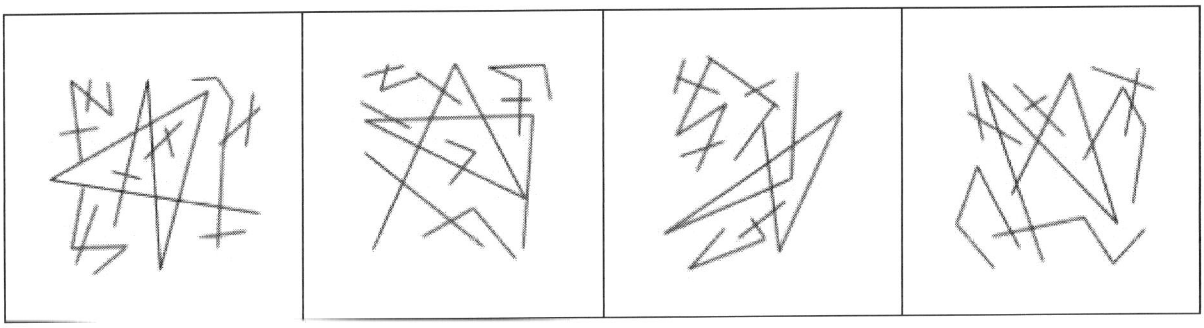

A. **B.** **C.** **D.**

50.

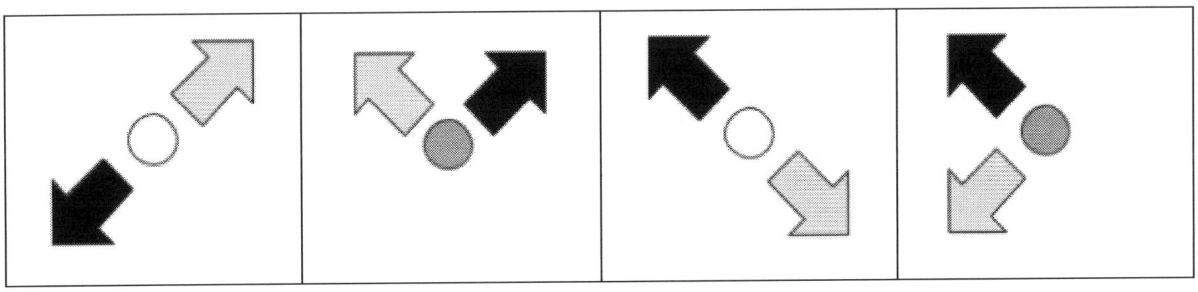

Which figure completes the series?

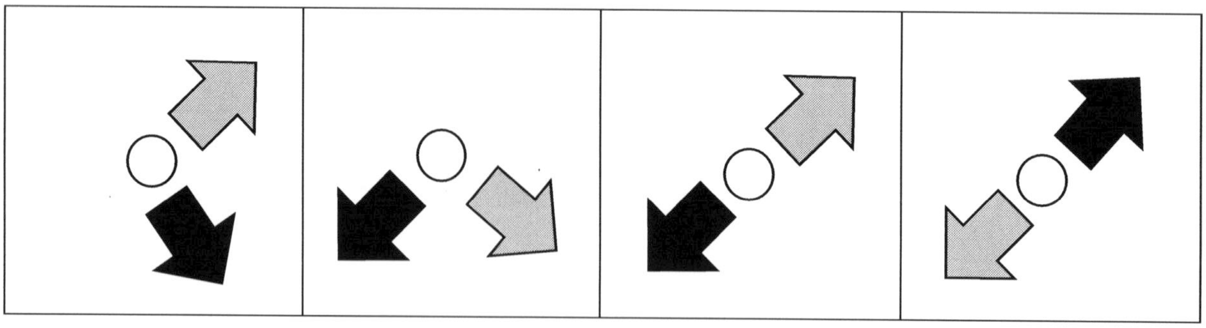

A. B. C. D.

51.

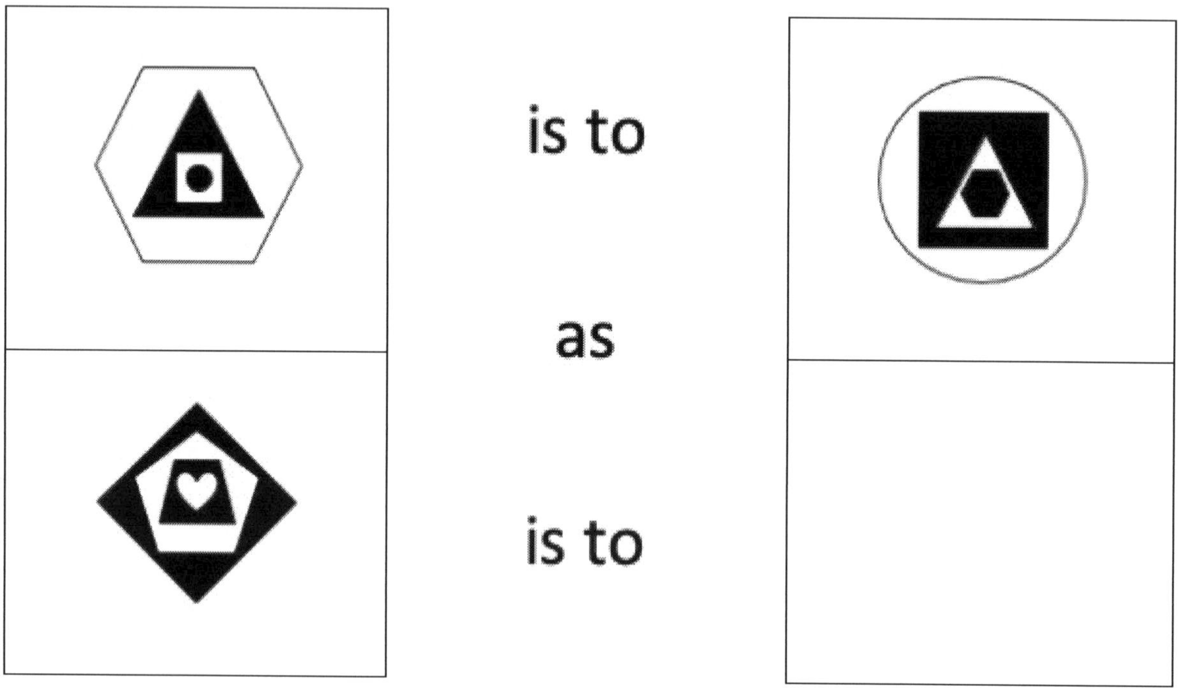

Which figure completes the statement?

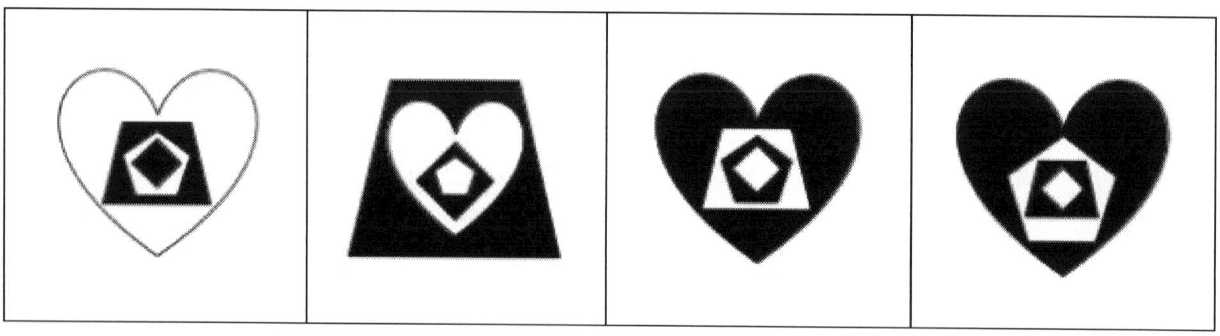

A. B. C. D.

52.

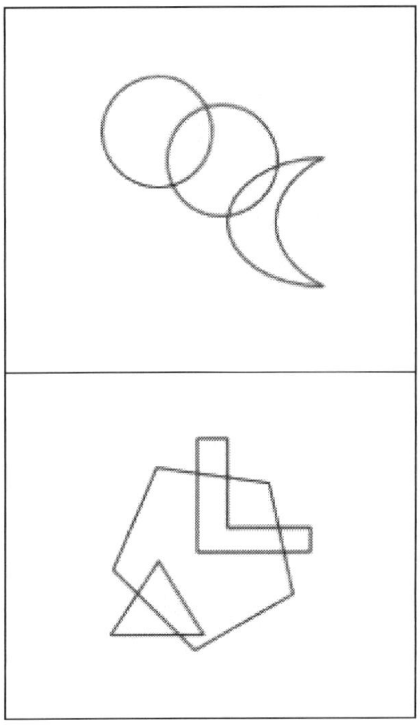

is to

as

is to

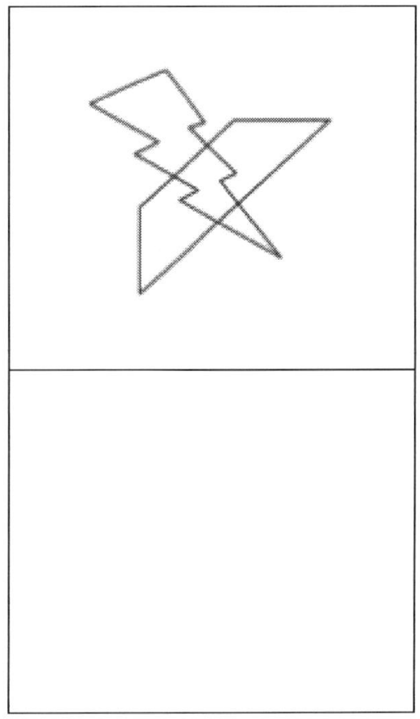

Which figure completes the statement?

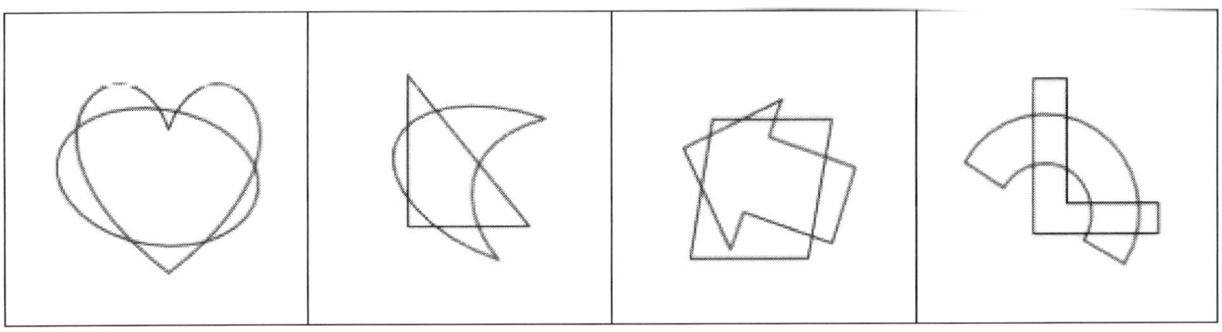

A. **B.** **C.** **D.**

53.

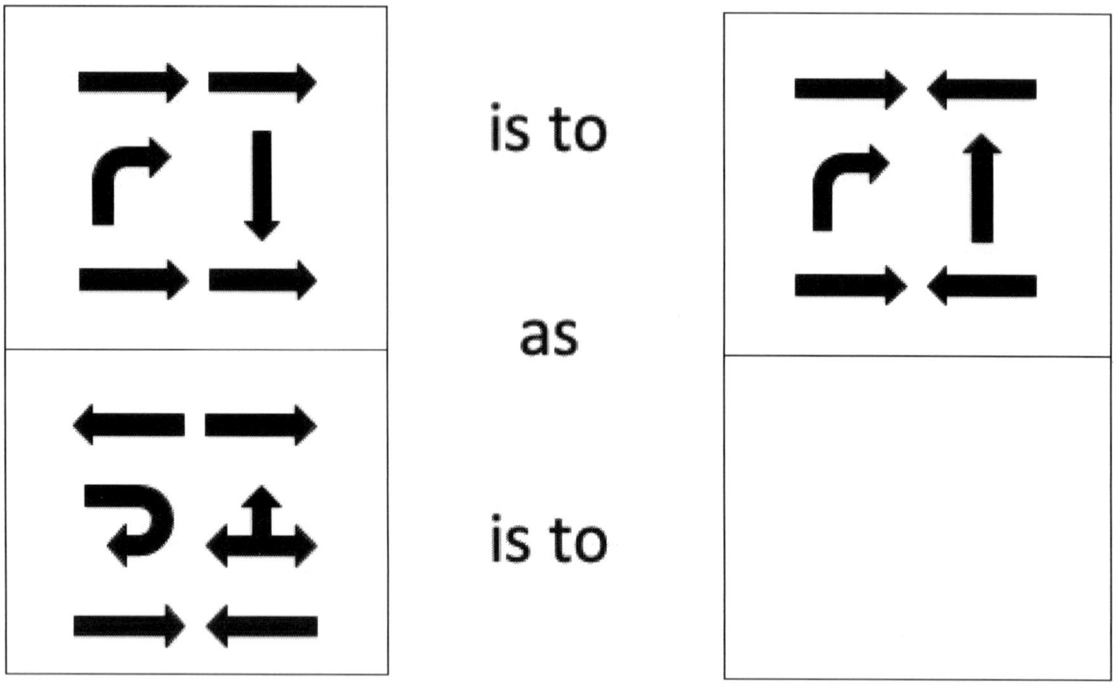

Which figure completes the statement?

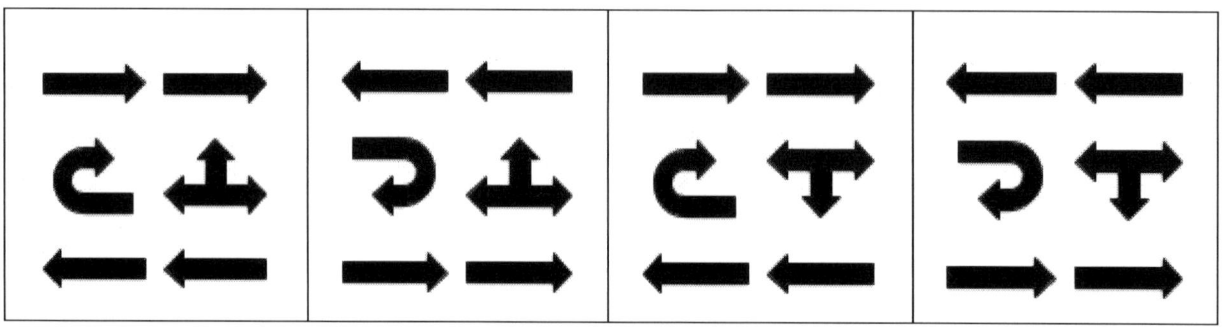

A. B. C. D.

54.

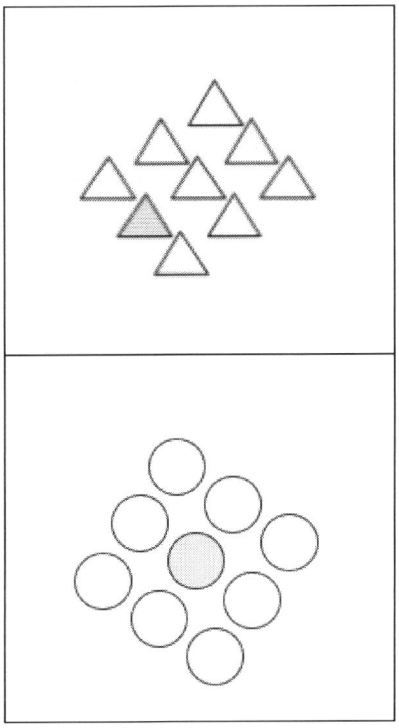

is to

as

is to

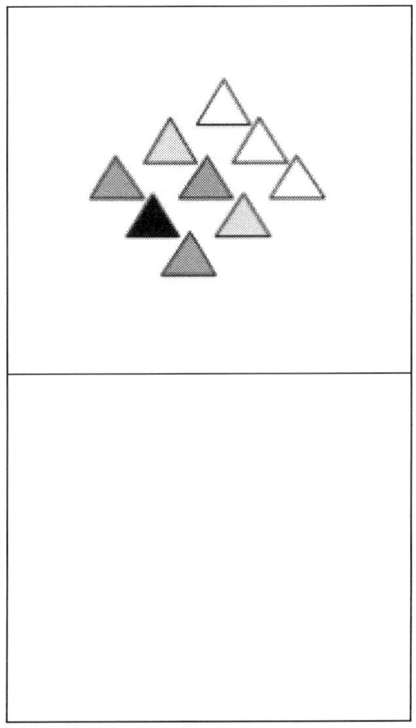

Which figure completes the statement?

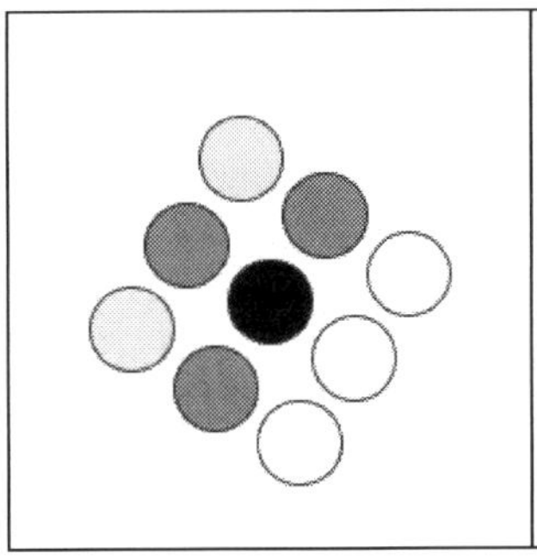

A.

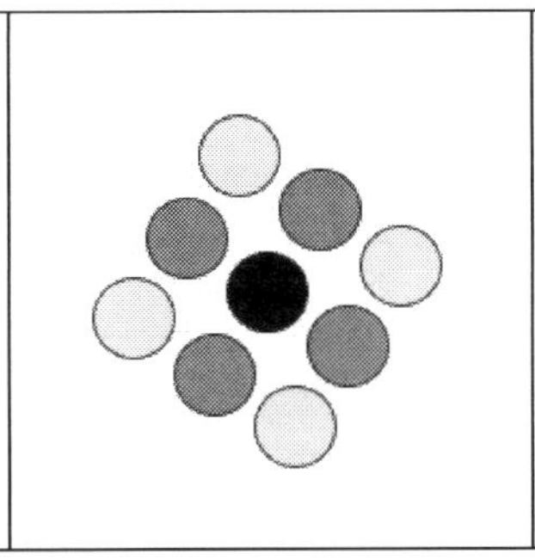

B.

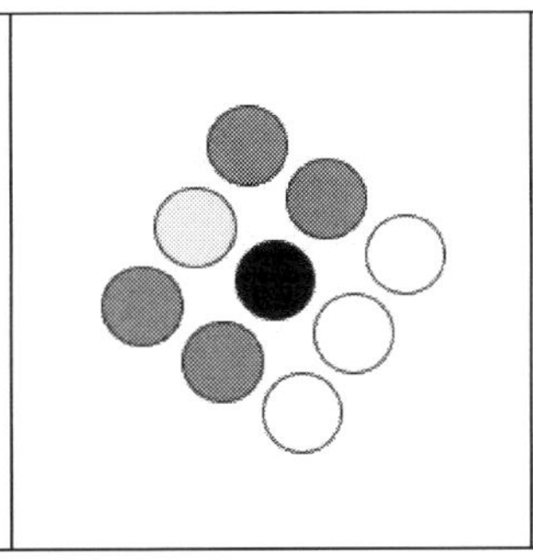

C.

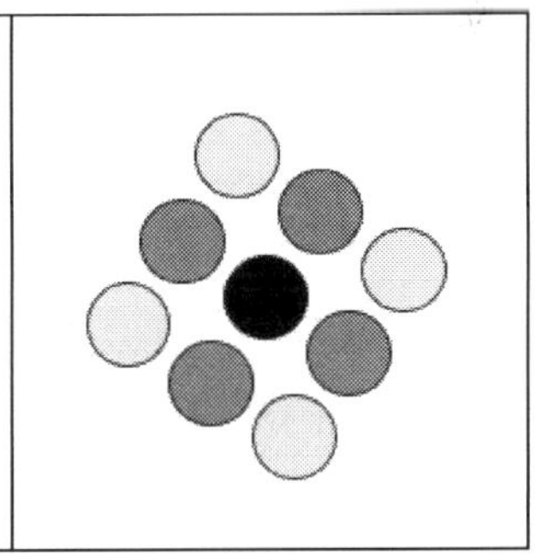

D.

55.

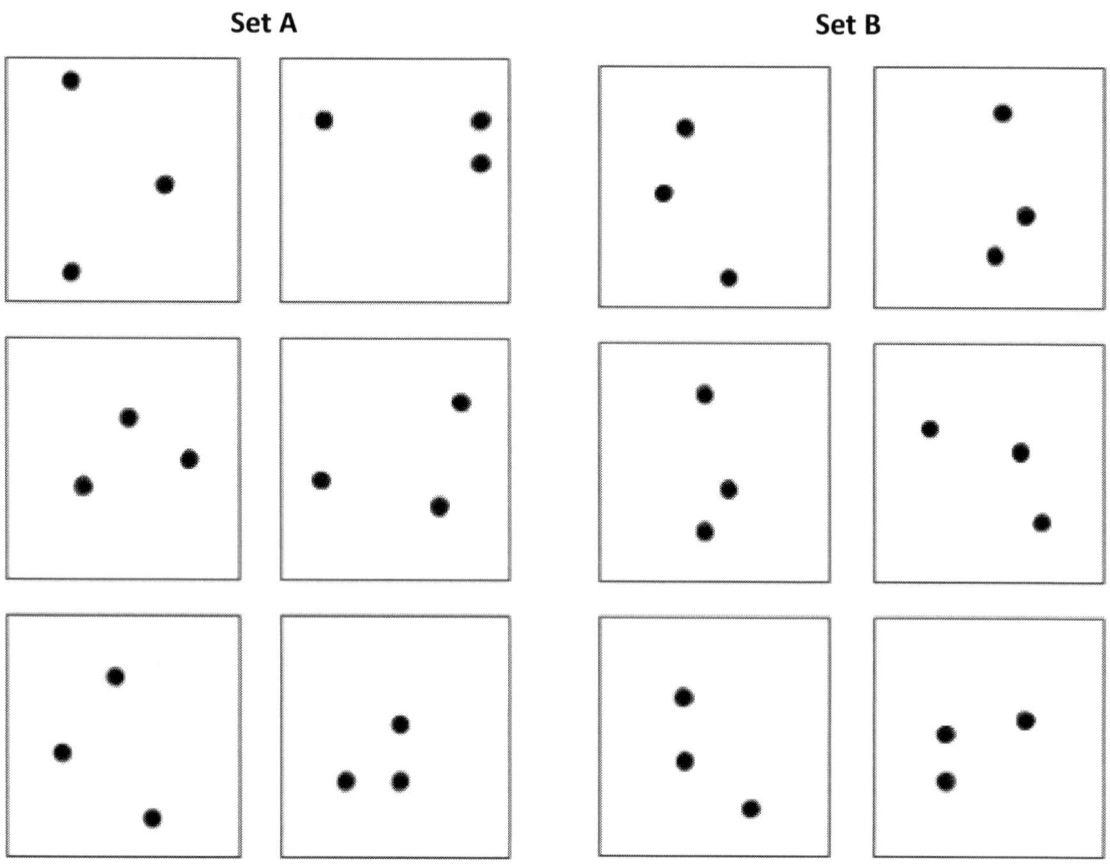

Which of the following test shapes belongs to Set A?

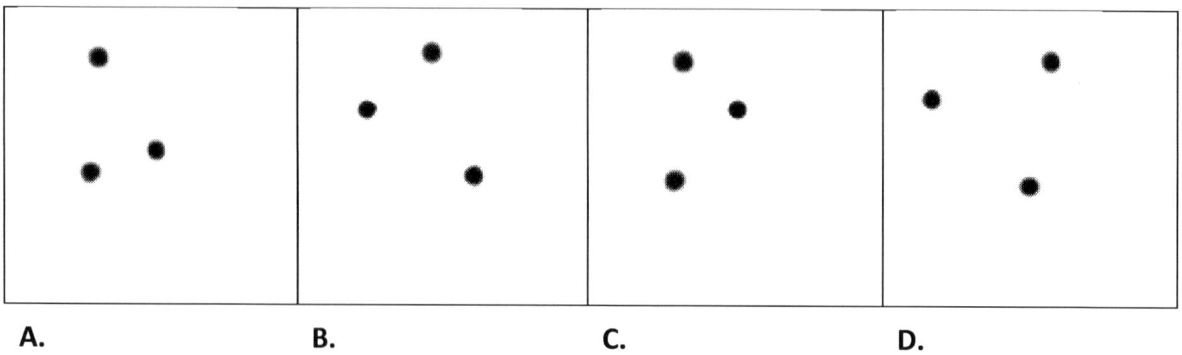

Situational Judgement Test

Scenario 1

James, a medical student, is taking a history from a patient. The patient mentions that she overheard racist remarks being made by a consultant regarding another member of staff. She feels deeply hurt and offended by what she heard and she wants to know what can be done about this.

How **appropriate** are the following responses by **James** in this situation?

1. Tell the patient that this is very out of character for the consultant and she probably misunderstood him.
   A. Very appropriate
   B. Appropriate, but not ideal
   C. Inappropriate, but not awful
   D. Very inappropriate

2. Apologise on behalf of the consultant and ask the patient for more information.
   A. Very appropriate
   B. Appropriate, but not ideal
   C. Inappropriate, but not awful
   D. Very inappropriate

3. Inform the patient that racism is not tolerated in their hospital trust and any such reports will be taken seriously.
   A. Very appropriate
   B. Appropriate, but not ideal
   C. Inappropriate, but not awful
   D. Very inappropriate

4. Ask the consultant to enter the room so they can discuss the matter.
   A. Very appropriate
   B. Appropriate, but not ideal
   C. Inappropriate, but not awful
   D. Very inappropriate

Scenario 2

Rajesh, a medical student, is unable to attend classes for a few days as he must travel to attend a family funeral. He does not want this to impact his attendance, so he asks his colleague, Anna, to sign his name on the register during this time. The classes are on important clinical skills that he will need as a doctor.

How **appropriate** are the following responses by **Anna** in this situation?

5. Sign him in as he can always learn the skills at a later date.
   A. Very appropriate
   B. Appropriate, but not ideal
   C. Inappropriate, but not awful
   D. Very inappropriate

6. Suggest that Rajesh talk to his course director to try to arrange a catch-up for what he will be missing.
   A. Very appropriate
   B. Appropriate, but not ideal
   C. Inappropriate, but not awful
   D. Very inappropriate

7. Refuse because it will affect her integrity.
   A. Very appropriate
   B. Appropriate, but not ideal
   C. Inappropriate, but not awful
   D. Very inappropriate

8. Tell him that he should not travel under any circumstances as he needs to attend his classes.
   A. Very appropriate
   B. Appropriate, but not ideal
   C. Inappropriate, but not awful
   D. Very inappropriate

Scenario 3

Amanda, a junior doctor, is asked to assist in sorting a list of operations in terms of priority. One of the inpatients informed her earlier that he was worried about staying in the hospital for longer than necessary due to the risk of hospital-acquired infections. He asked Amanda to make sure that he would be getting his operation quickly.

How **important** to take into account are the following considerations for **Amanda** when deciding how to respond to the situation?

9. How healthy and well the patient is.
    A. Very important
    B. Important
    C. Of minor importance
    D. Not important

10. The urgency of the patient's operation.
    A. Very important
    B. Important
    C. Of minor importance
    D. Not important

Scenario 4

Elizabeth, a junior doctor, is working on the wards. The registrar disagrees with her treatment plan for a patient. She has had some issues with this particular registrar in the past.

How **appropriate** are the following responses by **Elizabeth** in this situation?

11. Go ahead with your treatment plan as you are also a qualified doctor and so have every right to do so
    A. Very appropriate
    B. Appropriate, but not ideal
    C. Inappropriate, but not awful
    D. Very inappropriate

12. Outline why you think your treatment plan works well and ask the registrar why he thinks you should do it a different way
    A. Very appropriate
    B. Appropriate, but not ideal
    C. Inappropriate, but not awful
    D. Very inappropriate

13. Go with the registrar's plan as he is more experienced than you and so knows best
    A. Very appropriate
    B. Appropriate, but not ideal
    C. Inappropriate, but not awful

D. Very inappropriate

Scenario 5

Jen, a medical student, is headed to a teaching session after her lunch break. On the way, she gets a phone call from her friend, Anthony, who needs her urgent help. He says that he is in trouble and wants her to reach him as soon as possible, ideally within the next 20 minutes. It will take her 15 minutes to get to Anthony, and she will have to miss her teaching session.

How **appropriate** are the following responses by **Jen** in this situation?

14. Go to Anthony as her tutor will understand that she would not be missing the session unless it was urgent.
    A. Very appropriate
    B. Appropriate, but not ideal
    C. Inappropriate, but not awful
    D. Very inappropriate

15. After unsuccessfully attempting to contact the tutor, head to Anthony knowing that she tried her best.
    A. Very appropriate
    B. Appropriate, but not ideal
    C. Inappropriate, but not awful
    D. Very inappropriate

16. Quickly head to the teaching session to explain the situation, then head to Anthony.
    A. Very appropriate
    B. Appropriate, but not ideal
    C. Inappropriate, but not awful
    D. Very inappropriate

Scenario 6

John, a GP, is seeing Mrs. Adams regarding her pregnancy. Ms. Adams is a heavy smoker and has never indicated a wish to stop smoking.

How **important** to take into account are the following considerations for **John** when deciding how to respond to the situation?

17. The impact of smoking on the foetus' health and development.
    A. Very important

B. Important
C. Of minor importance
D. Not important at all

18. Mrs. Adams' autonomy to make her own decisions regarding her lifestyle choices.
    A. Very important
    B. Important
    C. Of minor importance
    D. Not important at all

19. Mrs. Adams' awareness of how smoking can impact her child's health.
    A. Very important
    B. Important
    C. Of minor importance
    D. Not important at all

Scenario 7

Chris, a medical student, shares a flat with Eleanor, another other medical student. Eleanor has recently become friends with a concerning group of students who Chris knows are heavily involved in drug abuse. Her attitude towards drugs has recently begun to change, and Chris is worried that she may also be abusing drugs.

How **important** to take into account are the following considerations for **Chris** when deciding how to respond to the situation?

20. The reason for Eleanor's recent changes.
    A. Very important
    B. Important
    C. Of minor importance
    D. Not important at all

21. How Eleanor's behaviour may impact her professional life.
    A. Very important
    B. Important
    C. Of minor importance
    D. Not important at all

22. Whether Eleanor is happy with her new friends.
    A. Very important
    B. Important
    C. Of minor importance

D. Not important at all

Scenario 8

Andrew, a dental student, has been allocated a group of four other dental students to work on a group presentation with. They divide the task fairly, but it becomes clear that two of the students, Javaid and Amy, have no desire to do the work required, affecting the whole group. The group is required to present on this topic in a week.

How **appropriate** are the following responses by **Andrew** in this situation?

23. Speak to Javaid and Amy together to help them understand that their lack of effort will impact the whole group.
    A. Very appropriate
    B. Appropriate, but not ideal
    C. Inappropriate, but not awful
    D. Very inappropriate

24. Mention at the start of the presentation that most of the work was conducted by the three group members not including Javaid and Amy.
    A. Very appropriate
    B. Appropriate, but not ideal
    C. Inappropriate, but not awful
    D. Very inappropriate

25. Speak to the other members of the group to try to work out how the three of them can do all of the work in the given timeframe.
    A. Very appropriate
    B. Appropriate, but not ideal
    C. Inappropriate, but not awful
    D. Very inappropriate

26. Write a detailed email to the course director to explain the situation.
    A. Very appropriate
    B. Appropriate, but not ideal
    C. Inappropriate, but not awful
    D. Very inappropriate

Scenario 9

Aryan, a medical student, is shadowing a consultant on a medical ward. The consultant prescribes a specific painkiller for a patient and asks Aryan to deliver the prescription to the nurse. The consultant then finishes his shift and heads home. Aryan notices prior to delivering the prescription that the patient in question has a previous addiction issue with that particular painkiller.

How **appropriate** are the following responses by **Aryan** in this situation?

27. Change the prescription to another type of painkiller.
    A. Very appropriate
    B. Appropriate, but not ideal
    C. Inappropriate, but not awful
    D. Very inappropriate

28. Ask the nurse for advice.
    A. Very appropriate
    B. Appropriate, but not ideal
    C. Inappropriate, but not awful
    D. Very inappropriate

29. Contact an on-call doctor to ask for advice.
    A. Very appropriate
    B. Appropriate, but not ideal
    C. Inappropriate, but not awful
    D. Very inappropriate

30. Apologise to the patient and explain that the medications will be reviewed the next day when the consultant returns.
    A. Very appropriate
    B. Appropriate, but not ideal
    C. Inappropriate, but not awful
    D. Very inappropriate

Scenario 10

Emma, a medical student, is on a train when the conductor starts asking if there is a doctor anywhere. She tells him that she is a medical student, but can try to help. He informs her that a child in another carriage swallowed part of a plastic fork and his mother is extremely worried that this will be harmful for him. Emma is not entirely sure how to solve this, but no one else on the train has come forward as a doctor.

How **important** to take into account are the following considerations for **Emma** when deciding how to respond to the situation?

31. The fact that nobody else has come forward.
    A. Very important
    B. Important
    C. Of minor importance
    D. Not important

32. The conductor is offering to move her to first class if she is able to help with the situation.
    A. Very important
    B. Important
    C. Of minor importance
    D. Not important

33. The conductor does not seem concerned about the child when he explains the situation to Emma.
    A. Very important
    B. Important
    C. Of minor importance
    D. Not important

Scenario 11

Dr Maxim is a cardiologist running a clinic. A patient comes into the clinic, clearly very angry. He complains that he has been waiting over an hour to be seen and that this is not the service he expects from the NHS.

How **appropriate** are the following responses by **Dr Maxim** in this situation?

34. Tell the patient that everybody has to wait and that there is not anything he can do.
    A. Very appropriate
    B. Appropriate, but not ideal
    C. Inappropriate, but not awful
    D. Very inappropriate

35. Ask the patient to calm down before they carry on with the consultation.
    A. Very appropriate

B. Appropriate, but not ideal
C. Inappropriate, but not awful
D. Very inappropriate

36. Tell the patient that they should be grateful that they do not have to pay to be seen by a doctor through the NHS.
    A. Very appropriate
    B. Appropriate, but not ideal
    C. Inappropriate, but not awful
    D. Very inappropriate

37. Tell the patient that he will pass the feedback on to the relevant department.
    A. Very appropriate
    B. Appropriate, but not ideal
    C. Inappropriate, but not awful
    D. Very inappropriate

Scenario 12

Yusuf, a medical student, is on a 4-week rotation at a GP practice. He must have his placement booklet signed each day to confirm his attendance. This is a requirement by his university, and failure to provide evidence for attendance can result in a professionalism issue. One day, he forgets his attendance booklet at home.

How **important** to take into account are the following considerations for **Yusuf** when deciding how to respond to the situation?

38. He has one week left of his rotation.
    A. Very important
    B. Important
    C. Of minor importance
    D. Not important

39. He has enough time during his lunch break to get his booklet from home.
    A. Very important
    B. Important
    C. Of minor importance
    D. Not important

Scenario 13

Harun, a junior doctor, is working in a hospice. He is asked to inform a patient, Carl, that treatment will now be withdrawn as he is on the end-of-life pathway. The focus of his care plan will now be to make sure that he is comfortable in his last few days. Carl was visited earlier by his daughter who informed him of a herbal remedy that she was certain would cure his condition. Carl asks Harun to look into the herbal remedy, but Harun doubts it would be of any medical benefit.

How **appropriate** are the following responses by **Harun** in this situation?

40. Tell Carl that the medical team's decision is final.
    A. Very appropriate
    B. Appropriate, but not ideal
    C. Inappropriate, but not awful
    D. Very inappropriate

41. Explain to Carl that any herbal remedy will not be beneficial to him.
    A. Very appropriate
    B. Appropriate, but not ideal
    C. Inappropriate, but not awful
    D. Very inappropriate

42. Discuss the herbal remedy with the consultant looking after Carl.
    A. Very appropriate
    B. Appropriate, but not ideal
    C. Inappropriate, but not awful
    D. Very inappropriate

Scenario 14

A junior doctor, Sharon, works in a renal unit. She has a medical student, Callum, shadowing her for the first time. Sharon has some difficulty balancing patient care and teaching the student at the same time. A fellow junior doctor jokingly makes a comment about Sharon's lack of capability managing a large workload, and Sharon appears to be upset at the remark.

How **appropriate** are the following responses by **Callum** in this situation?

43. Take the other junior doctor aside immediately and inform them that their comment was very offensive.
    A. Very appropriate
    B. Appropriate, but not ideal

C. Inappropriate, but not awful
D. Very inappropriate

44. Apologise to Sharon.
    A. Very appropriate
    B. Appropriate, but not ideal
    C. Inappropriate, but not awful
    D. Very inappropriate

45. Get a third party involved.
    A. Very appropriate
    B. Appropriate, but not ideal
    C. Inappropriate, but not awful
    D. Very inappropriate

Scenario 15

Gracie, a medical student, asks Dr Adams, a GP, to look at the blood test results of a patient in the waiting room. She says that it is her sister-in-law who was feeling unwell last week, so she wants to know how she is doing.

How **appropriate** are the following responses by **Dr Adams** in this situation?

46. Report Gracie to her course supervisor at medical school for attempting to breach confidentiality.
    A. Very appropriate
    B. Appropriate, but not ideal
    C. Inappropriate, but not awful
    D. Very inappropriate

47. Allow Gracie to access the files as her sister-in-law had previously informed her that she was unwell.
    A. Very appropriate
    B. Appropriate, but not ideal
    C. Inappropriate, but not awful
    D. Very inappropriate

48. Advise her that he is not the GP treating her sister-in-law, so she should ask the GP in charge if she can access the blood test results.
    A. Very appropriate
    B. Appropriate, but not ideal

C. Inappropriate, but not awful
D. Very inappropriate

49. Ask Gracie to speak to her sister-in-law in the waiting room and ask for permission to access the files.
    A. Very appropriate
    B. Appropriate, but not ideal
    C. Inappropriate, but not awful
    D. Very inappropriate

Scenario 16

Mikhail is a junior doctor on a respiratory ward. He is at the end of his shift and waiting for the next shift's junior doctor, Joe, to come take over. When Joe finally comes in late, Mikhail attempts to hand over the patients in his care to Joe. He notices that Joe seems very distracted and unable to concentrate. He also thinks that he can smell alcohol in Joe's breath.

How **important** to take into account are the following considerations for **Mikhail** when deciding how to respond to the situation?

50. The danger posed to the patients.
    A. Very important
    B. Important
    C. Of minor importance
    D. Not important

51. The reason that his colleague has come into work drinking.
    A. Very important
    B. Important
    C. Of minor importance
    D. Not important

52. Joe may lose his job for attending work intoxicated.
    A. Very important
    B. Important
    C. Of minor importance
    D. Not important

Scenario 17

Jake, a dental student, is assigned a group for a project. One of the group members, Mike, suggests a topic for the presentation that no one else seems to agree with. He is insistent that it is the best topic, and fills out the project proposal form with his chosen topic. No one else seems to have a say in this. Jake does not feel comfortable with the way Mike is handling the group project.

How **appropriate** are the following responses by **Jake** in this situation?

53. Speak up in front of the group and inform Mike that this is not appropriate.
    A. Very appropriate
    B. Appropriate, but not ideal
    C. Inappropriate, but not awful
    D. Very inappropriate

54. Accept the idea as it will avoid conflict, even though it makes him feel uncomfortable.
    A. Very appropriate
    B. Appropriate, but not ideal
    C. Inappropriate, but not awful
    D. Very inappropriate

55. Discuss the issue with the group supervisor after everyone has left.
    A. Very appropriate
    B. Appropriate, but not ideal
    C. Inappropriate, but not awful
    D. Very inappropriate

Scenario 18

Lily, a medical student, is talking to a young patient in the emergency room, who came in with severe injuries and bruising. The patient tells Lily that she gets these injuries at home, but asks Lily to keep it to herself and to not tell anybody.

How **important** to take into account are the following considerations for **Lily** when deciding how to respond to the situation?

56. The patient did not give Lily permission to discuss this with anyone else.
    A. Very important
    B. Important
    C. Of minor importance

D. Not important

57. Lily is planning to go back home this evening.
    A. Very important
    B. Important
    C. Of minor importance
    D. Not important

58. Lily does not know the correct procedure for dealing with cases of abuse.
    A. Very important
    B. Important
    C. Of minor importance
    D. Not important

Scenario 19

Yvonne, a dental student, received comments from her tutor stating that she should work on being more empathetic in her patient interactions. Yvonne already feels that she comes across as empathetic.

How **appropriate** are the following responses by **Yvonne** in this situation?

59. Tell her tutor that these comments are unfair and unfounded.
    A. Very important
    B. Important
    C. Of minor importance
    D. Not important

60. Ask for more details on how she should improve her patient manner.
    A. Very important
    B. Important
    C. Of minor importance
    D. Not important

Scenario 20

Sara, a dental student, is scrolling through her Instagram when she finds a video that Alex, another student on her course, has made. He recorded himself and his friends in clinic, and the video briefly showed a patient's face in the background.

How **appropriate** are the following responses by **Sara** in this situation?

61. Forward the video to the dental school without consulting Alex.
   A. Very appropriate
   B. Appropriate, but not ideal
   C. Inappropriate, but not awful
   D. Very inappropriate

62. Ask Alex to remove the video right away.
   A. Very appropriate
   B. Appropriate, but not ideal
   C. Inappropriate, but not awful
   D. Very inappropriate

63. Remind Alex that breaching patient confidentiality can get him kicked out of dental school.
   A. Very appropriate
   B. Appropriate, but not ideal
   C. Inappropriate, but not awful
   D. Very inappropriate

Scenario 21

Dr Markham, a hepatologist, is working in the transplant unit. A liver has just become available by a donor. There are two patients who require a transplant – a 38-year-old alcoholic man and an otherwise healthy 50-year-old woman.

How **important** to take into account are the following considerations by **Dr Markham** when deciding how to respond to the situation?

64. The alcohol consumption of each patient.
   A. Very important
   B. Important
   C. Of minor importance
   D. Not important
65. The number of Quality Adjusted Life Years available to each patient post-transplant.
   A. Very important
   B. Important
   C. Of minor importance
   D. Not important
66. The organ compatibility of each patient.
   A. Very important
   B. Important
   C. Of minor importance

D. Not important

Scenario 22

Humayra, a medical student, lives with three other medical students. One of her flatmates, Ella, is usually late to lectures, and often does not attend at all. She has also become increasingly withdrawn from her flatmates. Humayra tries to wake her up and ensure that she makes it to their lecture on time, but Ella refuses, claiming that she is tired and needs more sleep.

How **appropriate** are the following responses by **Humayra** in this situation?

67. Remind Ella that as a doctor, she will need to know everything that is being taught in the lectures that she is missing.
    A. Very appropriate
    B. Appropriate, but not ideal
    C. Inappropriate, but not awful
    D. Very inappropriate

68. Ask Ella if everything is okay.
    A. Very appropriate
    B. Appropriate, but not ideal
    C. Inappropriate, but not awful
    D. Very inappropriate

69. Leave Ella alone, as she is clearly tired.
    A. Very appropriate
    B. Appropriate, but not ideal
    C. Inappropriate, but not awful
    D. Very inappropriate

- END OF TEST. ANSWERS ON THE NEXT PAGE -

Verbal Reasoning Answers

Passage 1

1. The correct answer is A. "The Ottomans exchanged fire with the Venetian ships as soon as the Venetian fleet approached Gallipoli, forcing the Venetians to withdraw."
2. The correct answer is B. "The Venetians then retired to Tenedos to replenish their supplies and rest."
3. The correct answer is B. "Despite assurances that the Ottomans would welcome the envoys..."
4. The correct answer is C. This can be inferred from the following sentences: "The Venetian fleet, under Pietro Loredan, was charged with transporting Venetian envoys to the Sultan, but was authorized to attack if the Ottomans refused to negotiate. The subsequent events are known chiefly from a letter written by Loredan after the battle. On the next day, the two fleets manoeuvred and fought off Gallipoli, but during the evening, Loredan managed to contact the Ottoman authorities and inform them of his diplomatic mission."

Passage 2

5. The correct answer is B. This can be proven by the first paragraph "Because coal takes millions of years to develop and there is a limited amount of it, it is a nonrenewable resource. "
6. The correct answer is B. The second and third paragraphs explain the process of coal formation, with initiates from plants and algae.
7. The correct answer is D. In paragraph 2, "300 million years ago... the Earth was covered in wide, shallow seas and dense forests."
8. The correct answer is A. This can be found in the second and third paragraphs.

Passage 3

9. The correct answer is B. The decline began in 1800 BC and Dilmun was absorbed entirely by Babylon in 600 BC. This is found in the second paragraph. Be careful not to use any outside knowledge, as this may lead you to selecting option A.
10. The correct answer is C. Although Dilmun means "noble", it was described as "paradise" in the Epic of Gilgamesh, the world's oldest poetic saga.
11. The correct answer is B. "When the copper trade declined around 1800 BC, Dilmun's strength fell with it."

12. The correct answer is D. This is described towards the end of the first paragraph "...suggest an enlightened civilisation of considerable social and economic development."

Passage 4

13. The correct answer is B. "Three astronauts were killed in the fire".
14. The correct answer is D. None of the missions in the passage landed on the moon. Be careful not to use outside knowledge, as this may lead you to selecting option A.
15. The correct answer is A. "At the time, the United States was still trailing the Soviet Union in space developments..."
16. The correct answer is C. "In 1966, after five years of work by an international team of scientists and engineers, the National Aeronautics and Space Administration (NASA) conducted the first unmanned Apollo mission."

Passage 5

17. The correct answer is B. "The majority of artists, however, limited their investigations to the surface of the body..."
18. The correct answer is C. Antonio Pollaiuolo is listed as "the great Florentine sculptor, painter and printmaker" but no information about Giorgio Vasari is given in this regard.
19. The correct answer is C. The qualifier of necessity "all" makes this statement difficult to prove. The passage suggests that the artists had better anatomy than was taught at universities, but does not indicate that this applied to each of the artists of the time.
20. The correct answer is A. "...printmaker Antonio Pollaiuolo (ca. 1432–1498) was the 'first master to skin many human bodies in order to investigate the muscles and understand the nude in a more modern way.'"

Passage 6

21. The correct answer is C. "As early as 1000 BC, they had covered nearly the entire continent. It is not known when the first people arrived in the Americas."
22. The correct answer is C. It is stated that they hunted deer and bison, but does not explicitly state that these were used for food.
23. The correct answer is A. "Ten thousand years ago, when the Ice Age ended, changes in climate and increasing populations inspired some Native American tribes to experiment with growing different crops."
24. The correct answer is B. "And they used cargo rafts and other boats to ship their goods from one trading point to another."

Passage 7

25. The correct answer is B. "Seeking greater glory and riches, de Soto embarked on a major expedition in 1538 to conquer Florida for the Spanish crown."
26. The correct answer is D. "In 1541, de Soto and his men became the first Europeans to encounter the great Mississippi River and cross it; de Soto died early the next year."
27. The correct answer is D. "Around the age of 14, de Soto left for Seville, where he got himself included on an expedition to the West Indies led by Pedro Arias Dávila in 1514."
28. The correct answer is A. "De Soto's family was of minor nobility and modest means..."

Passage 8

29. The correct answer is D. "The Algerian (sometimes called the Algero-Provençal or Balearic) Basin, east of the Alborán Basin, is west of Sardinia and Corsica, extending from off the coast of Algeria to off the coast of France."
30. The correct answer is B. "Mediterranean Sea, an intercontinental sea that stretches from the Atlantic Ocean on the west..."
31. The correct answer is B. "The western extremity of the Mediterranean Sea connects with the Atlantic Ocean by the narrow and shallow channel of the Strait of Gibraltar."
32. The correct answer is A. This can be directly inferred from: "its average north-south extent, between Croatia's southernmost shores and Libya, is about 500 miles (800 km)."

Passage 9

33. The correct answer is B. "In repeat-blooming roses, the timing of the blooming process begins with the removal of an aged flower."
34. The correct answer is D. "When we cut off a dead spent bloom (deadheading) we signal to that stem to grow a new flower-producing stem."
35. The correct answer is A. This conclusion can be drawn from the following: "Roses with a lot of petals (45 – 50) take longer to re-bloom, usually 6 weeks. While densely-petaled roses like Belinda's Dream and Quietness (100+ petals) take the longest to rebloom..." 42 days is equivalent to 6 weeks, and it is a logical inference to make that Quietness will take over 6 weeks to bloom. Watch out for qualifiers of necessity in other options.

36. The correct answer is C. "Most modern roses sold today bloom somewhat regularly throughout the growing season... Roses that bloom on a regular basis are called 'repeat' bloomers."

Passage 10

37. The correct answer is C. This is evidenced throughout the passage with the mention of various countries.
38. The correct answer is B. "Early Chinese candles are said to have been molded in paper tubes, using rolled rice paper for the wick, and wax from an indigenous insect that was combined with seeds."
39. The correct answer is A. "Emperor Constantine is reported to have called for the use of candles during an Easter service in the 4th century."
40. The correct answer is A. "...the ancient Romans are generally credited with developing the wicked candle before that time by dipping rolled papyrus repeatedly in melted tallow or beeswax. The resulting candles were used to light their homes, to aid travelers at night, and in religious ceremonies." Be careful not to use any outside knowledge.

Passage 11

41. The correct answer is A. Watch out for options suggesting causation rather than correlation, as well as over-generalisation. For example, "poor law enforcement" in option D is not specific to traffic laws.
42. The correct answer is B. This shows how an individual can change their response to traffic laws based on how they perceive their likelihood of being caught. A is simply rewording the question; C only refers to speeding; D does not answer the question, as POBC is not discussed.
43. The correct answer is A. This can be inferred from the statement "Our enforcement of traffic laws has been lackadaisical, inefficient, corrupt and seasonal..." This demonstrates that traffic enforcement is greater in festive seasons, and the statement "We have to raise the POBC rate to a high level to instil discipline among Malaysian drivers and to do this we have to drastically improve our culture of enforcement..." demonstrates that POBC can be increased by stricter law enforcement.
44. The correct answer is B. "Motorists simply do not fear being caught as traffic summonses are often not paid, can be negotiated or cancelled through corruption and even discounts can be officially given." This sentence explains why the POBC is low, and option B counters this. The rest may be viable options but are not reinforced by the passage.

Decision Making Answers

Question 1

1. The correct answer is No. This graph shows cancer registrations, rather than cancer deaths. Further, it is of "24 major sites" rather than the entire UK population.
2. The correct answer is No. There is no information given in this graph to suggest that the cancers are non-contagious. Remember not to use any outside knowledge.
3. The correct answer is Yes. The total bar for "melanoma", including males and females, surpasses the 10,000 mark on the x-axis. If there are more than 10,000 registrations for melanoma, logically, there must be more than 10,000 people diagnosed with melanoma.
4. The correct answer is Yes. The blue bar, representing males, is largest for prostate cancer. This conclusion can be made as it refers to diagnoses in the population of the graph, rather than extrapolating data to include a larger population, such as the entire UK. Further, it can logically be inferred that cancers at these sites are registered, and so, the conclusion can be drawn that prostate cancer was the most commonly diagnosed cancer in males within the population of the study.
5. The correct answer is Yes. The bar for colorectal cancer is evidently the third largest.

Question 2

The correct answer is B. The blue circle (A) represents smart people; The orange circle (B) represents artistic people; The green circle (C) represents athletic people; The yellow circle (D) represents musicians.

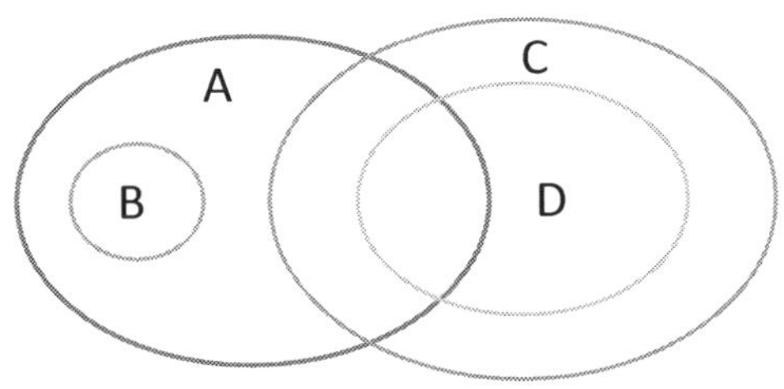

Question 3

The correct answer is C.

The equations deducted from the paragraph are as follows:

1. $3p + 6m + 4g = 231$
2. $p = m - 2$
3. $2p + g = 51$
4. $p - m = \frac{1}{2}(m - g)$

Equation 2 rearranged: $m = p + 2$
Equation 3 rearranged: $g = 51 - 2p$
Substitute these into equation 1:

$$3p + 6(p+2) + 4(51-2p) = 231$$
$$3p + 6p + 12 + 204 - 8p = 231$$
$$1p + 216 = 231$$
$$\mathbf{p = 15}$$

Substitute into equation 3 to find the length of g.

$$g = 51 - 2p$$
$$g = 51 - 2(15)$$
$$\mathbf{g = 21}$$

Question 4

1. The correct answer is Yes. “All bees are insects.”
2. The correct answer is No. There is not enough information given to draw this conclusion.
3. The correct answer is No. “No insects crawl”.
4. The correct answer is No. Bees are insects and therefore do not crawl.
5. The correct answer is Yes. All insects with wings are bees, so if it does not have wings, it is not a bee.

Question 5

The correct answer is B. This answer references studies so it is factual. It mentions engagement, which can be likened to interest. It also mentions attention span, which is important in maintaining interactivity and interest both. Option A mentions no evidence base and discusses “higher grades” which are not the focus of the question. Option C mentions no evidence base. Option D is also irrelevant to the question.

Question 6

The correct answer is D. If Harvin's height is double that of Jaspreet's, Jaspreet must be 112cm and Harvin must be 224cm, to make a total of 336cm. You can calculate this by dividing 336cm into 3 portions – 2 for Harvin, and 1 for Jaspreet. The average height of a male in Canada is 170cm + 10% of 170cm (17cm) = 187cm. Harvin is 224cm, thus option D must be true.

Question 7

A. The correct answer is Yes. Based on the information, all apple are red. If all apples are red, then *some* of them will definitely be red. Thus, this conclusion can be drawn.
B. The correct answer is Yes. If some strawberries are yellow, and all of the other items are red, strawberries must be either red or yellow.
C. The correct answer is No. "All baskets are strawberries."
D. The correct answer is No. There is not enough information given to make this conclusion. Syllogisms do not always make sense. It is possible that even though all baskets are strawberries, some mangoes might be baskets, or all mangoes might be baskets while all baskets are strawberries. For a conclusion to be drawn, there needs to be 100% certainty based on the information given, and in this case, there is not.
E. The correct answer is No. All baskets are strawberries, and strawberries are either red or yellow, thus baskets will be either red or yellow.

Question 8

The correct answer is C. The answer is evidence based and is related to the issue at hand, i.e. increasing the number of voters. The other options are either unrelated or lack an evidence base, thus making them weaker arguments than option C.

Question 9

The correct answer is B. The order from first in line to last in line is as follows: Huzaifa, Demetrius, Fabrice, Sky, Jared, Billy.

Question 10

The correct answer is A. The orange circle (A) represents "food", the blue circle (B) represents "taste good", the green circle (C) represents "fruit", and the yellow circle (D) represents "apples".

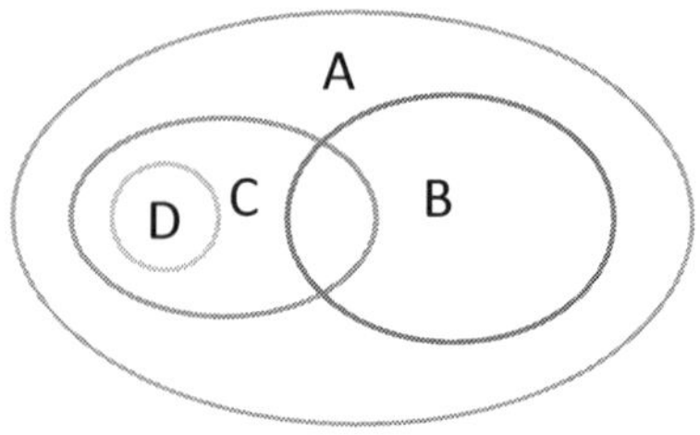

Question 11

The correct answer is D. Remember not to use outside knowledge. This is the strongest argument as it focusses on weight and brings up evidence, i.e. "no correlation found". Option A is not relevant, as it is focussed on making bicycles affordable. Option B uses evidence but is centred around allowing exercise, with no mention of weight or reducing obesity. Option C is a statement with no evidence given.

Question 12

A. The correct answer is No. Some of Dora's cards are blue, but there is no indication that all of them are blue.
B. The correct answer is No. There is no mention of whether Dora might have black playing cards.
C. The correct answer is Yes. Armani has no black playing cards, regardless of whether they are shiny, while Dora has no shiny playing cards, regardless of whether they are black.
D. The correct answer is No. There is no mention of whether Armani has any blue cards.
E. The correct answer is No. There is not enough information to draw this conclusion. While Dora's blue playing cards are not shiny, there is nothing to indicate that no blue playing cards can be shiny.

Question 13

The correct answer is A. The circle represents cricket; The square represents tennis; The triangle represents football; The rectangle represents hockey. Don't forget the numbers overlapping other shapes to calculate the total number contained within each shape.

Question 14

The correct answer is A. Add up the numbers in the areas with 3 or more shapes overlapping, i.e. 9 and 16.

Question 15

A. The correct answer is No. There is no information given to suggest this.
B. The correct answer is Yes. The testing capacity is represented by the grey line, which is always higher than the blue line which represents the number of tests processed.
C. The correct answer is Yes. The highest bar on the graph is two days before 02 Aug, which is the final day of July.
D. The correct answer is No. There is no information given about the number of infections.
E. The correct answer is No. There is no bar on 29th March, suggesting that there were no tests conducted on that day. Further, there is no information about whether testing began during the dates on this graph, or whether this is merely a sample of time when testing was taking place.

Question 16

The correct answer is A. The circle on the left represents badminton, the circle on the right represents soccer, and the circle at the bottom represents tennis. Outside the circles, 12 represents rugby, 8 represents running club, and 5 represents those who don't participate in any sports.

Question 17

The correct answer is A.

h = heart, t = triangle, d = diamond

Equation 2: 2d = h
Equation 3: 2h = t + d
Substitute equation 2 into equation 3:

$$2(2d) = t + d$$
$$4d = t + d$$
$$t = 3d$$

Substitute t into the final equation (2t = 2h + ?):

$$2(3d) = 2h$$

Substitute equation 2 into the final equation:

$$2(3d) = 2(2d) + ?$$

$6d = 4d + ?$

2d is needed to satisfy the equation, and we know that $h = 2d$.

Question 18

The correct answer is C. This addresses the fact that studying history is not guaranteed to lead to exposure of Britain's colonial past.

Question 19

The correct answer is B. This provides a logical argument for how this action could lead to reduced crime rates. Option A is focussed on the number of citizens arrested for crime, rather than crime itself, and is a weaker argument due to the word "may". Option C mentions that the impact may not be "large", although the question does not specify that it's looking to reduce crime rates by a large amount. Further, option C is weakened by the word "likely". Option D does not discuss whether legalising marijuana could reduce crime rates.

Question 20

The correct answer is C. If a percentage of students from overseas are positive for COVID-19, it can be concluded that students have made some contribution to the infection rates. There is not enough evidence to support option A, primarily due to the world "mainly". Option B is possible, but cannot definitely be concluded based on the information in the passage. It is worded as a definite statement, yet we cannot be 100% certain that this would be true. There is no evidence for option D.

Question 21

The correct answer is B.

Stari bought Blue Freeze:

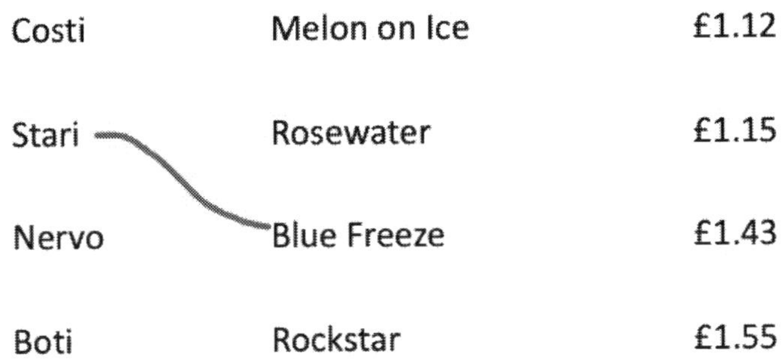

Melon on Ice and Blue Freeze cost £1.15 and £1.55 in any order:

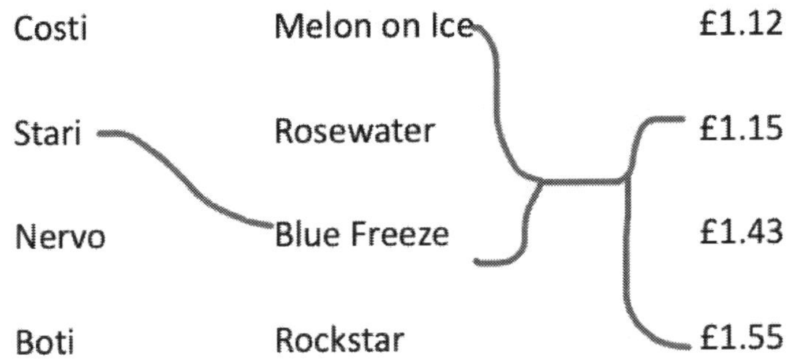

Nervo bought Rosewater or Rockstar

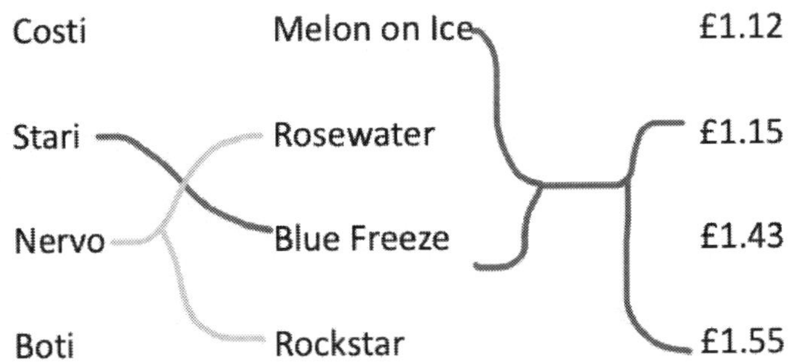

Rockstar costs £1.12:

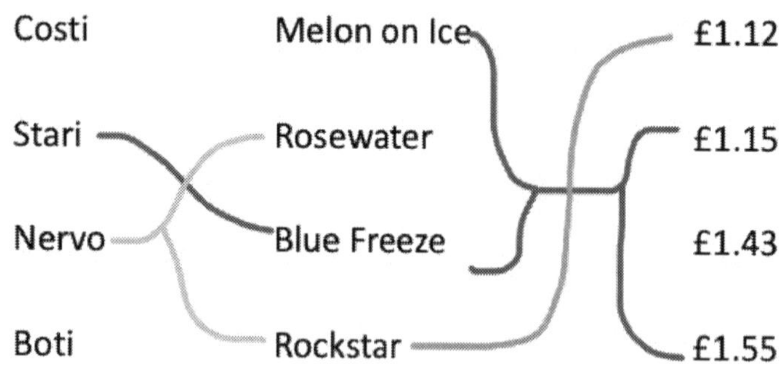

Costi bought the more expensive of £1.15 and £1.55, so they bought the £1.55 ice cream:

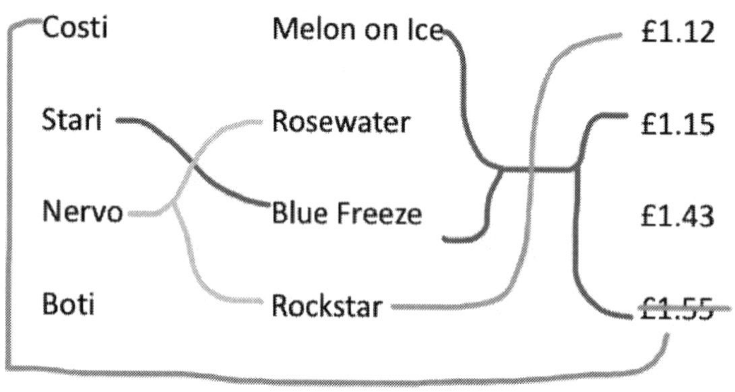

Stari bought Blue Freeze, and Costi bought the more expensive of Blue Freeze and Melon on Ice. Therefore, Blue Freeze must cost £1.15 (the lower of the two), and Melon in Ice must cost £1.55. Costi must have bought Melon on Ice.

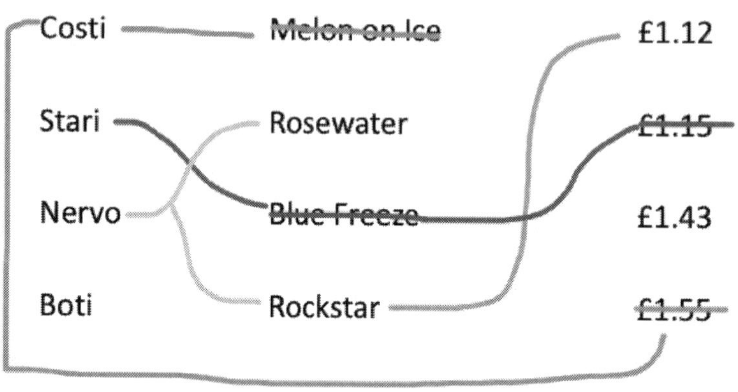

Question 22

The correct answer is D. The total number of patients who use a brown inhaler is 19. There are 10 patients who use a brown inhaler and another inhaler as well. 19-10=9, so there are 9 patients who use only a brown inhaler. The total number of participants is 110, so 9/110 use only a brown inhaler.

Question 23

25 products:

Rugs = 3
Cupboards = chairs - 2
Chairs = tables

If chairs = x, then tables also = x and cupboards = x - 2

Therefore, 25 (total) = 3 (rugs) + x (chairs) + x (tables) + x - 2 (cupboards)
25 = 1 + 3x
x = 8

So, there are 8 chairs, 8 tables, 6 cupboards (x - 2), and 3 rugs.

A. The correct answer is No. There are 3 rugs and 6 cupboards.
B. The correct answer is No. There is no information given about how many of the chairs are wooden. It is equally possible based on the information that all chairs are wooden, or that only 1 chair is wooden. Thus, we cannot draw a conclusion about the number of wooden chairs.
C. The correct answer is Yes.
D. The correct answer is No. Only chairs and tables are wooden.
E. The correct answer is No. There is no information given regarding the material of the rugs.

Question 24

The correct answer is A. A biased coin simply means that the chance of landing on either heads or tails is not equal, i.e. there is a greater than 50% chance of landing on one of the sides. This does not lead to a change in probability based on the results of previous coin tosses.

Question 25

A. The correct answer is No. All black cases are shiny, but there is nothing to suggest that shiny cases have to be black.

B. The correct answer is No. All black cases are shiny, but there is nothing to suggest that they cannot also be clear. Syllogisms will not always make sense, as you will have seen by now.
C. The correct answer is Yes. No grey cases are shiny, as evidenced by the text.
D. The correct answer is Yes. Although there is no mention of blue cases, there is nothing excluding other colours from being shiny.
E. The correct answer is No. Many grey cases are clear, but clear cases are not exclusively grey based on the information given.

Question 26

The correct answer is B. This focusses specifically on disadvantaged students, whereas option A focusses on students in general. Option C is opinionated, whereas option D is an argument without a premise.

Question 27

The correct answer is D. Although this one may look complicated, and you may automatically begin to draw your table, try to read the question first. You can easily answer this question by a process of elimination. It cannot be option A, as the question states that Habib did not go on a skyscraper. It cannot be option B, as the question states that Aaqib and Sadiq went on the same ride, and only one person went on a skyscraper. It cannot be option C as Mahdi did not go on a rollercoaster or a skyscraper. Therefore, by process of elimination, the answer must be D.

Question 28

Based on the information given, we can work out some numbers as follows:

Fruits: 3 apples, 6 bananas, 3 strawberries.
Frozen foods: 4 garlic breads, at least 1 pizza
Drinks: 6

A. The correct answer is No. There are 6 drinks and 12 fruits.
B. The correct answer is Yes. There are 12 drinks and 6 fruits.
C. The correct answer is No. There is at least 1 pizza, and there may be other frozen foods.
D. The correct answer is Yes. There are 3 strawberries and no fizzy drinks, as all of the drinks are not fizzy.

E. The correct answer is No. Although there are 26 items, there is nothing to suggest that the trolley is at its maximum capacity.

Question 29

The correct answer is D. Add up all of the areas with 2 shapes overlapping.

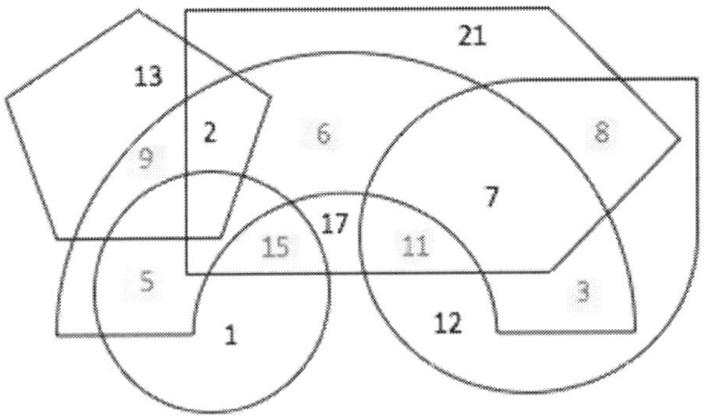

Quantitative Reasoning Answers

Scenario 1

1. The correct answer is B. There are 4 adults and 1 child. (4 x 436) + 212 = £1956. To convert this into KWD, multiply by 0.4 = 782.4 KWD.
2. The correct answer is B. 1650 CAD / 1.75 = 942.86 GBP. 942.86 x 50% = 471.43 GBP. 471.43 - 15% = £400.71. This is how much the ticket would cost. The total savings would be 942.86 - 400.71= £542.15
3. The correct answer is B. Hotel cost: 42 x 1.025 = 43.05 x 6 nights = 258.30 HKD. Cup final ticket per person = 2900/15 = 193.33 HKD. Total in HKD = 451.63 + (100 x 6 additional cost) = 1051.63 HKD. To get this in GBP, divide by 10.12 = 103.92 GBP. Flight cost converted to GBP = 455/1.11 = 409.9. £409.9 + £103.9= £513.82
4. The correct answer is C. 1310 USD = 1000 GBP = 1110 EUR

Scenario 2

5. The correct answer is B. This looks at your ability to interpret simple data in a table.
6. The correct answer is A. 5645 - 4316 = 1329. Take the difference and divide it by the original value: 1329/5645 = 23.54%
7. The correct answer is A. The total number of bookings is 13637. 2088/13637 = 15%

8. The correct answer is B. The total number of bookings in 2016 was 13305. 13305-6763 = 6542. Take the difference and divide it by the first value: 6542/6763= 96.7% You could also do 13305/6763= 96.7% increase.

Scenario 3

9. The correct answer is D. The area of the living room is 8x8=64m^2, and the surface area of the kitchen is (7x8)/2=28m^2. This gives a total of 92m^2. Each tile is 0.5m^2 so Yaqoob will need 92x2=184 tiles. Each tile costs £2.30, so 184x2.3=£423.20
10. The correct answer is C. We already know the living room is 64m^2. If extended by 3m, the front room would be (8 + 3) x 8 = 88m^2. (88 - 64) / 64= 37.5%
11. The correct answer is A. Each piece covers 0.96m^2 and the area of the extended front room is 88m^2. 88 / 0.96 = 91.67. This would need to be rounded up to 92 in order to cover the full floor, as you cannot purchase 0.67 of a piece.
12. The correct answer is B. The volume of the living room is 8 x 8 x 8 = 512m^3. Each box is 0.2 x 0.3 x 0.5 = 0.03m^3. Half of the volume of the living room is 256m^3. 256 / 0.03 = 8533 boxes. Remember not to round up as he's unable to take up more than half of the volume of the living room.

Scenario 4

13. The correct answer is A. First calculate his annual income. £12.50 x 8 hours x 5 days x 52 weeks = £26000. This falls into the second tax bracket. He will pay 22000 x 12% = £2640 tax for the first tack bracket, and (26000 - 22000) x 20% = £800 for the second tax bracket. This gives a total of £3440 per year. Divided by 12 = £286.67 per month
14. The correct answer is E. Alfonso earns £26,000 per year, as we know from the previous question. Bella earns 16 hours x £13.00 x 52 weeks = £10816 per year. 276000 - (26000+10816) = 239184 left over. The tax he pays on this would be 12% of 22000 + 20% of (50000 - 22000) + 32% of (75000 - 50000) + 40% of (239184 - 75000) = 2640 + 5600 + 8000 + 65673.60 = £81913.60.
15. The correct answer is E. If he pays £1250 in tax every month, he must pay £15000 in tax every year.
    - We know from the previous question that £2640 of tax is paid within the first tax bracket, £5600 in the second tax bracket, and £8000 in the third tax bracket. 2640 + 5600 + 8000 = 16240, therefore, as he pays £15000 in tax, he must fall within the third tax bracket and earn between £50,001 and £75,000 a year.
    - The next question is: How far into this tax bracket is he? £15000 - £8240 (total of the last 2 tax brackets) = £6760, so the tax he pays at a rate of 32% is £6760 per year.

- To calculate how much income would lead to a tax of £6760 in the third tax bracket, use the equation "32% of x = £6760" so 0.32x = 6760. x = 21125.
- This is how far into the third tax bracket he is, i.e. how much more than £50,000 he earns. So his total annual earnings are 50000 + 21125 = £71125

16. The correct answer is B. We know his annual income from the previous question. 71125 x 1.07 = £76,103.75 which is his new annual income. This makes him eligible for the final tax bracket of 40%, but only on everything he earns above £75,000. So, he pays 40% tax on £1103.75 of his income, which equates to £441.50 (1103.75 x 0.4). Now add up all of the taxes from each bracket:
    - Tax on first tax bracket: 22000 x 0.12 = 2640
    - Tax on second tax bracket: 28000 x 0.2 = 5600
    - Tax on third tax bracket: 25000 x 0.32 = 8000
    - Tax on fourth tax bracket: 441.50

    The total tax from each bracket = £16,681.50
    - 16681.50 / 12 = £1390.13 (monthly tax).
    - Previously, he was paying £1250 a month.
    - Monthly increase in tax = 1390.13 - 1250 = £140.13.

Scenario 5

17. The correct answer is D. His driving time was 3 hours + 0.5 hours + 3 hours = 6.5 hours. Convert 521km to miles to get the average speed in mph. 521/1.6=325.625. Average speed = 325.625 miles / 6.5 hours = 50.1 miles/hour
18. The correct answer is A. 6 hours and 20 minutes subtract 32 minutes equals 5 hours and 48 minutes. 48/60 = 0.8 so it took 5.8 hours to arrive in Saskatoon. If he travelled at 120 miles/hour and the time taken was 5.8 hours, you can calculate the miles travelled with the following equation: 120 miles/hour x 5.8 hours = 696 miles
19. The correct answer is E. 2:30 PM + 5 hours = 7:30 PM Toronto time when she lands. This is 3 hours ahead of Calgary time, so it'll be 4:30 PM in Calgary.
20. The correct answer is C. Calgary → Edmonton = 299 km. Edmonton → Saskatoon = 521 km. 6442 miles x 1.6 = 10,307.2 km. 299 + 521 + 10307.2 = 11127.2 km

Scenario 6

21. The correct answer is C. In 4 weeks, there are 2 bank holiday Mondays, 2 normal Mondays, 4 Wednesdays, and 8 weekend days.
    - Bank holiday Mondays: 2 days x 2 (double rate) x £7.65 x 10 hours = £306
    - Normal Mondays and Wednesdays: 6 days x £7.65 x 10 hours = £459
    - Weekends: 8 days x £8.65 x 10 hours = £692
    - Total: £1457

22. The correct answer is E. 99,999 x 0.9 = £89,999.10 is the amount she would need to pay for the car. There are 120 months in 10 years. 89,999.10/120 = £749.99.
23. The correct answer is C. Olive works 4 days a week and 10 hours on each day. If she works 40 hours a week for 52 weeks, that's 2080 hours. 4 cakes + 8 tarts = 12. 12 per hour x 2080 hours = 24,960.
24. The correct answer is E. Olive works 40 hours a week, so she bakes 160 cakes a week (4/hour x 40 hours). 160 x 1.07 = 171.2. The question asks how many more she would need to bake to reach this target. 171.2 - 160 = 11.2.

Scenario 7

25. The correct answer is A. Total number of students studying medicine = 72 + 59 + 125 + 16 + 80 = 352. 352 / 5 = 70.4
26. The correct answer is C. There are 331 students studying in Luton. It's quite easy to narrow this down by scanning for universities which appear to have a small number in comparison to others. For example, the physiotherapy students in Plymouth are limited to 5, and there are only 9 in Liverpool. If you have a look at the rest of Plymouth and Liverpool, they appear to be less populated than Luton. Sutton also appears to be far less populated just looking at the numbers. Likely, you won't have the time to work out the total of each university, so it's best to make an educated guess through scanning the table in order to save time.
27. The correct answer is C. Sutton radiography students next year: 12 x 1.25 = 15. Luton will still have 21 students. The difference is 6.
28. The correct answer is E.

Scenario 8

29. The correct answer is D. Wellington is 11 hours ahead of London. When it's 7:30 PM in London, it should be 6:30 AM in Wellington. 6:30 + 3 hours = 9.30 AM on Sunday.
30. The correct answer is A. Cameron sends the text message at 10:30 PM on Saturday in Dakar, and Abigail opens it at 11:30 PM in Dakar. Abigail is in Tokyo, which is 9 hours ahead of Dakar. 11:30 PM + 9 hours = 8.30 AM on Saturday.
31. The correct answer is B. 12 PM – 1.5 hours = 10:30 AM in Islamabad. Buenos Aires is 8 hours behind Islamabad, so the time there was 2.30 AM on Friday.
32. The correct answer is E. The journey is 8 + 3 + 14 = 25 hours. 6 PM + 25 hours = 7 PM in Tokyo. Tokyo is 13 hours ahead of Montreal. 7 PM – 13 hours = 6:00 AM.

Scenario 9

33. The correct answer is E. Gymnastics has a joining fee of £14.99 plus an annual fee of £95. Total = £109.99. Runners only has an annual fee of £200. (200-109.99)/200 = 0.45 or 45%.
34. The correct answer is A. Runners is clearly the most expensive 3-month pass by far, so this can be ruled out. The prices of the rest are as follows:
    - Muscle House: 40 x 0.8 = £32
    - Gymnastics: 14.99 + (35 x 0.75) = £41.24
    - All-time Fitness: 7.99 + (39.99 x 0.8) = £39.98
35. The correct answer is B. Gymnastics earned 89000 - (89000 x 0.18) = £72980 in 2020. 72980 + 150000 = £222,980.
36. The correct answer is E. The prices are as follows:
    - Muscle House: Cheapest 10 years = 5 x 2 yearly passes = 5 x 150 = £750
    - Gymnastics: 14.99 + (7 x 95) = £679.99
    - All-time Fitness: 7.99 + (20 x £39.99) = £807.79
    - Runners: 5 x £200 = £1000

Abstract Reasoning Answers

Question 1

Pattern:

- Set A: There is a grey oval when there are an odd number of boxes and a white circle when there are an even number of boxes.
- Set B: There is a white circle when there are an odd number of boxes and a grey oval when there are an even number of boxes.

Answers:

Test shape 1: The correct answer is A.
Test shape 2: The correct answer is A.
Test shape 3: The correct answer is C.
Test shape 4: The correct answer is B.
Test shape 5: The correct answer is C.

Question 2

Pattern:

- Set A: The grey triangle is always to the right of the moon. There is always at least 1 black box and 1 white circle present.

- Set B: The grey triangle is always to the left of the white moon. There is always at least 1 black box and 1 white circle present.

Answers:

Test shape 6: The correct answer is B.
Test shape 7: The correct answer is C.
Test shape 8: The correct answer is C.
Test shape 9: The correct answer is A.
Test shape 10: The correct answer is A.

Question 3

Pattern:

- Set A: When there are an odd number of overlapping circles, the first and last circles are grey and the middle circles are white. When there are an even number of overlapping circles, the first and last circles are white and the middle circles are grey.
- Set B: When there are an odd number of overlapping circles, the first and last circles are white and the middle circles are grey. When there are an even number of overlapping circles, the first and last circles are grey and the middle circles are white..

Answers:

Test shape 11: The correct answer is A.
Test shape 12: The correct answer is C.
Test shape 13: The correct answer is B.
Test shape 14: The correct answer is B.
Test shape 15: The correct answer is A.

Question 4

Pattern:

- Set A: The total number of sides of the black shapes is always 5 more than the total number of sides of the white shapes.
- Set B: The total number of sides of the black shapes is always 3 less than the total number of sides of the white shapes.

Answers:

Test shape 16: The correct answer is C.
Test shape 17: The correct answer is A.
Test shape 18: The correct answer is C.
Test shape 19: The correct answer is B.

Test shape 20: The correct answer is C.

Question 5

Pattern:

- Set A: When the colours of both of the "antennas" match the colours of the "eyes", there will be a "happy face". When neither match, there will be a "sad face". When only 1 of the antenna colours is present in the eyes, there will be a neutral face.
- Set B: The total number of sides of the black shapes is always 3 less than the total number of sides of the white shapes.

Answers:

Test shape 21: The correct answer is A.
Test shape 22: The correct answer is B.
Test shape 23: The correct answer is B.
Test shape 24: The correct answer is A.
Test shape 25: The correct answer is B.

Question 6

Pattern:

- Set A: In each row, the sum of the sides of the left and right shapes equals the number of sides of the middle shape.
- Set B: In each row, the sum of the sides of the middle and right shapes equals the number of sides on the left shape.

Answers:

Test shape 26: The correct answer is B.
Test shape 27: The correct answer is B.
Test shape 28: The correct answer is A.
Test shape 29: The correct answer is A.
Test shape 30: The correct answer is C.

Question 7

Pattern:

- Set A: The large shape in each box is white. There are an even number of shapes per box.
- Set B: The large shape in each box is black. There are an odd number of shapes per box.

Answers:

Test shape 31: The correct answer is C.
Test shape 32: The correct answer is A.
Test shape 33: The correct answer is B.
Test shape 34: The correct answer is C.
Test shape 35: The correct answer is C.

Question 8

Pattern:

- Set A: The pentagon is always below the circle.
- Set B: The pentagon is always above the circle.

Answers:

Test shape 36: The correct answer is A.
Test shape 37: The correct answer is A.
Test shape 38: The correct answer is B.
Test shape 39: The correct answer is C.
Test shape 40: The correct answer is C.

Question 9

Pattern:

- Set A: The number of small circles is the same as the sum of the right angles present in the box.
- Set B: The number of small circles is one less than the sum of the right angles present in the box.

Answers:

Test shape 41: The correct answer is B.
Test shape 42: The correct answer is B.
Test shape 43: The correct answer is C.
Test shape 44: The correct answer is A.
Test shape 45: The correct answer is A.

Single Questions

46. The correct answer is B. From the first to the second box, the bottom left and top right shapes swap position and colour. From the second to the third box, all of the

shapes rotate clockwise around the box. From the third to the fourth box, the bottom left and top right once again swap position and colour. The next step would be to rotate clockwise around the box.

47. The correct answer is D. Each successive box has 1 more straight line than the box before it. The final box in the pattern has 3 straight lines, so the next box in the series must have 4 straight lines.
48. The correct answer is B. Each box has 1 more line of symmetry than the box before it. The final box in the series has 4 lines of symmetry, so the next box must have 5 lines of symmetry.
49. The correct answer is A. Each box has 1 more enclosed space than the box before it. The final box in the series has 4 enclosed spaces, so the next box must have 5 enclosed spaces.
50. The correct answer is D. The middle circle alternates between white and grey in each successive box. From the first to the second box, the black arrow rotates 180° clockwise, then rotates a further 90° with each successive box – so it rotates 270° from the second to the third box, and so on. Similarly, the grey arrow rotates 90° anti-clockwise from the first box to the second, then rotates an additional 90° with each successive box – 270° from the second box to the third, then 360° from the third box to the fourth. From the fourth to the fifth box, the black arrow must rotate 450° clockwise and the grey arrow must rotate 360° anti-clockwise.
51. The correct answer is C. The smallest and largest shapes swap, and the two middle shapes swap. All of the white colours become black, and all of the black colours become white.
52. The correct answer is A. The number of intersections stays constant. If a box has all curved lines, the next box will have all straight lines. Therefore, if a box has all straight lines, the next box will have all curved lines.
53. The correct answer is D. All of the arrows on the right-hand side of the box turn 180°.
54. The correct answer is D. The coloured shape turns black and all those immediately adjacent to it within straight lines turn dark grey. The shapes next to the new dark grey shapes, which are not separated by the original coloured shape by any other shape, will turn light grey. Any shapes which are separated from the original shape by other shapes will not change in colour.
55. The correct answer is C. Connecting the dots in each box in Set A makes right-angled triangles. Connecting the dots in Set B makes scalene triangles.

Situational Judgement Test Answers

Scenario 1

1. The correct answer is D. This is a very inappropriate resolution as it trivialises the patient's concerns. Racism is a serious issue that needs to be dealt with. The patient should feel listened to and should be assured that the matter will be taken seriously.
2. The correct answer is B. By apologising on behalf of the consultant, James would be accepting that this situation took place and partially taking the blame. James is hearing of this for the first time, and should take the matter seriously, but it is not ideal to apologise on behalf of someone else. However, it is still appropriate as James is asking for more information, which demonstrates that he cares about the patient's issue and wants to help resolve it.
3. The correct answer is A. The patient wants to know what can be done about this matter, and it is reassuring of James to inform her that any form of racism will not be tolerated and that her complaint will be taken seriously. He may not have any more information regarding the reporting procedure, but as a medical student, he should be aware that it is important to respond to such reports.
4. The correct answer is D. Bringing the consultant into the room will make the situation more uncomfortable for both the patient and the consultant. James should get more information from the patient prior to bringing the consultant inside, as the patient may be unwilling to discuss this in front of the person who was responsible for the situation. Further, it can result in conflict between James and the consultant, or between the patient and the consultant. Because the patient confided in James, each side should first be heard individually.

Scenario 2

5. The correct answer is D. Signing him in is fraudulent and dishonest, so it must be very inappropriate. Further, this would mean Rajesh may never learn the important skills required. Most medical schools require attendance unless exempted, so signing him in would go against the medical school's rules and code of conduct.
6. The correct answer is A. This is a good resolution as Rajesh can speak directly to the course director and work out another time for him to learn the relevant skills. This will help him to gain permission to take the time off and to ensure that his learning is not impacted.
7. The correct answer is A. Although there are more steps that should be taken to resolve the issue at hand, this action does deal with the issue of integrity. For an option to be

"very appropriate", it does not need to be the only step that is taken. It is adamant that Anna does not do what Rajesh asked her to do.

8. The correct answer is D. This option presents no resolution whatsoever and could make Rajesh feel guilty about attending the funeral, demonstrating a lack of empathy on Anna's part. The funeral is likely very important for Rajesh, so Anna should respect this, rather than responding in such a manner.

Scenario 3

9. The correct answer is A. If the patient is generally unwell or has a poor immune system, their risk of contracting hospital-acquired infections is greater. It is important to consider the health of the patient when determining how long to keep them in hospital.
10. The correct answer is A. If the operation is urgent, it should be dealt with quickly. If it is not urgent, and there are more urgent operations that need to be carried out, this patient may be further down the list.

Scenario 4

11. The correct answer is D - Whilst in this situation the person in question is a qualified doctor, there is a reason that the registrar doesn't agree with your treatment plan. Going ahead with it anyway could put the patient at risk and also impact your relationship with your registrar or other doctors on the ward.
12. The correct answer is A - By doing this, you are able to explain to the registrar why you think your treatment plan is effective and hopefully you will also learn why the registrar thinks that it is not. By discussing it, you can work together to find a better plan for the patient.
13. The correct answer is C - Whilst the registrar is indeed more experienced than you in this situation, the registrar may not know all of the necessary information or history about the patient and so could put the patient in harm's way. Discussing your ideas and their ideas and finding a common resolution would be the best way to tackle this.

Scenario 5

14. The correct answer is D. It is not appropriate to miss a scheduled session without informing the relevant people in charge. Jen should make an effort to either contact her university or the tutor to report her absence.
15. The correct answer is B. It is most ideal to get in contact with the tutor so they are aware of why she is not present. However, if Jen has made an attempt and needs to rush out for an emergency, she can later explain herself. Although the tutor may be

unaware of her absence during the session, they will likely understand when she explains that she tried to get in contact prior to missing the session.

16. The correct answer is A. This is ideal, as Anthony needs her in 20 minutes, and it will take her 15 minutes to get there. She can likely explain the situation within the extra 5 minutes that she has, then head to Anthony.

Scenario 6

17. The correct answer is A. Smoking has a hugely detrimental effect on the health of a foetus, and so is one of the most important things to consider in this situation. It is also necessary to advise Mrs. Adams of the detrimental impact of her smoking.
18. The correct answer is A. It is always essential to consider the autonomy of patients. Regardless of what decisions they are making, you must remember that the patient has the right to make their own decisions.
19. The correct answer is A. If Mrs. Adams is not fully aware of the risks of smoking in pregnancy, she is more likely to continue smoking. Informing her of these risks is very important.

Scenario 7

20. The correct answer is A. As a flatmate, friend, and colleague, it is important to understand the reason for her recent changes. This will help Chris to deal with the matter empathetically and offer her the support that she may need. If he does not consider the reasons behind these changes, he may not be able to deal with them effectively.
21. The correct answer is A. Illegal substance abuse can have a significant impact on Eleanor's career, and she may be disqualified from university if she is found to be abusing drugs. It is very important for Chris to consider this so that he can remind her of the consequences.
22. The correct answer is B. Eleanor may be very happy with her new friend group, and it is important for Chris to be sensitive of this. However, the main issue at hand is the possibility of Eleanor abusing drugs as a result of her new influences. If Chris considers her attitude towards her new friends, it will help him to deal with the problem at hand. However, it is not an absolutely vital consideration.

Scenario 8

23. The correct answer is C. This resolution has good intention – conflict resolution. However, speaking to them together is not ideal, as conflicts are better resolved when discussed one-to-one. Javaid and Amy may have completely different reasons for not

participating, and having a discussion with both of them together may not be comfortable for them and may seem confrontational, thus they may not open up about the underlying issues. Thus, it is inappropriate to have the discussion with both of them.

24. The correct answer is D. This option has no resolution, embarrasses Javaid and Amy, and and presents opportunity for conflict.
25. The correct answer is C. This way, the work is completed and Andrew's grades are not affected. However, it does not solve the issue of Javaid and Amy not putting effort into the group project.
26. The correct answer is D. It is not an appropriate method of conflict resolution – you must deal with conflicts internally prior to escalating the situation. This will lead to further conflict within the group, and will likely impact the relationships between colleagues.

Scenario 9

27. The correct answer is D. As a medical student, Aryan has no right to prescribe medication. As he is not qualified, there is a significant risk of harm here and so this option would be very inappropriate.
28. The correct answer is B. Some nurses are qualified to prescribe medications, but they are not in charge of making decisions regarding patient care. As such, the nurse would have to seek another doctor's advice, and so, it would be more ideal to go directly to a doctor.
29. The correct answer is A. Asking another doctor to help is the most appropriate resolution as they will have the best knowledge of medications and will be better equipped to deal with the situation.
30. The correct answer is C. Although there is some attempt at resolving the situation, as evidenced by the apology given, this does not solve the issue that the patient will be in pain until the next day. The issue should be resolved more immediately so the patient can have their required prescription.

Scenario 10

31. The correct answer is A. The fact that nobody has come forward probably means that there is nobody more qualified than her on the train.
32. The correct answer is D. This is completely irrelevant to the situation at hand. If she considers this, she may have an inappropriate intention when responding. She may act outside of her limitations if there are incentives being offered, therefore, she should focus on the issue at hand and ignore any incentives.

33. The correct answer is D. The conductor likely does not have a medical background. If Emma considers that he is not concerned, she may act less urgently, potentially putting the child at risk.

Scenario 11

34. The correct answer is D. This response does nothing to address the patient's concerns. It is very impersonal and would likely make the patient feel undervalued and unable to voice their concerns.
35. The correct answer is C. This provides no resolution, as simply saying "calm down" will not help the patient to calm down. However, it is not awful as there is a correct intention in place, although it could be dealt with in a better manner.
36. The correct answer is D. A comment like this is unnecessary and leads to a more fractured doctor-patient relationship. This could compromise the quality of care and lead to the patient feeling as if their concerns are not valued.
37. The correct answer is A. It is important to pass on such feedback so it can be addressed appropriately. Perhaps the administration staff have been overbooking clinics, and reporting this would allow any necessary changes to be made.

Scenario 12

38. The correct answer is B. The main concern is the professionalism issue. He is present, so he is not doing anything wrong – he simply made a mistake by forgetting his booklet. By considering how much time he has left on the placement, he can arrange for his GP to sign the booklet at a later date. However, it is not essential to consider this, as the issue should be dealt with regardless of how much time he has left.
39. The correct answer is A. If he is able to deal with the matter during his lunch break, that is ideal, as he will still be able to receive a signature in his booklet for that day. If he considers that he has enough time, he can make the decision to retrieve his booklet during his break to avoid any further issues.

Scenario 13

40. The correct answer is D. This completely disregards Carl's concerns and revokes his right to autonomy.
41. The correct answer is C. Harun does not yet know any details about the herbal remedy, as evidenced by Carl's request for him to look into it. By generalising and explaining that no herbal remedy will be beneficial, Harun is doing a disservice to his patient. If there is something that Carl is requesting which will not harm him in any way, and may be able to ease his anxiety or help him feel calm, even via a placebo effect, this can be

considered. Immediately disregarding his request is inappropriate. However, the response is not awful as Harun is still attempting to explain things to Carl and keeping him informed of the care plan.

42. The correct answer is A. This would give the medical team an opportunity to evaluate their options and decide how to best care for their patient. A junior doctor may not be qualified to make complex decisions about a patient's care, thus it is always appropriate to ask a senior for advice.

Scenario 14

43. The correct answer is C. It is important to address the issue, but it is not appropriate to do so in this manner. Taking the junior doctor aside in front of Sharon may cause her to feel worse, as it would be evident that she was clearly upset. Further, it may make the junior doctor feel bad for unintentionally making an offensive remark. It would be best to discuss this privately, rather than pulling them aside in front of Sharon.
44. The correct answer is B. An apology is required, but this is not ideal as it should be coming from the doctor who made the comment, not from Callum. However, it may help to de-escalate the situation if at least some form of apology is given, and the junior doctor may realise his mistake if Callum steps in with an apology.
45. The correct answer is D. There are already three people in this situation. Conflict resolution should be conducted internally before involving anyone else. Bringing a third party into the situation could make it worse.

Scenario 15

46. The correct answer is D. There was no malicious intent behind her actions, and confidentiality was no actually breached, so the situation does not yet need to be escalated. A reminder of patient confidentiality rules would be most appropriate.
47. The correct answer is D. This is a direct violation of patient confidentiality. The patient did not give permission for Gracie to access her files, regardless of whether Gracie knew the reason behind her illness.
48. The correct answer is C. This is not awful, as confidentiality is not actually being breached. However, it is inappropriate to even suggest breaching confidentiality, and Dr Adams should know that the GP in charge will also not be able to show the files to Gracie.
49. The correct answer is C. This is inappropriate as Gracie should not approach someone she knows in the waiting room. They may not want her to know that they are there. She also should not be asking for any form of consent in a public place. Further, the patient may feel obliged to give consent given that Gracie is a medical student on placement with the doctors, whereas she otherwise may not have informed her of her

blood test results. However, it is not awful as confidentiality is not actually being breached, and a good-willed attempt is being made to resolve the issue at hand, which is Gracie's concern for her sister-in-law. It would be best to advise her to speak to her outside of a clinical setting and ask how she is, rather than in a waiting room.

Scenario 16

50. The correct answer is A. Patient safety is always a primary concern. The danger to patients is very high as alcohol will affect Joe's ability to make rational, thought-out decisions.
51. The correct answer is A. Assuming that this is not normal behaviour for Joe, there may have been something going on outside of his work life that is causing him to behave like this. By considering the reason for this, Mikhail can help to resolve the situation and remove Joe from the workplace in an empathetic manner.
52. The correct answer is C. The main concern here is patient safety. Regardless of whether or not Joe may lose his job, Mikhail needs to act urgently for the safety of the patients. However, by considering this, Mikhail may better assess the situation and confirm his thoughts before responding or taking it further. Therefore, considering this may help to resolve a minor problem, i.e. the consequences to Joe for his actions.

Scenario 17

53. The correct answer is D. This can make Mike feel very attacked, and is not an appropriate form of conflict resolution. For Mike to better understand what he is doing wrong, he should be spoken to privately about the situation, rather than in front of a large group.
54. The correct answer is C. This is not appropriate as Jake is feeling uncomfortable, and is likely not the only person feeling like this, thus it should be addressed. However, it is not awful as it does not make the situation worse.
55. The correct answer is D. It is not appropriate to escalate a concern prior to handling it internally. This should be discussed with Mike before discussing it with a supervisor.

Scenario 18

56. The correct answer is A. Patient confidentiality is always essential to consider. This does not mean that Lily should not tell someone. For the patient's safety, she must first seek permission from the patient to disclose this information. If the patient refuses, Lily must disclose it only to a person or persons who will help bring the patient to safety. This information should not be disclosed to anyone who will not be involved in the patient's care.

57. The correct answer is A. If the young patient is being abused at home, her safety and wellbeing are directly at risk, thus action needs to be taken. If she has nowhere else to safely stay, the medical team can make the decision to admit her to hospital to keep her in safe hands while arrangements are made and investigations are conducted.
58. The correct answer is A. The main concern here is patient safety. This is a very sensitive topic that needs to be dealt with accordingly. Lily must recognise her limitations to avoid acting outside of her capabilities. As a medical student, her role is to report this to a senior. She must seek further guidance if she is unclear on what else she is able to do. Because she is unaware of the protocol, she should not be making further phone calls to the police, social services, or any other organisation or person without first discussing this with a senior member of staff.

Scenario 19

59. The correct answer is D. It is important to be open to receiving both positive and negative feedback. To immediately claim that the comments are unfair is an immature and unprofessional approach. Healthcare professionals should seek to better themselves as much as possible, taking on board any feedback they receive.
60. The correct answer is A. To ensure high quality of care, it would be best to find out what prompted these comments. This will allow her to improve her manner with patients. This is a constructive and ideal approach.

Scenario 20

61. The correct answer is C. Patient confidentiality is a serious matter. This is not about getting Alex in trouble, but about ensuring that the video is taken down as soon as possible. Alex needs to be reminded of patient confidentiality, and this may require mentioning it to the dental school, but it is essential to first speak to Alex and ask him to take it down. It is possible that he was not aware of the patient's face in the background of his video.
62. The correct answer is A. This is ideal. He may need a further reminder of patient confidentiality, and to avoid taking pictures or videos in clinics with patients present. However, the response does not need to be complete in order to be "very appropriate".
63. The correct answer is C. The intent here is correct – a reminder of patient confidentiality. However, this does nothing to address the urgent matter at hand, which is the video on the internet. Further, this kind of reminder can lead to conflict between Sara and Alex. It is best to be more clear and refer to the video directly.

Scenario 21

64. The correct answer is A. Although Dr Markham cannot decide who to give the liver to purely based on alcohol consumption, it is important to consider all aspects of each patient when making this important decision. This includes alcohol consumption, as excessive consumption can be very detrimental to the liver. It is permissible to offer a transplant to patients with a high level of alcohol consumption, but it is essential to provide lifestyle advice and ensure that the patient is willing to decrease consumption to allow success of the new organ.
65. The correct answer is A. Quality Adjusted Life Years (QALYs) can demonstrate the benefit of a treatment, such as a transplant, to a patient. It is important to consider how many QALYs each patient will be able to obtain from the liver, as this can help determine which patient will take the most benefit from it.
66. The correct answer is A. If one patient is incompatible with the liver, they should not receive it, as it would be a waste of NHS resources and potentially be harmful to the patient.

Scenario 22

67. The correct answer is B. There is correct intent here, but this does not address the root of the problem.
68. The correct answer is A. This is an empathetic approach which will help to find the root of the issue and to further respond to it.
69. The correct answer is D. There appears to be an underlying problem, and as her flatmate and colleague, Humayra should be more empathetic and help to address the issue. Leaving Ella alone in a potentially vulnerable time can be detrimental to her.

- END OF BOOK -

Printed in Great Britain
by Amazon

64570238R00285